Child Development and Behavior: Role of Nutrition and Physical Activity

Child Development and Behavior: Role of Nutrition and Physical Activity

Editor: Duncan Bayer

AMERICAN
MEDICAL PUBLISHERS
www.americanmedicalpublishers.com

AMERICAN
MEDICAL PUBLISHERS
www.americanmedicalpublishers.com

Cataloging-in-Publication Data

Child development and behavior : role of nutrition and physical activity / edited by Duncan Bayer.
p. cm.
Includes bibliographical references and index.
ISBN 978-1-63927-628-8
1. Child development. 2. Child psychology. 3. Children--Nutrition. 4. Exercise for children. 5. Physical fitness for children.
6. Children--Health and hygiene. I. Bayer, Duncan.
RJ131 .C45 2023
618.92--dc23

American Medical Publishers,
41 Flatbush Avenue,
1st Floor, New York,
NY 11217, USA

ISBN 978-1-63927-628-8 (Hardback)

Contents

Preface

The health of children can be maintained and improved through a balanced diet and regular physical activity. Young children are more likely to engage in physical activity, which is important for their physical, emotional, cognitive and social development. Healthy eating habits and physical activity behaviors during the first five years of life are critical for children's health. One of the key factors affecting immunity and growth is adequate nutrition. A well-balanced diet must include adequate amounts of vitamins, carbohydrates, fiber, proteins, minerals and fats. Each of these nutrients is essential for children's overall development and growth. Children who are physically active perform better in school and have better brain function compared to children who are less physically active. This book unravels the recent studies on child development and behavior. It also aims to shed light on the importance of nutrition and physical activity for children. Those in search of information to further their knowledge will be greatly assisted by this book.

This book has been the outcome of endless efforts put in by authors and researchers on various issues and topics within the field. The book is a comprehensive collection of significant researches that are addressed in a variety of chapters. It will surely enhance the knowledge of the field among readers across the globe.

It gives us an immense pleasure to thank our researchers and authors for their efforts to submit their piece of writing before the deadlines. Finally in the end, I would like to thank my family and colleagues who have been a great source of inspiration and support.

Editor

1

Participatory Approaches to Understand Dietary Behaviours of Adolescents in the Secondary School Setting

Sarah Browne [1,*], Carol Barron [2], Anthony Staines [2] and Mary Rose Sweeney [2]

1 School of Public Health, Physiotherapy & Sports Science, University College Dublin, Dublin 4, Ireland
2 School of Nursing, Psychotherapy and Community Health, Dublin City University, Dublin 9, Ireland; carol.barron@dcu.ie (C.B.); anthony.staines@dcu.ie (A.S.); maryrose.sweeney@dcu.ie (M.R.S.)
* Correspondence: sarah.browne1@ucd.ie

Abstract: Acknowledgement of wider socio-ecological factors that influence dietary behaviours needs greater consideration in nutrition research with young people. Additionally, children and adolescents have a right to have their voices heard in research that concerns them. The aim of this methods paper is to describe and evaluate participatory methodologies undertaken as part of a dietary behaviour study with adolescents in the school setting in Ireland. Photovoice and peer-led focus groups were the key participatory methodologies, undertaken alongside food diaries and anthropometry. These methodologies were evaluated through discussion with peer researchers, qualitative surveys and in the context of the wider study process and outcomes. Peer researchers reported learning new skills including research, facilitation, listening and social skills and many felt they gained confidence, as well as an awareness about healthy and unhealthy practices at school. The findings were found to be authentic according to students, except for two limitations. Students believed body image was not adequately represented in the findings, and alternative focus group compositions could have influenced discussion content. Youth participants were afforded genuine opportunities to have their voices heard as part of a diet and nutrition research and the methodologies were acceptable and enjoyable. They demonstrated agency in valuable contributions at project design, data collection, analysis and interpretation stages of the research process. Furthermore, the participatory methodologies complemented quantitative data by providing environmental, behavioural, and socio-cultural insights into food choice in the school setting.

Keywords: adolescent health; participatory research; peer led research; photovoice; focus groups; school food; dietary behaviours; food choice; food environments

1. Introduction

The adolescent years represent a time of rapid growth and development, with high nutritional needs. Dietary patterns, however, disimprove compared to childhood, as access, social routines, and autonomy around food choice change [1,2]. Overweight and obesity in this age group is an immediate global concern, with socio-environmental factors linked to the rapid increase in prevalence in recent decades [3,4]. Everyday settings like schools, therefore, are important spaces for health promotion initiatives with young people and the sector has responsibilities in providing healthy eating education and food environments that can support healthy choices [3,5].

Adolescents source more free sugars, saturated fats, and sodium outside the home compared to inside [6]. Schools can be a source of low quality foods and beverages; however, local food outlets also need to be incorporated into our current concept of the school food setting [1,7–10]. A common thread in the literature is the influence of fast food within 1 km of schools, associated with greater consumption of low nutrient, energy dense foods and less high quality foods such as fruits and vegetables [9,11,12]. Competition with local food outlets, therefore, is a challenge to nutrition policies in secondary or high schools [1,7–12]. Additional considerations that school food reform can sometimes ignore are individual, interpersonal, social and temporal factors that are important to students [1,7,8,13–15]. Wider socio-ecological factors, therefore, need ongoing consideration in nutrition research that intends to understand and influence adolescent behaviour in the school setting.

In this study, a rights-based approach to research with young people was taken. The United Nations Convention on the Rights of the Child (UNCRC) outlines how children should be treated and that children and young people are 'rights holders' [16]. By ratifying the UNCRC in 1992, Ireland made a commitment under international law to respect, protect and fulfil children's rights as they are set out in the Convention. Article 12 of the UNCRC is important in relation to the rights of young people to have their voices heard about matters that concern them:

> "States Parties shall assure to the child who is capable of forming his or her own views the right to express those views freely in all matters affecting the child, the views of the child being given due weight in accordance with the age and maturity of the child".
>
> Article 12 of the UNCRC, 1989 [16]

The rights-based approach in this study follows the work of Lundy amongst others [17]. The methodology focuses on research with, rather than research about, children and young people. Participatory methodologies have contributed to research that can better influence practices and policies which are youth-centred and appropriate to adolescent's contemporary circumstances. There is a growing body of literature that incorporates participatory approaches with young people in food and nutrition research [14,18–21]. A number of researchers report on the importance of engaging sensitively and reflexively, which can lead to reduced power imbalances in the research process and can provide insight and understanding into experiences that are not easily conveyed or captured using traditional methodologies [22–25]. However, there is minimal literature which evaluates differing research techniques with young people by young people.

This methodology paper describes a study with an adult-led research question in which adolescents were invited to take up meaningful roles. Lundy's conceptualization of Article 12 of the UN Convention on the Rights of the Child was designed specifically for an examination of children's participation and focuses on four components of space, voice, audience and influence [17]. The application to this study means that: (1) safe and inclusive opportunities were provided to adolescents to form and express their views, (2) adolescents were facilitated in expressing their views, (3) adolescents were listened to and (4) their views were acted upon.

The aim of this paper is to describe participatory methodologies undertaken as part of a larger dietary behaviour study with adolescents in the school setting in Ireland, to describe participant evaluations of the methodologies, and to share insights on the process in the context of dietary behaviour research.

2. Materials and Methods

2.1. Study Design

A cross-sectional observation study with a sample of six Irish secondary schools was conducted. The aim of the study was to understand the socio-ecological factors influencing food choice for adolescents in this setting. Students, teachers and principals took part in qualitative methodologies [1], and students also participated in quantitative methodologies with regard to dietary behaviour and anthropometry [6]. In line with a rights-based approach to research with young people, a sub-sample of students participated as 'peer researchers', which involved moderating focus groups with peers and conducting observations of the school and local food environments through photovoice. Peer researchers also took part in debrief and feedback sessions with the adult researcher.

2.2. *School Recruitment*

Active student involvement in the research study was a key piece of information provided by the researchers to principals and link teachers when recruiting schools. Public secondary schools with a transition year programme were eligible because dedicated curriculum time for social and community projects is provided during the programme, and this aligns well with a participatory research approach. Additionally, to capture local food environments students would need permission to leave school grounds at lunch time, and this permission is typically in place by transition year. School characteristics and participants are outlined in Table 1.

2.3. *Student Recruitment*

The various aspects of the study were comprehensively explained to students in an assembly. Students were provided with information leaflets for themselves and their parents that outlined the participatory processes and other aspects of the study clearly. Students were given the option on their consent and assent form to opt-in for some or all aspects of the study, including as food diary and anthropometry participants, peer researchers (focus group moderators and photovoice researchers) and focus group participants. Where there were more volunteers than required for peer-led data collection, peer researchers were randomly selected using a random numbers table. Students returned parental consent and individual assent forms to the liaison teacher. Table 1 describes school characteristics and student participation in the different strands of the study.

2.4. *Quantitative Methodologies*

2.4.1. Food Diaries

The rationale for conducting food diaries was to capture quantitative information on food and nutrient consumption and sources of food at school with the objective of comparing nutrition quality of food intake from three sources—home packed lunches, school sourced lunches and lunches sourced in the local retail environment. Methods and results have been published elsewhere [6]. To briefly summarise, participants recorded the time of day, eating location, foods and beverages consumed, portions sizes of items consumed and food source over four days.

2.4.2. Anthropometry

Anthropometric measures were used to classify the sample according to weight, height, BMI and waist circumference for age. Additionally, direct measures of body weight were used to assess the accuracy of food records using methodologies outlined by Black [26]. Trained researchers with healthcare backgrounds (physicians, nurses, dietitian) conducted the weight, height and waist circumference measurements adhering to best practice [27]. The anthropometric protocols were evaluated with students via semi-quantitative self-report survey with students indicating either a 'positive', 'negative' or 'neither positive or negative' experience and providing reasons for their choice in an open comment box. The responses were analysed for frequencies and open comments analysed for content and categorised into themes.

Table 1. Characteristics of participating secondary schools and students participating in each photovoice, focus group, food diary and anthropometry methodologies.

School	Gender	Eligible Students *n*	Peer Researchers Photovoice Participants *n* M/F	Peer Researchers Focus Group Moderators *n* M/F	Focus Group Participants *n* M/F	Food Diary Participants *n* M/F	Anthropometry Participants *n* M/F
School A	Urban Male only	55	2/0	2/0	8/0	21/0	1/0
School B	Urban Female only	116	0/2	0/2	0/8	0/85	0/1
School C	Rural Male only	46	2/0	3/0 ∞	7/0	37/0	0/1
School D	Rural Female only	78	0/2	0/2	0/6	0/60	0/1
School E	Urban Male & female	209	2/2 **	2/3 **,∞	10/9	34/68	0/1
School F	Urban DEIS * Male & female	80	0/2	$\frac{1}{2}$ ∞	2/6	0/0	0/0
	Total	584	6/8	8/9	27/27	92/213	1/4

* Delivering Equality of Opportunity in Schools (DEIS)—Disadvantaged Status; ** Two focus and photovoice groups were conducted owing to larger student body in school; ∞ Three peer focus group moderators were preferred by three groups—two shared the moderator role, while one assisted with note taking. All participants were between 15.2 and 17.3 years at the time of data collection.

2.5. Development of Participatory Methodologies for the School Setting

Two key participatory methodologies will be the focus here: (1) Photovoice and (2) Peer led focus groups. A key step in developing the methodologies included preplanning consultation with secondary schools and students, and thereafter piloting peer-led focus groups and photovoice. In line with recommended practice, a youth advisory panel was consulted from the design stage [28]. Youth panel members (aged 15–17 years) represented urban and rural schools and met with the researcher on three occasions. The terms of reference included consultations on study design, procedures, and language used for tools and resources. They advised on the choice of recruitment process for "peer researchers", preferring volunteering to teacher/student nominations. They suggested incentives for peer researchers and online music vouchers were recommended as an acceptable compensation for their time and effort. Their review of the language and phrasing of questions for use in written material and focus group questions was valuable in implementing acceptable language. Furthermore, a degree of flexibility was incorporated into the study design so that participants could later influence data collection in their respective schools—e.g., adding new focus group questions or suggesting alternative settings for photovoice data collection. All methodologies were interactive, participatory, creative, and youth-friendly while being focused on the study aim.

2.6. Survey Instruments/Qualitative Approaches

2.6.1. Photovoice

The use of image-based data originates in the fields of anthropological and ethnographic studies [29] and has transferred to childhood studies in various disciplines. Photography is a part of most adolescents' daily lives through social networking and, therefore, is a methodology that they are very familiar with. Our approach was informed by previous work [23,30,31], and was further adapted for local school setting factors informed by participants in the youth advisory panel and pilot studies.

Peer researchers attended a short workshop for $1\frac{1}{2}$ hours at school, at which they were instructed on using the disposable cameras provided, and on annotating photographs. Information was provided about ethical issues, including respecting the privacy of students and staff (i.e., avoid identifiable imagery) and being transparent about their activity with peers. Peer researchers were informed that food availability, food pricing, food service and dining infrastructures, food marketing, nutrition messaging, and relevant student behaviours in both the school and local food settings were relevant to the study. They were asked to record additional descriptive notes about their school and local food environments on a form provided.

Peer researchers, working in pairs, were provided with blank observation forms, clip-boards, pens and disposable cameras and arrived at school early. They had permission to miss classes over one day to complete the research and continue observations through break and lunch times. At the end of the school day, the researcher met with the students to discuss their experience. Notes of their feedback were written down, and peer researchers filled in a qualitative evaluation questionnaire.

Visual content analysis following Bell [32] was used to analyse photographs and the process is described in more detail elsewhere [33]. Bell describes visual content analysis as an "*empirical and objective procedure for quantitatively recording visual representations using reliable and explicitly defined categories*" [32]. Content in photographs was supplemented by peer researchers' annotations, fieldwork notes and audio-records of debrief discussions. Feedback sessions were held with peer researchers to discuss their views of the dominant themes.

2.6.2. Peer Led Focus Groups

Peer led focus groups, where adolescents become the moderators, are based on a premise of minimizing adult influence within shared social networks and the method attempts to address power imbalances inherent in youth focused research [34]. A strong rationale for community involvement is that, in certain groups, an outside researcher may not be able to elicit in-depth, inside data that a peer or community member could [35]. This is relevant for adolescents, who are in a transition stage between parental/adult control and independence. However, there are few published studies evaluating this method among children or adolescents. We were guided by existing work on peer-led focus groups by Murray [34], who explored offending behaviour among adolescents. We sought to evaluate how this methodology could be adapted to dietary behaviour research.

A training workshop for students who volunteered to lead focus groups was designed for this study. The content of the training was informed by literature on traditional focus group moderation [35,36] and participatory methodologies [34,37,38], as well as input from the youth advisory panel described earlier.

Six to eight student volunteers attended a 3 h training workshop at each school with the researcher (SB). The workshops were conducted in a focus group style whereby chairs were set up in a circle and the session was audio-recorded. The content of the workshop included how to set 'group agreements' at the outset, learning about open and closed questions, probing for greater discussion, tools on dealing with difficult behaviours in groups, and time for skills practice. After the training students decided who would go on to moderate the focus group, who would assist, and who would prefer neither role. Some students opted to share moderation so that they could support each other. Extra students attended the training workshop to allow for drop-outs and absenteeism. Students were responsible for running focus groups in the school setting, which were audio-recorded for later transcription and analysis.

Greater detail of the analysis is described elsewhere [1]. In brief, conventional content analysis [39] was used to analyse the focus groups through a socio-ecological lens. Peer researchers listened to their respective recording and highlighted/noted important dialogue on a hard-copy of the transcript, which was accounted for in the analysis conducted by two researchers (SB, CB). Feedback sessions were held with students to discuss their views of the dominant themes.

2.7. Ethics

The project was granted full ethical approval from the research ethics committee at Dublin City University (DCUREC/2012/114). All students provided informed parental consent and individual assent before participating in the study.

3. Results

3.1. Student Evaluation of Methodologies

All peer researchers reported learning new skills that included research, facilitation, listening and social skills and many felt they gained confidence through the process. Matthew, for example valued "learning when to listen more and take in information people feel strongly about". Awareness-raising was appreciated and widely reported whereby students learned more about their school and the behaviours of peers. It made them take notice of healthy and unhealthy practices and some students reflected on their own behaviours as a result: "I realise I should eat healthy and exercise more after my experience" (Lisa). The 'fun' aspect was also important, and students enjoyed taking time from the usual school routine to be involved in a novel project.

Students moderating focus groups thought that they 'worked' and, for them, small group discussions without the presence of an adult allowed people to open up comfortably. They viewed the discussions as accurate because they could relate to what they were hearing from peers, as reflected in Sophie's comment: "They opened up and confessed some thoughts to us and maybe more than usual because we're all equal".

3.2. Limitations Identified by Students

In training, peer moderators were advised not to ask leading questions or share their own opinions as this might give the impression there were 'right' answers, particularly since peers would be aware that moderators had attended training. Some found it difficult not to do this and talked this through in debrief sessions. In the recordings, some examples were found where leading questions, attempts to build full consensus, assumptions or ill-timed interruptions seemed to limit discussion flow. Peer moderators did find silences or lulls in conversations a challenge. However, more examples were obvious where peer moderators used their insider knowledge in a natural way to advance or deepen discussions. Additionally, at the transcription review stage, peer moderators highlighted discussion points that concurred closely with the overall dominant themes being conducted in analysis by the researchers with focus group recordings across all schools. These latter two points strengthen the argument for providing flexibility in participatory research and offering young people opportunities to influence the research process at all stages, including data collection and analysis.

Student feedback on ways to improve the research process showed critical evaluation skills. Focus group moderators advised that more diverse discussion would be possible by changing group composition. In mixed gender schools some felt that single gender groups would have elicited a better discussion. Some groups generated very little conversation about physical activity and sport, which they acknowledged would be important, and their explanation was the absence of 'sporty' students within the group. They felt a mix of 'sporty' and 'non-sporty' students would have generated better conversation on how this individual-level identity would influence dietary behaviour. The students undertaking photovoice observations suggested carrying out the data collection for longer than one day, setting up agreements with managers from local food retailers to capture this setting more comprehensively, and some found school canteen management suspicious of their activity.

When the researcher (SB) met students to share the study findings, feedback indicated they agreed with key findings, however also identifying an important gap. Body image did not feature as a theme or within any themes in results and students believed this was inaccurate given their lived experience. They believed that body image plays a big role in influencing dietary behaviours, even in the school setting. Healthy or clean eating and fitness had become very trendy for many in the previous one to two years. One student suggested: "maybe people were just embarrassed to say that they wanted to look well" when we explored why it might not have been discussed more during the focus groups. It is important to highlight, therefore, the limitations of participatory research in this instance and how other approaches were needed to explore this topic meaningfully.

3.3. Student Views on Participating in Anthropometry

The majority of students (88%, $n = 268$) who participated in anthropometry reported it as a positive experience and their reasons fit into one of three categories: (1) interest in finding out their measurements, (2) satisfaction with communication and study protocol (i.e., privacy), and (3) taking part was enjoyable. Comments from students who found it 'neither positive or negative' (18%, $n = 55$) indicated that either they had no strong reaction to being measured or satisfaction with how measurements were conducted, but dissatisfaction with their body. A minority of students (2%, $n = 7$) reported being unhappy with their weight or height and this was the reason they reported anthropometric participation as a negative experience.

4. Discussion

This paper describes an evaluation of participatory methodologies undertaken as part of a wider dietary behaviour study to understand socio-ecological influences on food choice of adolescents in the Irish secondary school setting. Peer-led focus groups and photovoice were enjoyed and acceptable to students, who reported new skills, insights, and awareness. Importantly, an authentic and accurate representation in findings was reported. The outcomes complemented a traditional quantitative food record and nutrient analysis approach by providing depth, context and understanding of environmental and behavioural factors that have relevance for future interventions. This discussion will explore the participatory approaches undertaken and the lessons learned.

4.1. Comparison with Prior Research

Participatory research literature emphasises that identifying problems is the first step in creating conditions for the generation of solutions and social action [17,30,40,41]. Our participatory work indicated that students could play a more active role in shaping their food experiences at school. However, genuine participation, where real opportunities for influence are available, can be challenging to fit into traditional education settings [40,42]. It is also still the case that physical spaces (e.g., school buildings, infrastructures, recreational spaces and so forth) designed for children and adolescents, what Rasmussen [43] terms "spaces for children", largely remain adult designated and designed spaces, which still largely reflect adult values [44]. An earlier publication from this study, where students' clear call for healthier food environments as a solution to improve dietary behaviours contrasted starkly with teachers and principals' views on traditional education-based solutions, suggests that adults are more influential with regard to school food environments [1].

Peer led focus groups are not well described or evaluated in published literature. Exceptions include work on offending behaviour by Murray [34] and a recent study around moral and social values by Djohari and Higham [45] and in both there are similarities with some of our experiences. Skills training and a discussion framework seem to help guide the process but flexibility that allows peer moderators to follow group priorities is also important. Djohari and Higham incorporated a system of lead and assistant peer moderators [45], which worked well in our study too and helped peer researchers feel supported. Traditional focus group moderation is based on a level of detachment so that leading enquiries are avoided to minimize response bias. However, our work and others show that adolescent moderators have an alternative role whereby they need to be both facilitator and participant in order maintain a natural rapport with peers [34,45].

The photo-elicitation method is widely used in child and adolescent research [23,31,46] and has been used by some to describe food environments in and around schools [14,47]. Our findings align with other evaluations, whereby self-confidence and competence, critical awareness, and self-realisation or empowerment are important outcomes for participants in health-related research [30,48]. Wang et al. encourage us to evaluate the process holistically by categorising the potential advantages of photovoice for "participants with most power" and "participants with less power" [30]. Innovating in the school food context and learning from student's expertise were key advantages for researchers, where student enquiries yielding contextual and nuanced findings added new understanding. As an example, one issue highlighted in photovoice, not identified through other methodologies, was location of free drinking water for students. Water fountains were captured in toilet facilities and taps on outside walls, with one in a refuse laden outdoor corner. None were in the dining areas of schools as recommended [49,50] and contrasted starkly with photographs of fridges stocked with brightly coloured sugar-sweetened beverage for sale. This raised awareness of conditions among students and led to critical discussion of the influence of environmental factors on behaviours. The "increase access to power" that Wang et al. [30] describe as a potential advantage for participants was evident when photovoice allowed students to convey meanings creatively and safely about their physical environments.

4.2. Practical Considerations for Translation

According to Lerner et al. youth participation is most likely to succeed when positive adult relationships are fostered, and skill building and opportunities for leadership in meaningful activities are offered [38]. Participant engagement at various stages, as well as workshops, training and research supports offered by the study, demonstrated a framework in which participatory research at school can happen effectively. Attention to practical aspects of communication pathways with schools is recommended after our experience. In this study, strong partnerships with link teachers greatly assisted in successfully navigating various study stages including parental and student consent, timetabling, and facilitating the use of school spaces for data collection. In terms of project planning, extra time was designated to consult with youth panels, run training workshops, and debrief and feedback sessions. Many of these activities are now accepted as integral patient and public involvement (PPI) recommended for research [29,51] and collaboration as a right for research participants is rapidly becoming a requirement in grant funding. There are a number of frameworks available to guide this process when working with young people and most agree on some core principles including listening to young people, supporting them to express their views, taking their views into account, involving young people in decision making processes and sharing responsibility and power in the decision making [52]. A key recommendation based on our evaluation would be to consult and collaborate with adolescents at as many stages as possible of the research process right up to interpretation and dissemination, in order to instill confidence that the authentic 'voice', opinions and experiences of participants are well captured.

A review of photovoice in diet and nutrition research published in 2010 found limited examples of the methodology in the field [48]. However, the use of the methodology is growing in the last 10 years, particularly with youth from minority communities [14,18,19,21], where it can more readily explore cultural, behavioural and environmental influences in a safe and accessible way. There are many examples of intervention studies that facilitate students to lead food changes in the school setting [40,53–55]. Published studies on problem identification and evaluation of study design are less well represented. Limited published studies on peer-led focus groups with adolescents were available when we designed our study and one paper guiding the methodology here was in the field of sociology and criminal behaviour [34]. The process translated well to dietary behaviour research, and represents a participatory methodology that can avoid tokenism, which is an inherent risk for researchers and youth participants [52,56].

4.3. Strengths and Limitations

A key strength is that principles of youth participatory research were upheld, and furthermore were authentic according to participants. The sample included adolescents from urban, rural and disadvantaged backgrounds; however, more diverse groups including ethnic minorities and students with intellectual or physical disabilities were not represented and further exploration of the methodologies with these groups is recommended. Students from a disadvantaged school opted not to participate in food diaries and anthropometry, adding a demographic limitation to quantitative outcomes. Indeed, known reporting errors in the food diary methodology [57] were evident in our sample, as well as a strong bias towards female representation compared to males [6]. The qualitative participatory methods, therefore, offered a real opportunity for students to use their voice as an alternative to traditional approaches. As a result, it is possible that the qualitative outcomes offer a more authentic representation of their dietary behaviours in this setting.

One limitation of photovoice is that issues raised are those that are easily photographed and that the participants value, rather than complete representations of peer perspectives in the same setting [47,58]. This limitation is applicable to peer-led focus groups too and, indeed, students identified it when consulted in feedback session in relation to sporty identities and body image influences, not well explored by the study. One potential consideration for addressing these limitations is that of recruitment strategies. Murray, for example, chose close friendship network recruitment for a peer-led approach, which may ensure that participants share a closer social world and address individual identities more closely [34]. Equally, however, we should not unquestionably assume that participatory research is more appropriate for conducting research with young people in all instances and it does not automatically make research 'better' [23]. Indeed, body image was a topic identified as challenging—both in relation to a safe space to discuss with peers and the importance of creating safe, communicative spaces when being measured as part of nutrition study.

Given the known body image sensitivities in the adolescent years, an alternative could have been to discuss this explicitly with young people earlier at the design stage. Body image was not named in the topic guide used by peer researchers, which included open questions on perceptions of health, how food choice is made, the influence of different settings, and sources of information on food and nutrition [1].

Furthermore, we did not observe references to body image by participants in audio-recordings so that no opportunities were obvious for peer researchers to pursue the topic further. It is possible that students inherently knew that body image was 'off limits' for discussion with peers in the space provided, which is interesting and needs interpretation as a possible outcome of this evaluation. Explicitly keeping topics off limits is one potential solution to avoiding sensitive topics suggested by Sim and Waterfield's paper on ethical challenges in focus groups [59]. However, our evaluation indicates that an alternative was needed for students to express their views. To maintain authenticity in youth participatory research, there is an important role for experienced researchers to match methodologies appropriately, provide support and evaluate at various timepoints. Careful consideration is needed, therefore, to avoid disempowering the youth voice when participatory methodologies are not well matched to the topic or group [60].

5. Conclusions

Article 12 of the UNCRC has prompted the shift from conducting researching on children and young people to research with children and young people thereby enabling the young person's voice to be heard more clearly and the methodologies described are faithful to this approach. We also acknowledge instances where alternatives to participatory methodologies need to be considered.

We propose that photovoice and peer led focus groups are valuable and effective methodologies to deepen our understanding of food choice and dietary behaviours. As adjuncts to a traditional quantitative approach, the participatory methodologies described and evaluated can access hard to reach information required for assessing healthy eating intervention needs in the school setting. Additionally, the importance of collaboration and co-design with young people cannot be underestimated so that we address their rights to participate, have their voices heard and have meaningful influence into how their spaces are shaped.

Author Contributions: Conceptualization, S.B., C.B., A.S., M.R.S.; methodology, S.B., C.B., M.R.S.; formal analysis, S.B., C.B., M.R.S.; investigation, S.B., C.B., M.R.S.; resources, S.B., C.B.; data curation, S.B.; writing—original draft preparation, S.B.; writing—review and editing, S.B., C.B., A.S., M.R.S.; supervision, C.B., A.S., M.R.S.; project administration, S.B.; funding acquisition, M.R.S. All authors have read and agreed to the published version of the manuscript.

Acknowledgments: The authors would like to acknowledge the schools and students who participated in this research.

References

1. Browne, S.; Barron, C.; Staines, A.; Sweeney, M.R. 'We know what we should eat but we don't ... ': A qualitative study in Irish secondary schools. *Health Promot. Int.* **2020**, *35*, 984–993. [CrossRef] [PubMed]
2. Fitzgerald, A.; Heary, C.; Kelly, C.; Nixon, E.E.; Shevlin, M. Self-efficacy for healthy eating and peer support for unhealthy eating are associated with adolescents' food intake patterns. *Appetite* **2013**, *63*, 48–58. [CrossRef] [PubMed]
3. Swinburn, B.B.; Vandevijvere, S. WHO report on ending childhood obesity echoes earlier recommendations. *Public Health Nutr.* **2016**, *19*, 1–2. [CrossRef]
4. Swinburn, B.A.; Kraak, V.I.; Allender, S.; Atkins, V.J.; Baker, P.I.; Bogard, J.R.; Brinsden, H.; Calvillo, A.; De Schutter, O.; Devarajan, R.; et al. The Global Syndemic of Obesity, Undernutrition, and Climate Change: The Lancet Commission report. *Lancet* **2019**, *393*, 791–846. [CrossRef]
5. Nelson, M.M.; Breda, J. School food and nutrition: Developing the evidence base for policy. *Public Health Nutr.* **2013**, *16*, 955–957. [CrossRef]
6. Browne, S.; Staines, A.; Barron, C.; Lambert, V.; Susta, D.; Sweeney, M.R. School lunches in the Republic of Ireland: A comparison of the nutritional quality of adolescents' lunches sourced from home or purchased at school or 'out' at local food outlets. *Public Health Nutr.* **2017**, *20*, 504–514. [CrossRef]

7. Caraher, M.; Lloyd, S.; Mansfield, M.; Alp, C.; Brewster, Z.; Gresham, J. Secondary school pupils' food choices around schools in a London borough: Fast food and walls of crisps. *Appetite* **2016**, *103*, 208–220. [CrossRef]
8. MacDiarmid, J.I.; Wills, W.J.; Masson, L.F.; Craig, L.C.; Bromley, C.; McNeill, G. Food and drink purchasing habits out of school at lunchtime: A national survey of secondary school pupils in Scotland. *Int. J. Behav. Nutr. Phys. Act.* **2015**, *12*, 98. [CrossRef]
9. Virtanen, M.; Kivimäki, H.; Ervasti, J.; Oksanen, T.; Pentti, J.; Kouvonen, A.; Halonen, J.I.; Kivimäki, M.; Vahtera, J. Fast-food outlets and grocery stores near school and adolescents' eating habits and overweight in Finland. *Eur. J. Public Health* **2015**, *25*, 650–655. [CrossRef]
10. Kelly, C.; Callaghan, M.; Molcho, M.; Nic-Gabhainn, S.; Thomas, A.A. Food environments in and around post-primary schools in Ireland: Associations with youth dietary habits. *Appetite* **2019**, *132*, 182–189. [CrossRef]
11. Smith, D.; Cummins, S.; Clark, C.; Stansfeld, S. Does the local food environment around schools affect diet? Longitudinal associations in adolescents attending secondary schools in East London. *BMC Public Health* **2013**, *13*, 70. [CrossRef] [PubMed]
12. He, M.; Tucker, P.; Gilliland, J.A.; Irwin, J.D.; Larsen, K.; Hess, P. The influence of local food environments on adolescents' food purchasing behaviors. *Int. J. Environ. Res. Public Health* **2012**, *9*, 1458–1471. [CrossRef] [PubMed]
13. Fletcher, A.; Jamal, F.; Fitzgerald-Yau, N.; Bonell, C. 'We've Got Some Underground Business Selling Junk Food': Qualitative Evidence of the Unintended Effects of English School Food Policies. *Sociology* **2013**, *48*, 500–517. [CrossRef]
14. Brembeck, H.; Johansson, B.; Bergström, K.; Engelbrektsson, P.; Hillén, S.; Jonsson, L.; Karlsson, M.A.; Ossiansson, E.; Shanahan, H. Exploring Children's Foodscapes. *Child. Geogr.* **2013**, *11*, 74–88. [CrossRef]
15. Lalli, G.S. School meal time and social learning in England. *Camb. J. Educ.* **2019**, *50*, 57–75. [CrossRef]
16. United Nataions; UN Convention on the Rights of the Child (UNCRC). *Office of the United Nations High Commissioner for Human Rights*; United Nations: Geneva, Switzerland, 1989.
17. Lundy, L. 'Voice' is not enough: Conceptualising Article 12 of the United Nations Convention on the Rights of the Child. *Br. Educ. Res. J.* **2007**, *33*, 927–942. [CrossRef]
18. Agaronov, A.; Entwistle, T.; Leung, M.M. From the Lunch Table, to the Family Table: A Grounded Theory Approach to Understanding Urban Adolescents' Experiences of Food Culture Mismatch between School and Home Environments. *Ecol. Food Nutr.* **2019**, *58*, 23–44. [CrossRef]
19. Heidelberger, L.L.; Smith, C. The Food Environment Through the Camera Lenses of 9- to 13-Year-Olds Living in Urban, Low-Income, Midwestern Households: A Photovoice Project. *J. Nutr. Educ. Behav.* **2015**, *47*, 437–445. [CrossRef]
20. Leung, M.M.; Agaronov, A.; Entwistle, T.; Harry, L.; Sharkey-Buckley, J.; Freudenberg, N. Voices through Cameras. *Health Promot. Pract.* **2017**, *18*, 211–220. [CrossRef]
21. Riggsbee, K.; Riggsbee, J.; Vilaro, M.J.; Moret, L.; Spence, M.; Steeves, E.A.; Zhou, W.; Olfert, M.D.; Franzen-Castle, L.; Horacek, T.M.; et al. More than Fast Food: Development of a Story Map to Compare Adolescent Perceptions and Observations of Their Food Environments and Related Food Behaviors. *Int. J. Environ. Res. Public Health* **2018**, *16*, 76. [CrossRef]
22. Liebenberg, L.; Ungar, M.; Theron, L. Using Video Observation and Photo Elicitation Interviews to Understand Obscured Processes in the Lives of Youth Resilience. *Childhood* **2013**, *21*, 532–547. [CrossRef]
23. Barron, C. Enabling children's voices in ethnographic writing: An evaluation of photographs by children as a data generating tool. *Ir. J. Anthropol.* **2011**, *14*, 32–39.
24. Punch, S. Research with children: The same or different from research with adults? *Childhood* **2002**, *9*, 321–341. [CrossRef]
25. Hill, M. Children's Voices on Ways of Having a Voice: Children's and young people's perspectives on methods used in research and consultation. *Childhood* **2006**, *13*, 69. [CrossRef]
26. Black, A.E. Critical evaluation of energy intake using the Goldberg cut-off for energy intake:basal metabolic rate. A practical guide to its calculation, use and limitations. *Int. J. Obes.* **2000**, *24*, 1119–1130. [CrossRef] [PubMed]
27. World Health Organisation. *Physical Status: The Use and Interpretation of Anthropometry*; Report of a WHO Expert Committee; World Health Organisation: Geneva, Switzerland, 1995.

28. Brett, J.; Staniszewska, S.; Mockford, C.; Herron-Marx, S.; Hughes, J.; Tysall, C.; Suleman, R. A systematic review of the impact of patient and public involvement on service users, researchers and communities. *Patient-Patient-Cent. Outcomes Res.* **2014**, *7*, 387–395. [CrossRef]
29. Mead, M. Anthropology among the sciences; visual anthropology in a discipline of words. *Am. Anthropol.* **1975**, *63*, 475–482. [CrossRef]
30. Wang, C.C.; Yi, W.K.; Tao, Z.W.; Carovano, K. Photovoice as a Participatory Health Promotion Strategy. *Health Promot. Int.* **2010**, *13*, 75. [CrossRef]
31. Nic Gabhainn, S.; Sixsmith, J. Children photoing well-being: Facilitating participation in research. *Child. Soc.* **2006**, *20*, 249–259. [CrossRef]
32. Bell, P. Content analysis of visual images. In *Handbook of Visual Analysis*; Sage Publications: London, UK, 2001.
33. Browne, S. Exploring the Impact of Schools on the Quality of Diet and Physical Activity in Their Students: A Mixed Methods Study in Irish Post-Primary Schools. Ph.D. Thesis, Dublin City University, Dublin, Ireland, 2017.
34. Murray, C. Peer led focus groups and young people. *Child. Soc.* **2006**, *20*, 273–286. [CrossRef]
35. Krueger, R.K.J. *Involving Community Members in Focus Groups*; Sage Publications Ltd.: London, UK, 1998.
36. Kreuger, R. *Moderating Focus Groups*; Sage Publications Ltd.: London, UK, 1998.
37. Christensen, P.; James, A. (Eds.) *Research with Children: Perspectives and Practices*, 2nd ed.; Routledge: Oxon, UK, 2008.
38. Lerner, R.M.; Almerigi, J.B.; Theokas, C.; Lerner, J.V. Positive Youth Development: A view of the issues. *J. Early Adolesc.* **2005**, *25*, 10–16. [CrossRef]
39. Hsieh, H.F.; Shannon, S.E. Three approaches to qualitative content analysis. *Qual. Health Res.* **2005**, *15*, 1277–1288. [CrossRef]
40. Carlsson, M.M.; Simovska, V. Exploring learning outcomes of school-based health promotion—A multiple case study. *Health Educ. Res.* **2012**, *27*, 437–447. [CrossRef] [PubMed]
41. Simovska, V. The changing meanings of participation in school-based health education and health promotion: The participants' voices. *Health Educ. Res.* **2007**, *22*, 864–878. [CrossRef] [PubMed]
42. Horgan, D.D.; Forde, C.; Parkes, A.; Martin, S. *Children and Young People's Experiences of Participation in Decision-Making at Home, in Schools and in Their Communities*; Department of Children and Youth Affairs, Government Publications: Dublin, Ireland, 2015.
43. Rasmussen, K. Places for Children—Children's Places. *Childhood* **2004**, *11*, 155–173. [CrossRef]
44. Barron, C. *Play and Recreation Needs of Children and Young People Growing Up in Co. Kildare, Ireland*; Dublin Campus Print: Dublin, Ireland, 2017; ISBN 978-1-873769-68.
45. Djohari, N.N.; Higham, R. Peer-led focus groups as 'dialogic spaces' for exploring young people's evolving values. *Camb. J. Educ.* **2020**, *50*, 1–16. [CrossRef]
46. Leonard, M.; McKnight, M. Look and tell: Using photo-elicitation methods with teenagers. *Child. Geogr.* **2015**, *13*, 629–642. [CrossRef]
47. Kontak, J.C.H.; McIsaac, J.-L.D.; Penney, T.; Kuhle, S.; Kirk, S.F.L. The picture of health: Examining school-based health environments through photographs. *Health Promot. Int.* **2017**, *32*, 322–330. [CrossRef]
48. Martin, N.; Garcia, A.C.; Leipert, B. Photovoice and its potential use in nutrition and dietetic research. *Can. J. Diet. Pract. Res.* **2010**, *71*, 93–97. [CrossRef]
49. Patel, A.I.; Hampton, K.E. Encouraging consumption of water in school and child care settings: Access, challenges, and strategies for improvement. *Am. J. Public Health* **2011**, *101*, 1370–1379. [CrossRef]
50. Department of Health and Children. *Guidelines for Developing a Healthy Eating Policy in Post-Primary Schools*; Department of Health and Children; Government Publications: Dublin, Ireland, 2008.
51. Prikken, I.; Burall, S. Doing Public Dialogue: A Support Resource for Research Council Staff. INVOLVE. 2012. Available online: https://www.involve.org.uk/sites/default/files/uploads/120727RCUKResource.pdf (accessed on 30 November 2020).
52. Larsson, I.; Staland-Nyman, C.; Svedberg, P.; Nygren, J.M.; Carlsson, I.-M. Children and young people's participation in developing interventions in health and well-being: A scoping review. *BMC Health Serv. Res.* **2018**, *18*, 507. [CrossRef] [PubMed]
53. Bogart, L.M.; Elliott, M.N.; Uyeda, K.; Hawes-Dawson, J.; Klein, D.J.; Schuster, M.A. Preliminary healthy eating outcomes of SNaX, a pilot community-based intervention for adolescents. *J. Adolesc. Health* **2011**, *48*, 196–202. [CrossRef] [PubMed]

54. Meininger, J.C.; Reyes, L.R.; Selwyn, B.J.; Upchurch, S.L.; Brosnan, C.A.; Taylor, W.C.; Villagomez, E.; Quintana, V.; Pullis, B.; Caudill, D.; et al. A structured, interactive method for youth participation in a school district-university partnership to prevent obesity. *J. Sch. Health* **2010**, *80*, 493–500. [CrossRef] [PubMed]
55. Hamdan, S.; Story, M.; French, S.A.; Fulkerson, J.A.; Nelson, H. Perceptions of adolescents involved in promoting lower-fat foods in schools: Associations with level of involvement. *J. Am. Diet. Assoc.* **2005**, *105*, 247–251. [CrossRef]
56. Hart, R. *Children's Participation: From Tokenism to Citizenship*; Unicef; United Nations Children's Fund: New York, NY, USA, 1992.
57. Livingstone, M.B.E.; Robson, P.J.; Wallace, J.M.W. Issues in dietary intake assessment of children and adolescents. *Br. J. Nutr.* **2004**, *92* (Suppl. S2), S213–S222. [CrossRef]
58. Wang, C.C.; Burris, M.A. Photovoice: Concept, methodology, and use for participatory needs assessment. *Health Educ. Behav.* **1997**, *24*, 369–387. [CrossRef]
59. Sim, J.; Waterfield, J. Focus group methodology: Some ethical challenges. *Qual. Quant* **2019**, *53*, 3003–3022. [CrossRef]
60. Schafer, N.; Yarwood, R. Involving young people as researchers: Uncovering multiple power relations among youths. *Child. Geogr.* **2008**, *6*, 121–135. [CrossRef]

2

Impacts of Dietary Macronutrient Pattern on Adolescent Body Composition and Metabolic Risk: Current and Future Health Status

Oh Yoen Kim [1,2], **Eun Mi Kim** [3] and **Sochung Chung** [4,*]

[1] Department of Health Science, Graduate School, Dong-A University, Busan 49315, Korea; oykim@dau.ac.kr
[2] Department of Food Science and Nutrition, Dong-A University, Busan 49315, Korea
[3] Dietetic Department, Kangbuk Samsung Hospital, Seoul 03181, Korea; em82.kim@samsung.com
[4] Department of Pediatrics, Konkuk University Medical Center, Konkuk University School of Medicine, Seoul 05030, Korea
* Correspondence: scchung@kuh.ac.kr;

Abstract: Obesity, particularly in childhood and adolescence, is one of the serious public health problems worldwide. According to the World Health Organization, 10% of young people aged 5–17 years are obese, which is rapidly increasing around the world. Furthermore, approximately 80% of adolescents who become obese develop bodyweight-related health problems in adulthood. Eating habits and lifestyles play important roles in forming body composition and metabolic status. Changes in body composition in adolescence, the period in which secondary sex characteristics begin to develop, can alter hormonal and metabolic status, can consequently affect health status and the risk of developing chronic diseases in adulthood, and moreover may have an impact on probable body composition and metabolic status in the next generation. Here, we reviewed cross-sectional and interventional studies to analyze the role of dietary patterns focusing on macronutrient intake in growth, body composition, and metabolic changes in adolescents. These findings provide insights into optimal dietary guidelines for healthy growth with accretion of adequate body composition in adolescence, and provide an effective strategy for preventing and managing the risk of obesity-related metabolic disease in adulthood, with the additional benefit of providing potential benefits for the next generation's health.

Keywords: adolescent obesity; dietary macronutrient modification; body composition; metabolic status

---

1. Introduction

The prevalence ratios of overweight and obesity continue to increase worldwide, with subsequent increases in the burden of health care costs [1,2]. Obesity in childhood and adolescence in particular is thought to be one of most serious global public health problems in the 21st century [3]. According to a World Health Organization (WHO) European report from 2017, 10% of children and adolescents aged 5 to 17 years are obese, with rapidly increasing proportions in many countries and regions [4]. Up to 80% of obese adolescents may develop bodyweight-related health problems that are traditionally more common in adulthood, such as metabolic syndrome, type 2 diabetes, sleep apnea, and cardiovascular disease [4–6].

Various behavioral and emotional aspects are related to the occurrence of obesity, which affects adolescents' quality of life [7–9]. In particular, dietary factors such as energy intake and expenditure, macronutrient proportion, food selection patterns, eating habits, and lifestyles play important roles in the formation of body composition and metabolic status [10–18]. Effective weight control in adolescents can reduce the risk of developing metabolic diseases commonly observed in adulthood. Recent studies have demonstrated that the composition of macronutrients in the diet and food selection patterns affect body fat and muscle composition and endocrine metabolism in children and adolescents [12–17,19]. However, several other studies reported that bodyweight reduction can be accomplished regardless of dietary macronutrient composition, and individualized dietary intervention with decreased total energy intake to achieve optimal compliance may be the key for proper weight reduction [20–24].

Changes in body composition such as body fat mass (BFM), fat-free mass (FFM), and the ratio between these two factors in adolescence by gender, the time period in which secondary sexual characteristics begin to develop, can alter hormonal and metabolic status, and consequently can affect the health status and risk of developing chronic diseases in adulthood [4–6]. Modulation of diet composition can affect the secretion of endogenous hormones related to satiety, as well as glucose and lipid metabolisms [14,15,25–27]. In addition, it was reported that maternal pre-pregnancy and life course nutrition rather than nutrition during pregnancy itself is more clearly linked to offspring fetal nutrition and growth, as well as bodyweight [28,29]. That is, fetal nutrition can be influenced by the mother's own early life nutrition, including the accumulated energy balance of the mother in the months and years prior to conception [28,29]. In summary, health and nutritional status during childhood and adolescence, which affect probable body composition and health status in adulthood, are expected to influence the body composition and metabolic status of future offspring.

Therefore, we reviewed articles including observational studies (i.e., cross-sectional, intervention and longitudinal studies) with the key words such as children and adolescent obesity, body composition, macronutrients, eating habits, maternal nutrition, off-spring published in English since 1990 through Pubmed (http://pubmed.ncbi.nlm.nih.gov). We also considered systematic reviews and meta-analysis performed in adults as well as children and adolescents. This narrative review aimed to analyze the role of dietary patterns, particularly of macronutrient intake in growth, body composition and metabolic changes in adolescents, and thereby providing novel insight into the establishment of optimal dietary guidelines for healthy growth with accretion of adequate body composition in the adolescent.

2. Trends in Obesity and Related Metabolic Disease in Childhood and Adolescence

Obesity in childhood and adolescence has become a major global public health concern [3,4]. According to the previously mentioned WHO report, one out of ten children and adolescents are obese, and this proportion is rapidly increasing in many parts of the world [1,2,4]. In particular, a higher prevalence of overweight and obesity has been reported among younger adolescents and boys, and the average prevalence of overweight and obesity was 19% across countries and regions included in the WHO survey of health behavior in school-aged children (HBSC), with the highest levels of overweight and obesity generally being in Southern European countries [4]. Based on data from the 2015–2016 National Health and Nutrition Examination Survey (NHANES) in the United States, the prevalence of obesity was 18.5% and affected approximately 13.7 million children and adolescents [30]. In that report, the prevalence of obesity was higher among youth aged 6 to 11 years (18.4%) and adolescents aged 12 to 19 years (20.6%) compared to the prevalence among children aged 2 to 5 years (13.9%) [30]. According to the 2017 report from the Organization for Economic Co-operation and Development (OECD) [31], the average ratio of overweight and obesity in boys was 25.6%, with higher ratios in Chile (46.2%), USA (41.3%), and New Zealand (32.8%). The incidence of childhood and adolescent obesity in the Republic of Korea increased steadily from 11.2% in 2008 to 25% in 2018; furthermore, the rate of increase for severe obesity is much higher (137.5%) than for moderate (30.6%) and mild (57.1%) obesity during the same period [32,33]. The prevalence of severe obesity is also increasing rapidly among Korean young adults aged 20 to 30 years, which may be due to the rapid increase in adolescent obesity during the last 20 years [32]. Moreover, four of every five obese adolescents are at risk for chronic diseases frequently observed in obese adults (i.e., type 2 diabetes, asthma, sleep apnea, and cardiovascular disease), as well as emotional (psychological) and social (school absenteeism and social isolation) problems [4–6]. Therefore, optimal strategies to reduce obesity are critical for slowing down and reversing the observed trends of increasing obesity prevalence and its related complications.

3. Factors Influencing Adolescent Obesity and Body Composition

Obesity affects adolescents' quality of life and can result from various factors, either alone or in combination, which include behavioral, emotional, and social factors, as well as genetic background [7–9] (Figure 1A,B). In general, obesity occurs due to an imbalance between energy intake and expenditure as a result of unhealthy diet and sedentary lifestyle [34–36]. Dietary pattern (i.e., energy intake, macronutrient composition, and food selection), eating habits, and lifestyle (including physical activity level) all play important roles in forming the body composition, including BFM, FFM, the ratio between these two factors, body mass index (BMI), and metabolic status [10–24] (Figure 1A). According to data from the WHO HBSC survey, the primary causes of obesity in children and adolescents can be traced to energy-related behaviors (i.e., physical activity, sedentary lifestyle, eating habits, and sleep patterns), which contribute to imbalances between energy intake and energy expenditure [4]. In addition, the report published by the WHO Commission on Ending Childhood Obesity identified obesogenic environments such as lower physical activity, higher sedentary behavior, and intake of energy-dense, nutrient-poor foods as key drivers for the development of obesity [37]. Furthermore, dietary patterns and lifestyle in maternal and infant periods, as well as in childhood and adolescence, may have impacts on health status and obesity-related disease risk throughout the lifetime [28,29] (Figure 1B).

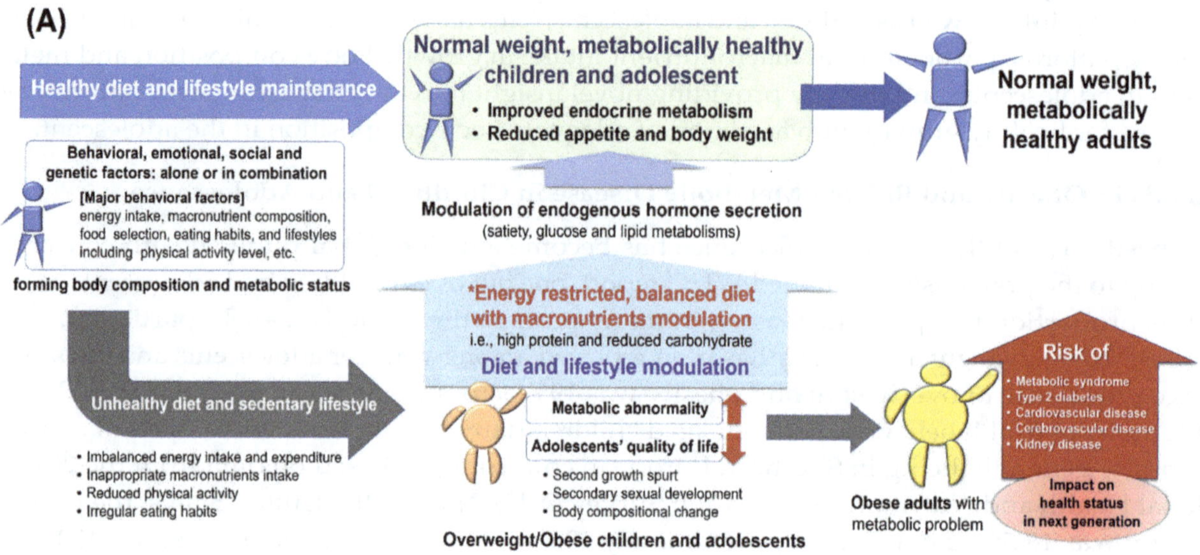

Figure 1. *Cont*'

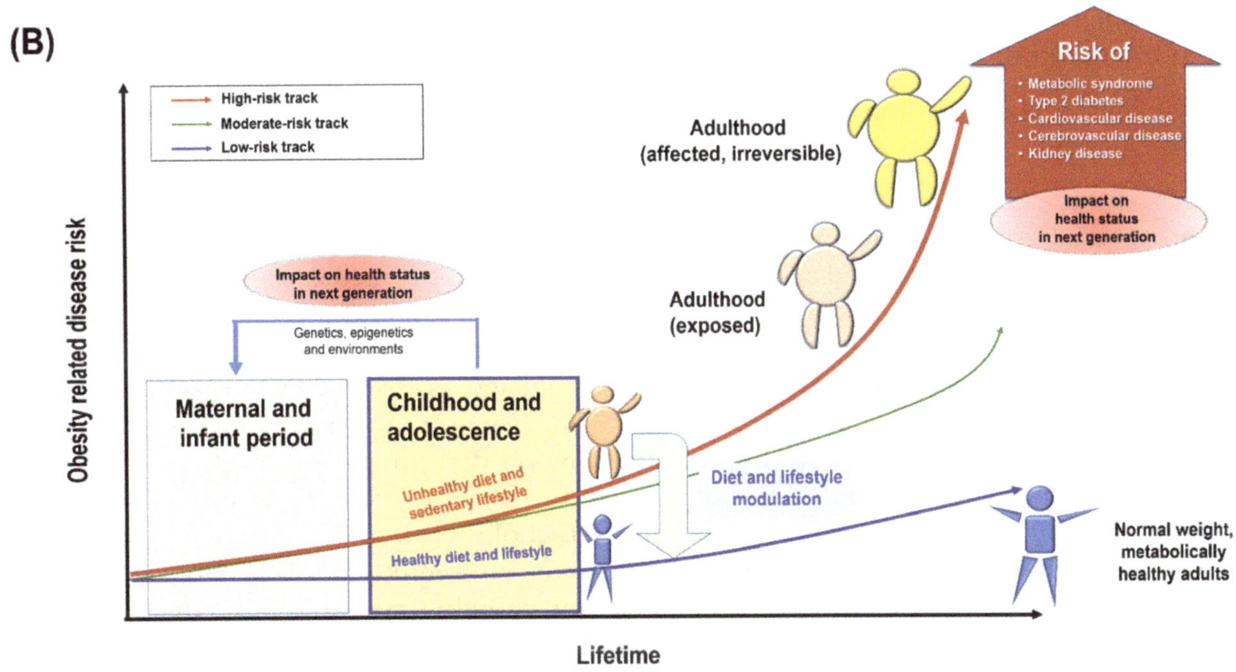

Figure 1. Effect of an energy-restricted, balanced diet with macronutrient modulation on body composition and metabolic status in children and adolescents, as well as throughout the lifetime. (**A**) Effect of dietary macronutrient modulation on children and adolescent body composition and metabolic status. *Energy restricted, balanced diets are effective in the treatment of obese adolescents and children, but the modulation effects of macronutrient composition on weight loss were inconsistent among the studies (**B**) Obesity-related disease risk throughout the lifetime [10,12–24,38].

4. Association between Dietary Macronutrient Intake Pattern, Obesity, and Related Metabolic Status in Children and Adolescents

Many interventions have been attempted to reduce bodyweight, maintain healthy bodyweight, and improve cardiometabolic risk factors by controlling dietary factors; for example, by reducing total energy intake, changing dietary macronutrient composition, and increasing energy expenditure [10–24]. Here, we summarize the effects of dietary pattern on body composition and metabolic status among children and adolescents, with a focus on dietary macronutrient modulation (DMM).

4.1. Definition of Low- or High-Macronutrient Dietary Compositions

Different studies apply a wide variety of definitions for low and high dietary composition of macronutrients. For example, macronutrient recommendations from 5 global institutions and governments (USA, Europe, Norway, Australia, New Zealand) have defined a balanced diet as one in which the proportions of total energy intake derived from carbohydrates, fat, and protein are between 45% and 65%, 25% and 35%, and 10% and 20%, respectively [39–43]. This means that a carbohydrate intake of over 65% of the total energy intake indicates high carbohydrate consumption, while a fat intake lower than 25% of the total energy intake indicates low fat consumption in the diet. Furthermore, the Akins diet, one of the most famous low-carbohydrate and high-fat diets, has an extremely restricted carbohydrate intake (5–20% of the total energy intake), and does not limit fat intake regardless of fat type (i.e., saturated or unsaturated) [44,45]. Another famous diet, named the zone diet, defines macronutrient dietary composition differently, promoting low carbohydrate (40%), high protein (30%), and high fat (25–35%) intake; this diet is also concerned with the quality of food ingredients consumed [46,47]. On the other hand, the Current Dietary Reference Intake for Korea (KDRI) defined a balanced diet as one composed of between 55% and 65% carbohydrates, 15% and 30% fats, and 7% and 20% protein; this definition differs from the Western definition [48]. The outcomes of studies can, therefore, be influenced by the definition used in the study. Therefore, this should be taken into consideration when drawing conclusions or comparing different studies.

4.2. Beneficial Effect of Dietary Macronutrient Modulation (DMM) on Body Composition and Metabolic Outcomes

Recently, the dietary macronutrient proportion in the diet and food selection patterns of children and adolescents were reported to affect body composition and metabolic status [10,12–17,19]. A short-term (12-week) randomized clinical trial for weight loss performed in obese adolescents showed that both a low-fat diet (55% carbohydrate; 20% protein; 25% fat) and modified-carbohydrate diet (35% carbohydrate; 30% protein; 35% fat) significantly improved body composition indicators, such as bodyweight, BMI, waist circumference, and body fat percentage, as assessed by bioelectrical impedance analysis and compared with a wait list control diet [17]. However, the improved body composition levels were not significantly different between the low-fat diet group and modified-carbohydrate diet group. In addition, the significant metabolic improvements were differently observed in the low-fat diet group (insulin resistance, total and LDL-cholesterol, and C-reactive protein) and in the modified-carbohydrate diet group (adiponectin and interleukin-6) [17]. On the other hand, a systemic review of 13 childhood studies compared low-carbohydrate, ad libitum diets with low-fat, energy-restricted diets and reported that the former were more effective for both weight loss and lowering of blood lipid levels at 6 months [10]. A meta-analysis of studies conducted among youth aged 6 to 18 years old also indicated that a low-carbohydrate diet showed a greater reduction in BMI immediately after dietary intervention than did a low-fat diet, even though cardiometabolic benefits from both diets were inconsistent [12].

Many studies have reported the effectiveness of low-carbohydrate and increased protein diets on weight reduction, weight maintenance, and improved cardiometabolic risk in obese adults [11,49–54]. Dietary protein is often considered as an important nutrient for diet-based weight management because it modulates neuro-endocrine signals related to satiety, thereby having a higher satiating effect than dietary carbohydrate and fat [6,15,55,56]. Moreover, a high-protein diet showed greater attenuation of a rebound of the relative change in ghrelin over time compared with a high-carbohydrate diet. This was observed in younger children [25] as well as in adults [38,54], although no effects were observed in another study [26]. In fact, sufficient protein intake and physical activity are important for forming body composition, particularly FFM [57]. Protein intake was significantly associated with BMI and FFM in young adults aged in their 20's [57], increased FFM in children and adolescents [58], and the maintenance of FFM in elderly people [59]. According to Rayman et al. [60,61], high-protein diets exceeding 25% of total energy intake or as protein intake ranging from 0.8 g/kg bodyweight (recommend dietary allowance, RDA) to 1.2–1.6 g/kg (up to double RDA values) in adults improve body composition by preserving lean mass and reducing BFM, especially when combined with training. In addition, Helms et al. suggested that protein intake in the range of 2.3–3.1 g/kg FFM was appropriate for lean, resistance-trained athletes in hypocaloric conditions in adults [62].

4.3. Non-Effectiveness of DMM on Body Composition and Metabolic Outcomes

As mentioned above, many studies have reported a beneficial effect of DMM on body composition and metabolic improvement. However, other evidence also suggests that improved weight status and body composition in overweight or obese children and adolescents can be achieved by reducing total energy in the diet and not by modulating macronutrient composition [20–24]. According to reports by Figueroa-Colon et al. [19] and Demol et al. [21], hypocaloric diets were effective in the treatment of obese adolescents and children, but the weight loss effect was not associated with macronutrient composition (low-carbohydrate–high-fat or high-carbohydrate–low-fat diets). In addition, several studies comparing the weight reduction effect of protein-increased diets in obese children and adolescents found the effect to be not significantly different from that of standard protein diet, regardless of the intervention periods (from 1 month to 2 years) [22–24,63]. These studies also showed no significant differences in the improvement of metabolic parameters such as blood pressure, lipid profiles, glucose concentrations, and insulin sensitivity [22–24,39]. According to a report by Sunehag et al. [14], obese adolescents had increased insulin secretory demands regardless of diet, and failure to increase insulin sensitivity while receiving a high-carbohydrate diet required a further increase in insulin secretion, which may lead to earlier β-cell failure. In addition, a high-fat (low-carbohydrate) diet could potentially increase the risk of fatty liver in obese adolescents [14]. These findings may indicate that neither the fat nor the carbohydrate composition in the diet have any effect on the improvement of insulin resistance in otherwise healthy adolescents who are obese [14]. Further investigations are needed to elucidate the macronutrient effect on weight loss and metabolic improvement in obese adolescents.

Table 1, presented on the next page, summarizes the descriptive information for the selected studies on the macronutrient effects on body composition and metabolic improvement in obese children and adolescents in terms of beneficial effects and non-effectiveness. More details are explained in Sections 4.2 and 4.3.

Table 1. Descriptive information for the selected studies on the macronutrient effects on body composition and metabolic improvement in obese children and adolescents.

Ref	Sources	Region	Subjects Characteristics	Study Design	Dietary Macronutrient Information	Main Outcome
[14]	J Clin Endocrinol Metab; 90: 4496–4502, 2005	Italy	Healthy obesity (boys $n = 6$; girls $n = 7$, 14.7 ± 0.3 y, BMI: 34 ± 1 kg/m^2, body fat: 42 ± 1%); normal weight adolescents in previous studies	Randomized crossover design (7-d)	Isocaloric/isonitrogenous diet; High-CHO: 60% CHO, 25% FAT; low-CHO: 30% CHO, 55% FAT	Increased total cholesterol, β-OH butyrate, and gluconeogenesis in the low-CHO group
[15]	Nutrients; 11: 340, 2019	Australia	Obesity ($n = 8$, 16.1 ± 0.4 y, BMI ≥ 95th percentile); healthy weight ($n = 12$, 16.0 ± 0.6 y, BMI: 5–85th percentile)	Double-blind crossover design	High-CHO: 79% CHO, 5% PRO, 16% FAT. High-PRO: 55% PRO, 30% CHO, 15% FAT	Higher ghrelin reduction in high-PRO group than high-CHO group; no differences in postprandial GLP-1 and PYY between the groups; higher postprandial glucose and insulin in high-CHO group than high-PRO group, particularly among obese subjects than normal weight subjects
[16]	Eur J Nutr; 58: 2327–2333, 2019	Australia	Obesity ($n = 13$, 15.4 ± 0.5 y, BMI ≥ 95th percentile); healthy weight ($n = 13$, 16.0 ± 0.6 y, BMI: 5–85th percentile)	Double-blind crossover design	High-CHO: 79% CHO, 5% PRO, 16% FAT. High-PRO: 55% PRO, 30% CHO, 15% FAT	Higher meal-induced thermogenesis in high-PRO group than high-CHO group; higher hunger in high-CHO group than high-PRO group
[17]	PLoS ONE; 11: e0151787, 2016	Australia	Hospitalized overweight /obesity (10–17 y, BMI ≥ 90th percentile): SMC ($n = 37$, 13.2 y), SLF ($n = 36$, 13.2 y), control ($n = 14$, 13.6 y)	Randomized, clinical trial (12-wk)	SMC: 35% CHO, 30% PRO, 35% FAT; SLF: 55% CHO, 20% PRO, 25% FAT	BMI z-score improvement in both SMC and, SLF groups; improvement of insulin resistance, total and LDL-cholesterol, and C-reactive protein in SLF group; improvement of adiponectin and interleukin-6 in SMC group

Table 1. *Cont.*

Ref	Sources	Region	Subjects Characteristics	Study Design	Dietary Macronutrient Information	Main Outcome
[19]	Am J Dis Child; 147: 160–166, 1993	USA	Obesity (n = 19, 7.5–16.9 y)	Intervention (14.5-m)	PSMFD: 2520 to 3360 J; HBD: 3360 to 4200 J	Significant weight reduction in both diet groups after 6 months; more weight reduction and fat-free mass maintenance in PSMFD group at 10-wk and 6-m
[21]	Pediatr Obes; 12; 179–194, 2017	Israel	Health obesity (boys n = 21, girls n = 34); 12–18 y (14.4 ± 1.7 y); BMI ≥ 90th percentile	Randomized clinical trial (12-wk) and follow-up (9-m)	LCLF (n = 18): 60g CHO (up to 20%), 30% FAT, 50% PRO; LCHF (n = 17): 60 g CHO (up to 20%), 20% FAT, 60% PRO; HCLF (n = 20): 50–60% CHO, 30% FAT, 20% PRO	No differences in the changes of BMI, BMI percentile, body fat %, and metabolic parameters among the all groups; reduction of insulin and insulin resistance in LCLF and LCHF groups
[22]	Obesity; 17;1808–1810, 2009	USA	Healthy obesity (boys n = 34, girls n = 61, 9–18 y)	Randomized trials (31-d)	SD (n = 49): 50–55% CHO, 15% PRO, 30–35% FAT; High-PRO (n = 46): 40–45% CHO, 25% PRO, 30–35% FAT	Reduction of BMI (−2 ± 0.25 kg/m^2) and other anthropometric parameters except body fat and systolic blood pressure in both groups; no differences of height or appetite between the two groups; increased desire for appetite in both groups
[23]	Am J Clin Nutr; 97; 276–285, 2013	Spain	Healthy obesity (boys n = 58, girls n = 55, 7–15 y), BMI ≥ 90th percentile	Randomized clinical trial (12-wk) and follow-up (2-y)	LGD (n = 57): 45–50% CHO-LG), 20–25% PRO, 30–35% FAT; LFD (n = 56): 55–60% CHO-no LGI, 15–20% PRO, 25–30% FAT	Significant reduction of BMI z-score in both groups; no significant differences in the changes of weight loss, insulin resistance, and metabolic syndrome risk factors between LGD and LFD groups

Table 1. *Cont.*

Ref	Sources	Region	Subjects Characteristics	Study Design	Dietary Macronutrient Information	Main Outcome
[24]	J Clin Endocrinol Metab; 98; 2116–2125	Australia	Overweight/obesity with prediabetes or insulin resistance (n = 111, boys 45, girls 66, 10–17 y)	Randomized clinical trials (12-m) and follow-up (24-m) *	HCLF (n = 55): 55–60% CHO-MGL, 30% FAT (≤10% saturated fat), 15% PRO; MCIP (n = 56): 40–45% CHO-MGL, 30% FAT(≤10% saturated fat), 25–30% PRO	Increased insulin sensitivity and reduced insulin to glucose in MCIP after 6-m; significant reductions of fasting insulin, SBP z-score, and DBP z-score in HCLF and MCIP groups, but not different between the two groups
[63]	Intern J Obes; 28; 514–519, 2004	France	Healthy obesity (boys n = 32, girls n = 89, 11–16 y, BMI ≥ 97 percentile)	Intervention (9-m) and follow-up (2-y)	Low-PRO (n = 53), 54% CHO, 15% PRO; High-PRO (n = 46), 50% CHO, 19% PRO with energy by breakfast 20%, lunch 31%, afternoon snack 16%, and dinner 33%	Reduction of BMI and BMI z-score in Low-PRO and High-PRO groups after the intervention, but yoyo effect observed after 2-y follow-up; no significant differences in the changes of weight loss (BMI z-score) between the two groups

CHO: carbohydrate; d: day, FAT: fat; HBD: hypocaloric balanced diet; HCLF: high-carbohydrate and low-fat diet; LCLF: low-carbohydrate and low-fat diet; LFD: low-fat diet MGL: moderate glycemic load; LGD: low glycemic diet; LGI: low glycemic index; m: month; MCIP: moderate-carbohydrate, increased protein diet %; SD: standard diet; SLF: structured low-fat diet; SMC: structured modified-carbohydrate diet; PRO: protein; PSMFD: protein-sparing modified fast diet; wk: week; y: year; * Metformin consumed during the intervention (start with 500 mg/day and end with 1000 mg/day).

5. Additional Factors Determining the Effectiveness of DMM on Body Adiposity and Metabolic Improvement

The effects of DMM-based interventions (i.e., a low-carbohydrate, increased-protein diet) on weight reduction and metabolic improvement in obese children and adolescents were inconsistent in the analyzed studies [10,12–24,61]. However, based on previous study results [19,21,22,64–66], we speculated that if the effects of several elements are taken into consideration, modulating macronutrient intake may improve body composition and specific cardiometabolic risk factors in obese children and adolescents.

5.1. Study Period

As with the study definition, the study period (short-term or long-term) should also be considered. For example, the beneficial effects of a low-carbohydrate diet compared with a standard low-fat diet on weight reduction and metabolic improvement in children and adolescents have usually been observed in the short term (10–12 weeks) and not in the long term (1 years or more) [19,21,22]. According to a report by Naude et al. [64], weight loss trials in overweight and obese adults showed weight reduction in the short term, irrespective of whether the diet is low in carbohydrate or balanced, and showed little or no difference in weight loss and changes in cardiovascular risk factors up to two years of follow-up. In fact, the study periods for weight reduction conducted in obese children and adolescents are typically shorter than those in obese adults. Therefore, to elucidate the weight loss effects of various dietary interventions in obese children and adolescents, long-term studies are needed. It should be noted, however, that body growth rate and hormonal changes should also be carefully considered, because secondary sexual characteristics begin to develop during this period. Furthermore, policies with a long-range view are needed in order to implement the optimal changes in the typical diets of children and adolescents to improve their health outcomes in real life.

5.2. Typical Eating Habits

Previous studies emphasized the importance of eating habits, such as regularity of breakfast intake and meal time, and the frequency of overeating and eating out in terms of healthy weight maintenance and improvement of metabolic abnormality [65,66]. For example, a randomized crossover trial with two 14-day isoenergetic diet periods separated by a 14-day habitual diet washout period compared the effects of regular (6 meals/day) and irregular (3–9 meals/day) meal patterns on the thermic effect of food (TEF), carbohydrate metabolism, subjective appetite, and gut hormones in healthy women [65]. The study findings showed that a regular meal pattern presented a greater TEF, greater insulin sensitivity, lower glucose responses, and beneficial subjective appetite changes, which may favor weight management and metabolic health. According to the cohort analysis of the National Survey for Health and Development, subjects with a more irregular intake of energy, especially at breakfast and lunch, appeared to have an increased cardiometabolic risk 10 and 17 years later [66].

Taken together, the findings of the studies analyzed in this narrative review suggest that DMM is an important part of therapeutic lifestyle intervention for weight control and healthy metabolic status. However, the effectiveness of DMM may not always be observed during the intervention period due to various influencing or confounding factors in the real world. Therefore, there is a need for persistence in maintaining the lifestyle modifications, including meal regularity and physical activity, over a long period, in order to accomplish the goal of achieving healthy body composition and metabolic status.

6. Effects of Adolescent Macronutrient Intake on Body Composition and Metabolic Status in Adulthood and Consequent Effects on the Health of the Next Generation

Previous studies suggested that maternal pre-pregnancy and life course nutrition rather than nutrition during pregnancy itself is more clearly linked to the offspring's fetal nutrition and growth and bodyweight [28,29]; that is, fetal nutrition can be influenced by the mother's own early life nutrition, including the accumulated energy balance of the mother in the months and years prior to conception [28,29]. Furthermore, the mother's own fetal life determines the germinal epithelium, where mature endometrial glands form, implying that the qualities of the endometrium may in part reflect the gestational nutritional conditions of the grandmother [29,67]. Of course, maternal macronutrient intake may influence the development and metabolic status of the offspring [55,56,68]. The Danish Fetal Origins Cohort study demonstrated that higher maternal dietary protein intake at the expense of carbohydrates during the second trimester of pregnancy was associated with a modest increase in offspring blood pressure in young adulthood [55]. On the other hand, maternal protein restriction in animal models throughout pregnancy and lactation, as well as during lactation only, was associated with placental dysfunction, offspring growth retardation, a generalized reduction in organ growth (with brain- and heart-sparing effects), and improved insulin sensitivity in the offspring [56,69–73], however protein restriction during the pregnancy only and not during lactation led to insulin resistance in the male offspring [73]. In addition, a lower protein-to-carbohydrate ratio (high-carbohydrate diet) in the maternal diet during pregnancy is associated with higher systolic blood pressure in childhood, which continues up to 4 years of age [74]. Consumption of diets including high saturated fats or refined sugars during pregnancy or lactation promote the pathogenesis of obesity, metabolic syndrome, and cardiovascular disorders in the offspring [75,76]. According to the Healthy Start study, maternal BMI and overnutrition due to a high-fat diet (30% of total energy intake from fat, with a high proportion of saturated fat) can induce obesity, insulin resistance, and impaired glucose utilization in the mothers [77,78]. These unfavorable maternal metabolic conditions may increase fetal growth and birth weight and expose offspring to the risk of obesity and type 2 diabetes in adulthood [77,78]. As briefly mentioned above, changes in body composition (i.e., the proportion and distribution of body FFM, FM, as well as BMI) in adolescence can alter the hormonal and metabolic status, consequently affecting adulthood health status and the risk of developing chronic diseases in adulthood. Based on the previous studies, we speculated that health and nutritional status during childhood and adolescence, which affect the probable body composition and health status in adulthood, are expected to influence the body composition and metabolic status of future offspring, i.e., the next generation (Figure 1B). In addition, changes in macronutrients ratios, especially in pregnancy, children, and adolescents, must be carried out very carefully and with contrasted scientific evidence, since this population is much more sensitive to changes of macronutrient proportions. Further studies are needed to clarify the relationship between adolescent health status and the health status of the next generation.

7. Summary

This study reviewed the effects of DMM on body composition and metabolic changes in adolescents and the consecutive influence on health status in adulthood, as well as on probable body composition and metabolic status in the next generation. Based on the findings of previous and recent reports, we suggest that DMM, including sufficient protein intake with slightly reduced carbohydrate intake, may be the most suitable way to improve body composition and metabolic status in obese adolescents, who should still grow up normally with the development of secondary sexual characteristics. However, this narrative review has some limitation. This is a narrative review that describes and appraises published articles so as to speculate on the new types of interventions and meta-analysis available, but may include potential selection and evaluation biases. This is in contrast to systemic reviews and meta-analyses, whose queries, criteria, and article selection processes are well-defined. In addition, this narrative review focused on the major types of macronutrients. The types of macronutrient subgroups (i.e., simple sugar, saturated fats) need to be considered in further studies. Despite these limitations, our review may provide novel insights into optimal dietary guidelines for healthy growth with accretion of adequate body composition during adolescence. It also provides guidance for effective strategies for prevention and management of the risk of obesity-related metabolic disease in adulthood and potential impacts on the health of the next generation.

Author Contributions: O.Y.K. and S.C. conceptualized and wrote the manuscript. O.Y.K., E.M.K., and S.C. revised the manuscript and finalized it. All authors have read and agreed to the published version of the manuscript.

References

1. World Health Organization. *WHO Obesity and Overweight Fact Sheet. No. 311*; World Health Organization: Geneva, Switzerland, 2016.
2. Bhupathiraju, S.N.; Hu, F.B. Epidemiology of Obesity and Diabetes and Their Cardiovascular Complications. *Circ. Res.* **2016**, *118*, 1723–1735. [CrossRef]
3. Gupta, N.; Goel, K.; Shah, P.; Misra, A. Childhood Obesity in Developing Countries: Epidemiology, Determinants, and Prevention. *Endocr. Rev.* **2012**, *33*, 48–70. [CrossRef] [PubMed]
4. Inchley, J.; Currie, D.; Jewell, J.; Breda, J.; Barnekow, V. (Eds.) *Adolescent Obesity and Related Behaviours: Trends and Inequalities in the WHO European Region, 2002–2014. Observation from the Health Behavior in School-Aged Children (HBSC) WHO Collaborative Cross-National Study*; World Health Organization Regional Office for Europe: Copenhagen, Denmark, 2017.
5. Biro, F.M.; Wien, M. Childhood obesity and adult morbidities. *Am. J. Clin. Nutr.* **2010**, *91*, 1499S–1505S. [CrossRef] [PubMed]
6. Freedman, D.S.; Khan, L.K.; Serdula, M.K.; Dietz, W.H.; Srinivasan, S.R.; Berenson, G.S. The Relation of Childhood BMI to Adult Adiposity: The Bogalusa Heart Study. *Pediatrics* **2005**, *115*, 22–27. [CrossRef]
7. Mustillo, S.; Worthman, C.; Erkanli, A.; Keeler, G.; Angold, A.; Costello, E.J. Obesity and Psychiatric Disorder: Developmental Trajectories. *Pediatrics* **2003**, *111*, 851–859. [CrossRef]
8. Strauss, R.S. Childhood obesity and self-esteem. *Pediatrics* **2000**, *105*, e15. [CrossRef]
9. Swallen, K.C.; Reither, E.N.; Haas, S.A.; Meier, A.M. Overweight, Obesity, and Health-Related Quality of Life among Adolescents: The National Longitudinal Study of Adolescent Health. *Pediatrics* **2005**, *115*, 340–347. [CrossRef]
10. Collins, C.; Warren, J.; Neve, M.; McCoy, P.; Stokes, B. Measuring effectiveness of dietetic interventions in child obesity: A systematic review of randomized trials. *Arch. Pediatr. Adolesc. Med.* **2006**, *160*, 906–922. [CrossRef]
11. Wycherley, T.P.; Moran, L.; Clifton, P.M.; Noakes, M.; Brinkworth, G.D. Effects of energy-restricted high-protein, low-fat compared with standard-protein, low-fat diets: A meta-analysis of randomized controlled trials. *Am. J. Clin. Nutr.* **2012**, *96*, 1281–1298. [CrossRef]
12. Gow, M.L.; Ho, M.; Burrows, T.L.; Baur, L.A.; Stewart, L.; Hutchesson, M.J.; Cowell, C.T.; Collins, C.E.; Garnett, S.P. Impact of dietary macronutrient distribution on BMI and cardiometabolic outcomes in overweight and obese children and adolescents: A systematic review. *Nutr. Rev.* **2014**, *72*, 453–470. [CrossRef]
13. Ervin, R.B.; Ogden, C.L. Trends in intake of energy and macronutrients in children and adolescents from 1999-2000 through 2009–2010. *NCHS Data Brief* **2013**, *113*, 1–8.
14. Sunehag, A.L.; Toffolo, G.; Campioni, M.; Bier, D.M.; Haymond, M.W. Effects of Dietary Macronutrient Intake on Insulin Sensitivity and Secretion and Glucose and Lipid Metabolism in Healthy, Obese Adolescents. *J. Clin. Endocrinol. Metab.* **2005**, *90*, 4496–4502. [CrossRef] [PubMed]
15. Nguo, K.; Bonham, M.; Truby, H.; Barber, E.; Brown, J.; Huggins, C.E. Effect of Macronutrient Composition on Appetite Hormone Responses in Adolescents with Obesity. *Nutrients* **2019**, *11*, 340. [CrossRef] [PubMed]
16. Nguo, K.; Huggins, C.E.; Truby, H.; Brown, J.; Bonham, M.P. Effect of macronutrient composition on meal-induced thermogenesis in adolescents with obesity. *Eur. J. Nutr.* **2019**, *58*, 2327–2333. [CrossRef] [PubMed]
17. Truby, H.; Baxter, K.; Ware, R.S.; Jensen, D.E.; Cardinal, J.W.; Warren, J.M.; Daniels, L.; Davies, P.S.W.; Barrett, P.; Blumfield, M.L.; et al. A Randomized Controlled Trial of Two Different Macronutrient Profiles on Weight, Body Composition and Metabolic Parameters in Obese Adolescents Seeking Weight Loss. *PLoS ONE* **2016**, *11*, e0151787. [CrossRef]
18. An, J.; Yoon, S.R.; Lee, J.H.; Kim, H.; Kim, O.Y. Importance of Adherence to Personalized Diet Intervention in Obesity Related Metabolic Improvement in Overweight and Obese Korean Adults. *Clin. Nutr. Res.* **2019**, *8*, 171–183. [CrossRef]

19. Figueroa-Colon, R.; Von Almen, T.K.; Franklin, F.A.; Schuftan, C.; Suskind, R.M. Comparison of Two Hypocaloric Diets in Obese Children. *Am. J. Dis. Child.* **1993**, *147*, 160–166. [CrossRef]
20. Schwartz, C.; King, N.A.; Perreira, B.; Blundell, J.E.; Thivel, D. A systematic review and meta-analysis of energy and macronutrient intake responses to physical activity interventions in children and adolescents with obesity. *Pediatr. Obes.* **2017**, *12*, 179–194. [CrossRef]
21. Demol, S.; Yackobovitch-Gavan, M.; Shalitin, S.; Nagelberg, N.; Gillon-Keren, M.; Phillip, M. Low-carbohydrate (low & high-fat) versus high-carbohydrate low-fat diets in the treatment of obesity in adolescents. *Acta Paediatr.* **2008**, *98*, 346–351. [CrossRef]
22. Duckworth, L.C.; Gately, P.J.; Radley, D.; Cooke, C.B.; King, R.F.; Hill, A.J. RCT of a High-protein Diet on Hunger Motivation and Weight-loss in Obese Children: An Extension and Replication. *Obesity* **2009**, *17*, 1808–1810. [CrossRef]
23. Mirza, N.M.; Palmer, M.G.; Sinclair, K.B.; McCarter, R.; He, J.; Ebbeling, C.B.; Ludwig, D.S.; A Yanovski, J. Effects of a low glycemic load or a low-fat dietary intervention on body weight in obese Hispanic American children and adolescents: A randomized controlled trial. *Am. J. Clin. Nutr.* **2013**, *97*, 276–285. [CrossRef]
24. Garnett, S.P.; Gow, M.L.; Ho, M.; Baur, L.A.; Noakes, M.; Woodhead, H.J.; Broderick, C.R.; Burrell, S.; Chisholm, K.; Halim, J.; et al. Optimal Macronutrient Content of the Diet for Adolescents with Prediabetes; RESIST a Randomised Control Trial. *J. Clin. Endocrinol. Metab.* **2013**, *98*, 2116–2125. [CrossRef]
25. Lomenick, J.P.; Clasey, J.L.; Anderson, J.W. Meal-related Changes in Ghrelin, Peptide YY, and Appetite in Normal Weight and Overweight Children. *Obesity* **2008**, *16*, 547–552. [CrossRef]
26. Smeets, A.J.; Soenen, S.; Luscombe-Marsh, N.D.; Ueland, O.; Westerterp-Plantenga, M.S. Energy Expenditure, Satiety, and Plasma Ghrelin, Glucagon-Like Peptide 1, and Peptide Tyrosine-Tyrosine Concentrations following a Single High-Protein Lunch. *J. Nutr.* **2008**, *138*, 698–702. [CrossRef]
27. Haroun, D.; Croker, H.; Viner, R.M.; Williams, J.E.; Darch, T.S.; Fewtrell, M.S.; Eaton, S.; Wells, J.C.K. Validation of BIA in Obese Children and Adolescents and Re-evaluation in a Longitudinal Study. *Obesity* **2009**, *17*, 2245–2250. [CrossRef]
28. Institute of Medicine, Subcommittee on Nutritional Status Weight Gain during Pregnancy, Subcommittee on Dietary Intake and Nutrient Supplements during Pregnancy. *Nutrition during Pregnancy: Part I, Weight Gain: Part II, Nutrient Supplements*; The National Academies Press: Washington, DC, USA, 1990.
29. Gray, C.A.; Bartol, F.F.; Tarleton, B.J.; Wiley, A.A.; Johnson, G.A.; Bazer, F.W.; Spencer, T.E. Developmental Biology of Uterine Glands. *Biol. Reprod.* **2001**, *65*, 1311–1323. [CrossRef]
30. Hales, C.M.; Carroll, M.D.; Fryar, C.D.; Ogden, C.L. Prevalence of Obesity Among Adults and Youth: United States, 2015–2016. *NCHS Data Brief* **2017**, *288*, 1–8.
31. Health at a Glance 2017. OECD Indicators. *OECD Library*. Available online: https://www.oecd-ilibrary.org/social-issues-migration-health/health-at-a-glance-2017_health_glance-2017-en (accessed on 16 May 2020).
32. Korean Health Promotion Institute. *Korea Health Promotion Forum*; Korean Health Promotion Institute: Wonju City, Korea, 2018.
33. Ministry of Education. *2018 School Health Statistics Report*; Ministry of Education: Sejong City, Korea, 2019.
34. Webb, V.L.; Wadden, T.A. Intensive Lifestyle Intervention for Obesity: Principles, Practices, and Results. *Gastroenterology* **2017**, *152*, 1752–1764. [CrossRef]
35. Fock, K.M.; Khoo, J. Diet and exercise in management of obesity and overweight. *J. Gastroenterol. Hepatol.* **2013**, *28*, 59–63. [CrossRef]
36. Ryan, D.H.; Frühbeck, G.; Ryan, D.H.; Wilding, J.P.H. Management of obesity. *Lancet* **2016**, *387*, 1947–1956. [CrossRef]
37. *Report of the Commission on Ending Childhood Obesity*; World Health Organization: Geneva, Switzerland, 2016. Available online: http://www.who.int/end-childhood-obesity/news/launch-final-report/en/ (accessed on 16 August 2020).
38. Bowen, J.; Noakes, M.; Trenerry, C.; Clifton, P.M. Energy Intake, Ghrelin, and Cholecystokinin after Different Carbohydrate and Protein Preloads in Overweight Men. *J. Clin. Endocrinol. Metab.* **2006**, *91*, 1477–1483. [CrossRef]
39. Institute of Medicine Food and Nutrition Board. *Dietary Reference Intakes for Energy, Carbohydrate, Fiber, Fat, Fatty Acids, Cholesterol, Protein, and Amino Acids (Macronutrients)*; National Academies Press: Washington, DC, USA, 2005.

40. European Food Safety Authority. Dietary Reference Values for Nutrients. Summary Report. EFSA Supporting Publication. 2017, e15121. Available online: https://www.efsa.europa.eu/en/supporting/pub/e15121 (accessed on 16 August 2020).
41. NNR Project Group. *Nordic Nutrition Recommendations 2004: Integrating Nutrition And Physical Activit*, 4th ed.; Nordic Council of Ministers: Copenhagen, Denmark, 2005.
42. Becker, W.; Lyhne, N.; Pedersen, A.N.; Aro, A.; Fogelholm, M.; Phorsdottir, I.; Alexander, J.; Anderssen, S.A.; Meltzer, H.M.; Pedersen, J.I. Nordic Nutrition Recommendations 2004—Integrating nutrition and physical activity. *Scandi J. Nutr.* **2004**, *48*, 178–187. [CrossRef]
43. Australian National Health and Medical Research Council and the New Zealand Ministry of Health. *Nutrient Reference Values for Australia and New Zealand: Including Recommended Dietary Intakes*; Australian National Health and Medical Research Council and the New Zealand Ministry of Health: Canberra, Australia, 2006.
44. Atkins Nutritionals. New Atkins. Atkins Nutritionals 2011. Available online: http://sa.atkins.com/ (accessed on 16 August 2020).
45. WebMD. The Atkins Diet. WebMD, 2012. Available online: http://www.webmd.com/diet/atkins-dietwhat-it-is (accessed on 19 November 2020).
46. Zone Labs. Dr Sears Zone Diet. Zone Labs Inc. 2012. Available online: http://www.zonediet.com/ (accessed on 16 August 2020).
47. Barnett, J. The Zone Diet Explained. Crossfit Impulse, 2009. Available online: http://crossfitimpulse.com/thezone-diet-explained-edited (accessed on 17 May 2020).
48. Ministry of Health and Welfare. *Korean Nutrition Society. Dietary Reference Intake for Koreans*; Ministry of Health and Welfare: Sejong City, Korea, 2015.
49. Westerterp-Plantenga, M.S.; Nieuwenhuizen, A.; Tomé, D.; Soenen, S.; Westerterp, K. Dietary Protein, Weight Loss, and Weight Maintenance. *Annu. Rev. Nutr.* **2009**, *29*, 21–41. [CrossRef] [PubMed]
50. Skov, A.R.; Toubro, S.; Rønn, B.; Holm, L.; Astrup, A. Randomized trial on protein vs carbohydrate in ad libitum fat reduced diet for the treatment of obesity. *Int. J. Obes.* **1999**, *23*, 528–536. [CrossRef]
51. Westerterp-Plantenga, M.S.; Lejeune, M.P.; Nijs, I.; Van Ooijen, A.; Kovacs, E. High protein intake sustains weight maintenance after body weight loss in humans. *Int. J. Obes. Relat. Metab. Disord.* **2004**, *28*, 57–64. [CrossRef]
52. Larsen, T.M.; Dalskov, S.M.; van Baak, M.; Jebb, S.A.; Papadaki, A.; Pfeiffer, A.F.; Martinez, J.A.; Handjieva-Darlenska, T.; Kunešová, M.; Pihlsgård, M.; et al. Diets with High or Low Protein Content and Glycemic Index for Weight-Loss Maintenance. *N. Engl. J. Med.* **2010**, *363*, 2102–2113. [CrossRef]
53. Gögebakan, Ö.; Kohl, A.; Osterhoff, M.A.; van Baak, M.A.; Jebb, S.A.; Papadaki, A.; Martinez, J.A.; Handjieva-Darlenska, T.; Hlavaty, P.; Weickert, M.O.; et al. Effects of weight loss and long-term weight maintenance with diets varying in protein and glycemic index on cardiovascular risk factors: The diet, obesity, and genes (DiOGenes) study: A randomized, controlled trial. *Circulation* **2011**, *124*, 2829–2838. [CrossRef]
54. Foster-Schubert, K.E.; Overduin, J.; Prudom, C.E.; Liu, J.; Callahan, H.S.; Gaylinn, B.D.; Thorner, M.O.; Cummings, D.E. Acyl and Total Ghrelin Are Suppressed Strongly by Ingested Proteins, Weakly by Lipids, and Biphasically by Carbohydrates. *J. Clin. Endocrinol. Metab.* **2008**, *93*, 1971–1979. [CrossRef]
55. Hrolfsdottir, L.; Halldorsson, T.I.; Rytter, R.; Bech, B.H.; Birgisdottir, B.E.; Gunnarsdottir, I.; Granström, C.; Henriksen, T.B.; Olsen, S.F.; Maslova, E. Maternal Macronutrient Intake and Offspring Blood Pressure 20 Years Later. *J. Am. Heart Assoc.* **2017**, *6*, e005808. [CrossRef]
56. Kereliuk, S.M.; Brawerman, G.M.; Dolinsky, V.W. Maternal Macronutrient Consumption and the Developmental Origins of Metabolic Disease in the Offspring. *Int. J. Mol. Sci.* **2017**, *18*, 1451. [CrossRef]
57. Correa-Rodríguez, M.; Rueda-Medina, B.; González-Jiménez, E.; Schmidt-RioValle, J. Associations between body composition, nutrition, and physical activity in young adults. *Am. J. Hum. Biol.* **2017**, *29*, e22903. [CrossRef] [PubMed]
58. Cameron, J.D.; Sigal, R.J.; Kenny, G.P.; Alberga, A.S.; Prud'Homme, D.; Phillips, P.; Doucette, S.; Goldfield, G.S. Body composition and energy intake—Skeletal muscle mass is the strongest predictor of food intake in obese adolescents: The HEARTY trial. *Appl. Physiol. Nutr. Metab.* **2016**, *41*, 611–617. [CrossRef] [PubMed]
59. Verreijen, A.M.; Engberink, M.F.; Memelink, R.G.; Van Der Plas, S.E.; Visser, M.; Weijs, P.J.M. Effect of a high protein diet and/or resistance exercise on the preservation of fat free mass during weight loss in overweight and obese older adults: A randomized controlled trial. *Nutr. J.* **2017**, *16*, 1–8. [CrossRef] [PubMed]

60. Layman, D.K.; Evans, E.M.; Erickson, D.; Seyler, J.; Weber, J.; Bagshaw, D.; Griel, A.; Psota, T.; Kris-Etherton, P. A Moderate-Protein Diet Produces Sustained Weight Loss and Long-Term Changes in Body Composition and Blood Lipids in Obese Adults. *J. Nutr.* **2009**, *139*, 514–521. [CrossRef]
61. Layman, D.K.; Evans, E.; Baum, J.I.; Seyler, J.; Erickson, D.J.; Boileau, R.A. Dietary Protein and Exercise Have Additive Effects on Body Composition during Weight Loss in Adult Women. *J. Nutr.* **2005**, *135*, 1903–1910. [CrossRef]
62. Helms, E.R.; Zinn, C.; Rowlands, D.S.; Brown, S.R. A Systematic Review of Dietary Protein during Caloric Restriction in Resistance Trained Lean Athletes: A Case for Higher Intakes. *Int. J. Sport Nutr. Exerc. Metab.* **2014**, *24*, 127–138. [CrossRef]
63. Rolland-Cachera, M.F.; Thibault, H.; Souberbielle, J.C.; Soulié, D.; Carbonel, P.; Deheeger, M.; Roinsol, D.; Longueville, E.; Bellisle, F.; Serog, P. Massive obesity in adolescents: Dietary interventions and behaviours associated with weight regain at 2 y follow-up. *Int. J. Obes. Relat. Metab. Disord.* **2004**, *28*, 514–519. [CrossRef]
64. Naude, C.E.; Schoonees, A.; Senekal, M.; Young, T.; Garner, P.; Volmink, J. Low carbohydrate versus isoenergetic balanced diets for reducing weight and cardiovascular risk: A systematic review and meta-analysis. *PLoS ONE* **2014**, *9*, e100652. [CrossRef]
65. Alhussain, M.H.; Macdonald, I.A.; Taylor, M.A. Irregular meal-pattern effects on energy expenditure, metabolism, and appetite regulation: A randomized controlled trial in healthy normal-weight women. *Am. J. Clin. Nutr.* **2016**, *104*, 21–32. [CrossRef]
66. Pot, G.K.; Hardy, R.; Stephen, A.M. Irregularity of energy intake at meals: Prospective associations with the metabolic syndrome in adults of the 1946 British birth cohort. *Br. J. Nutr.* **2016**, *115*, 315–323. [CrossRef]
67. Thayer, Z.M.; Rutherford, J.; Kuzawa, C.W. The Maternal Nutritional Buffering Model: An evolutionary framework for pregnancy nutritional intervention. *Evol. Med. Public Health* **2020**, *2020*, 14–27. [CrossRef]
68. Chen, L.-W.; Aris, I.M.; Bernard, J.Y.; Tint, M.-T.; Colega, M.; Gluckman, P.D.; Tan, K.H.; Shek, L.P.-C.; Chong, Y.-S.; Yap, F.; et al. Associations of maternal macronutrient intake during pregnancy with infant BMI peak characteristics and childhood BMI. *Am. J. Clin. Nutr.* **2017**, *105*, 705–713. [CrossRef]
69. Fernandez-Twinn, D.S.; Wayman, A.P.; Ekizoglou, S.; Martin, M.S.; Hales, C.N.; Ozanne, S.E. Maternal protein restriction leads to hyperinsulinemia and reduced insulin-signaling protein expression in 21-mo-old female rat offspring. *Am. J. Physiol. Regul. Integr. Comp. Physiol.* **2005**, *288*, R368–R373. [CrossRef]
70. Gonzalez, P.N.; Gasperowicz, M.; Barbeito-Andres, J.; Klenin, N.; Cross, J.C.; Hallgrimsson, B. Chronicprotein restriction in mice impacts placental function and maternal body weight before fetal growth. *PLoS ONE* **2016**, *11*, e0152227. [CrossRef]
71. Ozanne, S.E.; Hales, C.N. For Debate: Fetal and early postnatal growth restriction lead to diabetes, the metabolic syndrome and renal failure. *Diabetologia* **2003**, *46*, 1013–1019. [CrossRef]
72. De Brito Alves, J.L.; de Oliveira, J.M.D.; Ferreira, D.J.S.; de V Barros, M.A.; Nogueira, V.O.; Alves, D.S.; Vida, H.; Leandro, C.G.; Lagranha, C.J.; Pirola, L.; et al. Maternal protein restriction induced-hypertension is associated to oxidative disruption at transcriptional and functional levels in the medullaoblongata. *Clin. Exp. Pharmacol. Physiol.* **2016**, *43*, 1177–1184. [CrossRef]
73. Zambrano, E.; Bautista, C.J.; Deás, M.; Martínez-Samayoa, P.M.; González-Zamorano, M.; Ledesma, H.; Morales, J.; Larrea, F.; Nathanielsz, P.W. A low maternal protein diet during pregnancy and lactation has sex-and window of exposure-specific effects on offspring growth and food intake, glucose metabolism and serum leptin in the rat. *J. Physiol.* **2006**, *571*, 221–230. [CrossRef]
74. Blumfield, M.L.; Nowson, C.A.; Hure, A.J.; Smith, R.; Simpson, S.J.; Raubenheimer, D.; MacDonald-Wicks, L.; Collins, C.E. Lower Protein-to-Carbohydrate Ratio in Maternal Diet is Associated with Higher Childhood Systolic Blood Pressure up to Age Four Years. *Nutrients* **2015**, *7*, 3078–3093. [CrossRef]
75. Pereira, T.J.; Fonseca, M.A.; Campbell, K.E.; Moyce, B.L.; Cole, L.K.; Hatch, G.M.; Doucette, C.A.; Klein, J.; Aliani, M.; Dolinsky, V.W. Maternal obesity characterized by gestational diabetes increases the susceptibility of rat offspring to hepatic steatosis via a disrupted liver metabolome. *J. Physiol.* **2015**, *593*, 3181–3197. [CrossRef]
76. Clausen, T.D.; Mathiesen, E.R.; Hansen, T.; Pedersen, O.; Jensen, D.M.; Lauenborg, J.; Schmidt, L.; Damm, P. Overweight and the Metabolic Syndrome in Adult Offspring of Women with Diet-Treated Gestational Diabetes Mellitus or Type 1 Diabetes. *J. Clin. Endocrinol. Metab.* **2009**, *94*, 2464–2470. [CrossRef]

77. Shapiro, A.L.B.; Ringham, B.M.; Glueck, D.H.; Norris, J.M.; Barbour, L.A.; Friedman, J.E.; Dabelea, D.; Glueck, D.H. Infant Adiposity is Independently Associated with a Maternal High Fat Diet but not Related to Niacin Intake: The Healthy Start Study. *Matern. Child Health J.* **2017**, *21*, 1662–1668. [CrossRef]
78. Shapiro, A.L.B.; Schmiege, S.J.; Brinton, J.T.; Glueck, D.; Crume, T.L.; Friedman, J.E.; Dabelea, D. Testing the fuel-mediated hypothesis: Maternal insulin resistance and glucose mediate the association between maternal and neonatal adiposity, the Healthy Start study. *Diabetologia* **2015**, *58*, 937–941. [CrossRef] [PubMed]

3

A Polish Study on the Influence of Food Neophobia in Children (10–12 Years Old) on the Intake of Vegetables and Fruits

Dominika Guzek [1,*], Dominika Głąbska [2], Ewa Lange [2] and Marzena Jezewska-Zychowicz [1]

1 Department of Organization and Consumption Economics, Faculty of Human Nutrition and Consumer Sciences, Warsaw University of Life Sciences (SGGW-WULS), 159C Nowoursynowska Street, 02-787 Warsaw, Poland; marzena_jezewska_zychowicz@sggw.pl

2 Department of Dietetics, Faculty of Human Nutrition and Consumer Sciences, Warsaw University of Life Sciences (SGGW-WULS), 159C Nowoursynowska Street, 02-787 Warsaw, Poland; dominika_glabska@sggw.pl (D.G.); ewa_lange@sggw.pl (E.L.)

* Correspondence: dominika_guzek@sggw.pl

Abstract: Adhering to the recommended intake of fruits and vegetables is an important habit that should be inculcated in children, whereas food neophobia is indicated as one of the most important factors creating food preferences that may interfere. The aim of the presented study was to analyze the association between the food neophobia level and the intake of fruits and vegetables in children aged 10–12 years. The study was conducted among a group of 163 children (78 girls and 85 boys). The assessment of the food neophobia level was based on the Food Neophobia Scale (FNS) questionnaire and the assessment of the fruit and vegetable intake was based on the food frequency questionnaire. A negative correlation between the food neophobia level and the vegetable intake was observed both for girls ($p = 0.032$; $R = -0.2432$) and for boys ($p = 0.004$; $R = -0.3071$), whereas for girls differences in vegetable intake were observed also between various food neophobia categories ($p = 0.0144$). It may be concluded that children with higher food neophobia level are characterized by lower vegetable intake than children with lower food neophobia level. For fruits and juices of fruits and vegetables, associations with food neophobia level were not observed.

Keywords: food neophobia; Food Neophobia Scale (FNS); children; fruits; vegetables; juices

---

1. Introduction

Inadequate intake of fruits and vegetables is indicated as a reason for 6.7 million deaths worldwide each year, which was estimated for the year 2010 [1]. The World Health Organization indicated in a report [2] that, if consumed in the recommended amounts, fruits and vegetables reduce the risk of noncommunicable diseases, including coronary heart disease, stroke, and some types of cancers.

Especially in the case of children, vegetable intake is perceived as beneficial, and consuming them in every meal is a positive behavior that may contribute to healthier dietary patterns [3]. Moreover, it was confirmed in a Polish study on a group of girls that the pattern associated with high fruit and vegetable intake was connected with greater restrictions in the intake of products high in sugar, fat, and starch [4].

In spite of the beneficial effects of fruits and vegetables, in a study of 52 countries taking part in the World Health Survey (2002–2003), the intake was stated to be lower than the lowest recommended number of five servings per day (80 g of fruits/vegetables per serving) for 77.6% of men and 78.4% of women from all the countries [5]. Similarly, in the Child and Adolescent Health Surveys (KiGGS wave 1), it was found that in the age group of 3–17 years, girls consumed 2.7 and boys consumed 2.4 servings of fruits and vegetables per day, whereas only 12.2% of girls and 9.4% of boys consumed five servings per day [6].

It is emphasized that even higher fruit and vegetable intake must be considered, as the World Health Organization recommends 600 g (7.5 servings) per day in adults and 480 g (6 servings) per day in children aged 5–14 years [7]. Achieving the recommended intake of fruits and vegetables in children is a challenge. On the one hand, established children's dietary patterns predict adulthood dietary patterns, but on the other, compared with adults, there are additional factors influencing children's fruit and vegetable intake [2]. Considering both factors, parental role modeling is important, as it is a significant predictor of children's dietary patterns [8]. In general, it may be indicated that the two determining factors, not observed in the case of adults, are parental intake and home accessibility, while the other most prominent determinants indicated for children are gender, age, socioeconomic position of the family, and preferences [9].

Among all the determinants of food choices indicated for children, only their preferences are directly dependent on them. However, children typically prefer familiar, bland, and sweet products, whereas in the case of unknown food products, aversion may occur [10]. Food neophobia is indicated as the most important factor creating food preferences in the case of younger children [11], but also, in the case of children aged 10–11 years, it is emphasized that they should be introduced to unfamiliar fruits and vegetables in order to increase their taste preferences [12].

The aim of the presented study was to analyze the association between the food neophobia level and the intake of fruits and vegetables in children aged 10–12 years.

2. Materials and Methods

2.1. Ethics Approval

The study was conducted according to the guidelines laid down in the Declaration of Helsinki, and all the procedures involving human subjects were approved by the Ethics Committee of the Faculty of Human Nutrition and Consumer Sciences of the Warsaw University of Life Sciences (SGGW-WULS) in Warsaw, Poland (No. 10/2016; 12.12.2016).

2.2. Study Participants

The study group was recruited in the group of children aged 10–12 years from Warsaw, who participated in the scientific nutrition workshops for children conducted in the Dietary Outpatient Clinic of the Faculty of Human Nutrition and Consumer Sciences of the SGGW-WULS. Inclusion criteria were children aged 10–12 years, not suffering from any developmental disorder affecting intellectual abilities, including various intellectual or cognitive deficits. The information about nutritional workshops for children aged 10–12 years was placed on the web page, and 258 children were signed up for the workshops by their parents. The workshops' participants were proposed to take part in the study for analyzing the association between food neophobia level and fruit and vegetable intake. One hundred and seventy-five children agreed to participate, and their parents or legal guardians also provided written consent to participate. The exclusion criterion was nonprovision of written consent to participate.

The participants were asked to fill in two questionnaires: the Food Neophobia Scale (FNS) questionnaire by Pliner and Hobden [13] and the food frequency questionnaire consisting of 31 questions about various groups of products. Because not all participants filled in both questionnaires and due to some missing data, 163 participants (78 girls and 85 boys) were included in the final analysis. The study design and number of participants are presented in Figure 1.

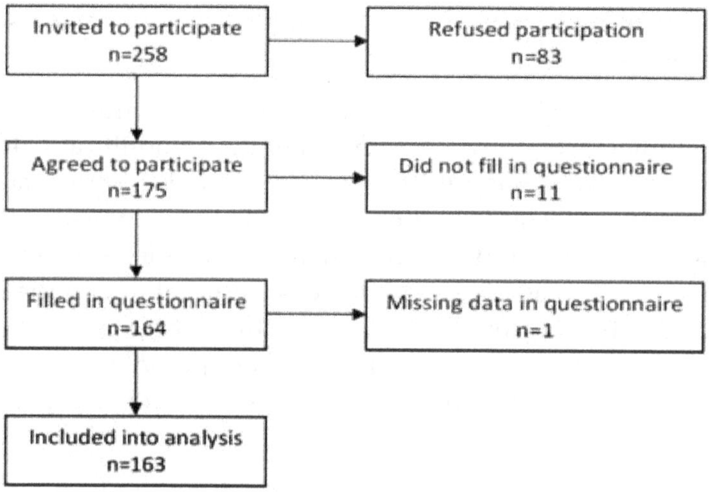

Figure 1. Study design and number of participants.

2.3. Assessment of the Food Neophobia Level

The FNS questionnaire was applied in order to assess the food neophobia level in the analyzed individuals. Each individual received the list of sentences and was asked to rate his or her level of agreement with each sentence, using one of the seven categories of answer (scale from strongly disagree to strongly agree). Because the 10-item FNS questionnaire of Pliner and Hobden [13] includes five positive items (indicating neophilic individuals) and five negative items (indicating neophobic individuals), negative responses were reversed during the analysis of data [14]. In the present group, Cronbach's alpha was at a respectable level (0.78; $n = 163$), and the same respectable level was observed for the group of boys (0.78; $n = 78$), whereas for the group of girls, it was stated to be very good (0.85; $n = 85$), indicating good internal consistency [15].

The calculated food neophobia level ranged from 10 to 70 and, on the basis of the level, the participants were divided into three tertiles characterized by various food neophobia levels: low values (first tertile) are attributed to a low neophobia level (neophilic), medium values (second tertile) are attributed to a medium neophobia level, and high values (third tertile) are attributed to a high neophobia level (neophobic) [16].

2.4. Assessment of the Fruit and Vegetable Intake

The food frequency questionnaire was applied in order to assess the typical intake of fruits and vegetables as well as fruit and vegetable juices among the analyzed individuals. In order to reduce overestimation due to high self-appraisal, the respondents were asked not only about fruits and vegetables, and fruit and vegetable juices, but also about all the most important food products groups, without giving any information as to which items would be assessed. Potatoes were also categorized as a separate group to avoid misinterpreting them as vegetables. The applied questionnaire was previously positively validated on the basis of a Bland-Altman plot in a group of 172 children.

Each individual received the list of food products groups with specified serving size and was asked about the exact number of servings (calculated not only in integers, but also decimal parts) of the products specified in the questionnaire consumed per day/week/month (depending on the product), according the methodology described previously [17]. In the case of fruits and vegetables, participants were asked to specify the number of servings consumed per day, whereas in the case of fruit and vegetable juices, they were asked to specify the number of servings consumed per week. In the case of fruits and vegetables, the described serving size was 100 g, so the numbers of servings were multiplied by 100 g to obtain the typical intake value per day. In the case of fruit and vegetable juices, the described serving size was 250 g, so the number of servings was multiplied by 250 g and divided by seven (days) to obtain a typical intake value per day. The serving sizes were not only expressed in terms of grams, but also described using typical household measures.

2.5. Statistical Analysis

The obtained data are presented as means ± standard deviation (SD) with minimum, maximum, and median values. The distributions of the analyzed factors were verified by using the Shapiro-Wilk test. Internal reliability of the FNS for the group was tested using the Cronbach's alpha coefficient. Differences between groups were identified by using the U Mann-Whitney test and Kruskal-Wallis ANOVA test (applied for nonparametric distribution). Analyses of the correlations were verified by using Spearman's rank correlation coefficient (applied for nonparametric distribution).

The accepted level of significance was set at $p \leq 0.05$. Statistical analysis was conducted using Statistica software version 8.0 (StatSoft Inc., Tulsa, OK, USA).

3. Results

The assessment of fruit intake observed for the analyzed groups of girls and boys in various food neophobia categories is presented in Table 1. No differences in fruit intake in the groups of children characterized by various neophobia levels were stated for both girls and boys. Also, no differences in fruit intake between girls and boys from the same neophobia level were observed.

Table 1. Fruit intake (g/day) for boys and girls in Food Neophobia Scale categories—mean ± SD, as well as median, minimum, and maximum values are presented, and compared between genders and between food neophobia categories.

Food Neophobia Category (Tertile of Food Neophobia Scale)	Girls; n = 78		Boys; n = 85		p-Value
	Mean ± SD	Median (Minimum–Maximum)	Mean ± SD	Median (Minimum–Maximum)	
Low (first)	198.1 ± 122.0	200.0 * (0.0–500.0)	202.1 ± 156.2	200.0 * (10.0–600.0)	0.7077
Medium (second)	180.8 ± 99.1	175.0 * (50.0–400.0)	187.9 ± 108.3	200.0 * (50.0–400.0)	0.7594
High (third)	163.5 ± 126.9	100.0 * (50.0–600.0)	175.9 ± 116.2	150.0 * (0.0–500.0)	0.4121
p-Value	0.8890		0.2736		

* distribution different than normal (verified using Shapiro-Wilk test—$p \leq 0.05$).

The assessment of vegetable intake observed for the analyzed groups of girls and boys in various food neophobia categories is presented in Table 2. No differences in vegetable intake in the group of boys characterized by various neophobia levels were found. In the group of girls, it was found that the differences in vegetable intake observed between various food neophobia categories were statistically significant ($p = 0.0144$). At the same time, no differences in vegetable intake between girls and boys from the same neophobia level were observed.

Table 2. Vegetable intake (g/day) for boys and girls in Food Neophobia Scale categories—mean ± SD, as well as median, minimum, and maximum values are presented, and compared between genders and between food neophobia categories.

Food Neophobia Category (Tertile of Food Neophobia Scale)	Girls; n = 78		Boys; n = 85		p-Value
	Mean ± SD	Median (Minimum–Maximum)	Mean ± SD	Median (Minimum–Maximum)	
Low (first)	165.4 ± 119.0	100.0 * (0.0–400.0)	158.2 ± 107.3	100.0 * (50.0–500.0)	0.9635
Medium (second)	167.3 ± 103.9	200.0 * (0.0–400.0)	161.2 ± 144.8	100.0 * (50.0–800.0)	0.3796
High (third)	118.8 ± 105.2	100.0 * (0.0–500.0)	97.5 ± 76.4	100.0 * (0.0–300.0)	0.4988
p-Value	0.0144		0.0983		

* distribution different than normal (verified using Shapiro-Wilk test—$p \leq 0.05$).

The assessment of fruit and vegetable juice intake observed for the analyzed groups of girls and boys in various food neophobia categories is presented in Table 3. No differences in fruit and vegetable juice intake in the groups of children characterized by various neophobia levels were stated for both girls and boys. Also, no differences in fruit and vegetable juice intake between girls and boys from the same neophobia level were observed.

Table 3. Fruit and vegetable juice intake (g/day) for boys and girls in Food Neophobia Scale categories—mean ± SD, as well as median, minimum, and maximum values are presented, and compared between genders and between food neophobia categories.

Food Neophobia Category (Tertile of Food Neophobia Scale)	Girls; $n = 78$		Boys; $n = 85$		p-Value
	Mean ± SD	Median (Minimum–Maximum)	Mean ± SD	Median (Minimum–Maximum)	
Low (first)	115.4 ± 106.6	89.3 * (0.0–428.6)	195.8 ± 225.0	107.1 * (0.0–1000.0)	0.3245
Medium (second)	140.1 ± 119.0	107.1 * (0.0–357.1)	153.9 ± 147.9	107.1 * (0.0–535.7)	0.7998
High (third)	136.7 ± 185.2	71.4 * (0.0–642.9)	154.3 ± 127.5	142.9 * (0.0–500.0)	0.1496
p-Value	0.9602		0.5550		

* distribution different than normal (verified using Shapiro-Wilk test—$p \leq 0.05$).

To verify the differences in fruit and vegetable intake observed between girls of various food neophobia categories, analysis of correlation between the food neophobia level and the intake of fruits, vegetables, and fruit and vegetable juices was conducted (Table 4). It was confirmed that neither for fruits nor for fruit and vegetable juices, the association between food neophobia level and intake exists, for both girls and boys. Simultaneously, the previously indicated association for vegetables was proven. It was stated that the negative correlation between the food neophobia level and vegetable intake exists in both girls ($p = 0.032$; $R = -0.2432$) and boys ($p = 0.004$; $R = -0.3071$); thus, it may be indicated that children with a higher neophobia level are characterized by lower vegetable intake than children with a lower neophobia level.

Table 4. Analysis of correlation between food neophobia level and fruit intake, vegetable intake, as well as fruit and vegetable juice intake.

	Girls; $n = 78$		Boys; $n = 85$	
	p	R	p	R
Fruits	0.069	−0.2071 *	0.842	−0.0219 *
Vegetables	0.032	−0.2432 *	0.004	−0.3071*
Fruit and vegetable juices	0.416	−0.0933 *	0.490	−0.0759 *

* Spearman's rank coefficient.

4. Discussion

Considering the low fruit and vegetable intake in children, indicating the factors that may influence it as well as suggesting the possible ways to overcome the observed trend may be crucial to improve the nutritional value of diet by increasing its variety [18]. Food neophobia (defined as reluctance or avoidance of unknown food products) and pickiness (defined as consuming an inadequate variety of food products, due to the rejection of substantial number of them) are indicated as the most important factors that may cause low vegetable intake [19]. Pickiness is not always reasoned by food neophobia [20] but, in the case of food neophobia, pickiness of unknown food products is common [21].

Food neophobia in children may be associated not only with pickiness, but also with unwillingness to even try unfamiliar food products, which might result in following an improperly balanced diet [18]. Because of food neophobia in adolescence, neophobic behaviors may be transferred to adulthood [22], as it was indicated that such behaviors often remain stable from the age of 13 years to adulthood [23]. At the same time, the age of 9 years is indicated as critical because before that age, the development of food behaviors takes place [24]. Taking this into account, the analysis of food neophobia, its determinants, and consequences among the group of children aged 10–12 years is of a great value, as at such an age there is still a possibility of creating preferences and to trying to reduce the level of neophobic behaviors.

It needs to be emphasized that, in spite of the fact that in preschool children (early childhood) parents can influence dietary patterns [25], in the late childhood, parental influence is reduced in comparison with early childhood, which is associated inter alia with not participating in family dinners [26]. However, the influence of peers is also an important factor, which was proven in the case of vegetable choices, as it was observed that eating vegetables with peers was associated not only with choosing nonpreferred ones, while peers did so, but also with changing preferences [27].

Fruit and vegetable choices in general are associated with children preferences and accessibility [14], which are related to the factors associated not only with the family but also with the country. In the Polish population, it is indicated that national traditions and customs may influence vegetable intake, as they may, for example, cause higher cabbage intake, which is associated with a number of traditional recipes of cabbage dishes that are commonly consumed [28]. However, among the most preferred and most frequently consumed vegetables in Poland in the group of school children are carrots, cucumbers, radishes, and tomatoes; among the most preferred fruits are strawberries, tangerines, oranges, and blueberries, whereas among the most frequently consumed fruits are apples, tangerines, bananas, and oranges [29]. At the same time, in a group of Spanish children and young people, among the most preferred fruits and vegetables are similar products such as apples, bananas, carrots, tomatoes, and lettuce [30].

Vegetable intake is important in the context of food neophobia, as it concerns mainly fruits and vegetables [31]. Moreover, it is indicated that in general, for children, vegetables are characterized by a lower acceptance level than fruits [32], and is even observed to be the lowest among the acceptance levels for all the food product groups [33]. This may partly explain the results of the present study, and the fact that vegetable intake was more prone than fruit intake to be reduced in the case of children characterized by a high food neophobia level. This may result from the fact that vegetables are not as sweet as fruits, and sometimes even have a bitter taste [34], and thus may be subjected to natural rejection evolved as an adaptive safeguard reaction to the potential toxicity of food products [35]. However, in the case of the analyzed group, who have had more experiences with a variety of food products compared to younger children, factors other than naturally evolved reactions must be rather taken into account.

Among the factors influencing vegetable intake, food neophobia and pickiness have been indicated as the important ones. In the study of Galloway et al. [36], it was indicated that girls characterized by high food neophobia and pickiness had higher vegetable intake than those characterized by low food neophobia and pickiness. However, in the mentioned study, in a comparison between the groups of girls with high food neophobia accompanied by low pickiness and those with low food neophobia accompanied by high pickiness, no differences between groups were indicated [36]. In the case of the present study, a similar association was observed; however, new conclusions may be formulated. It may be supposed that food neophobia not only influences vegetable intake when combined with pickiness but, in the population of Polish children, may also be the strong independent factor that may influence it alone. However, to draw more general conclusions, further studies should be conducted also in countries other than Poland.

Another new insight into the area of food neophobia is associated with the fact that, in the study of Galloway et al. [36], only a group of girls was analyzed. It is well known that among girls and boys, food preferences may differ, wherein girls are characterized by a higher general preference of fruits and vegetables compared to boys [33]. Moreover, it is indicated that not only boys are characterized by a higher food neophobia level than girls, but also adult males than females [37]. However, concerning food neophobia, in the majority of studies on the association between food neophobia level and intake of fruits and vegetables in children, the authors analyze data for the combined groups of boys and girls [38–42], whereas only a few studies present data for boys and girls separately or for only one gender [33,36,43].

Although the attitude toward food products may differ between boys and girls, analyzing them as one combined group may result in changing observed associations. For example, a study by Falciglia et al. [18] reported that no relationship between food neophobia level and vegetable intake was observed, however, this finding may have resulted from analyzing boys and girls together.

At the same time, in the study of Tsuji et al. [43], a high food neophobia level in Japanese boys was associated with low vegetable intake, which was not observed in the group of girls. On the one hand, it is in agreement with the results of Galloway et al. [36], as in the mentioned study not a high food neophobia level alone, but only that combined with a high level of pickiness was associated with low vegetable intake in girls. However, on the other hand, it should be mentioned that vegetable intake in the Japanese diet is different from that in the Western diet, while, for example, a higher level of soya intake must be considered [43].

The results of the conducted study indicated that both girls and boys, aged 10–12 years, with a higher food neophobia level may be characterized by lower vegetable intake than children with a lower food neophobia level. It must also be emphasized that, in the case of girls, the association was stronger than that found in boys, as was observed in both the analysis of correlations and comparison between the groups of various food neophobia levels.

Such an observation may be useful for public health purposes. In order to obtain the recommended vegetable intake in children, the reduction of the food neophobia levels may be essential. It may be achieved by taste education and food exposures, which may lead to creating new dietary habits [44,45]. However, it is also observed that implementing taste education and food exposures has produced contradictory results; for vegetables, either a successful education [27] or lack of success was observed [45] in various studies. Taking this into account, not only the association between food neophobia level and vegetable intake must be assessed, but also the most efficient ways of education must be analyzed in order to achieve the reduction of food neophobia levels.

In spite of the promising results of this study, some limitations exist. On the one hand, the general heterogeneity of the analyzed group is positive, as it represents a group representative of the Polish population of children aged 10–12 years more realistically than a homogeneous group. However, on the other hand, it may be argued that in a heterogeneous group, the observed associations may be influenced by the existing variations between individuals. Moreover, in spite of the fact that the food frequency questionnaire is one the most commonly applied methods in dietary research, this tool is also limited by specific error associated with fact that it is a retrospective method, based on the memory of respondents [46]. However, the applied food frequency questionnaire was a previously validated and comprehensive questionnaire, in which respondents were asked not only about fruit and vegetable intake, but also about all food products groups, without specifying which items would be assessed. Applying a self-administrated questionnaire is also a well-known method to reduce a social desirability bias, and is thus considered better than other methods of questionnaire administration. Such an approach may reduce the effect of desirable bias, but it is still not completely eliminated [47]. Taking into account the aim of this study, it may be indicated that the systematic errors resulting from the applied method did not influence the association between the food neophobia level and the observed intake of fruits and vegetables in children aged 10–12 years.

Simultaneously, it must be emphasized that the varying results of the studies conducted worldwide may result from differences in the applied methodology, as well as from cultural differences between children from analyzed countries. The previously indicated differences of the most commonly chosen fruits and vegetables between Asian and European countries, as well as the indicated similarities of the most commonly chosen fruits and vegetables between European countries, are confirmed by the broad data from international comparisons. Taking into account the data from 2013, it must be indicated that fruit intake in Poland was similar to those in countries in the geographical proximity, such as Czech Republic, Slovakia, Hungary, Latvia, Ukraine, Republic of Moldavia, Romania, and the Russian Federation [48], and vegetable intake in Poland was also similar to those in countries such as Hungary, Lithuania, Slovenia, Serbia, Croatia, Republic of Moldavia, as well as Germany and Austria [48].

Given the abovementioned data, it must be emphasized that the obtained results could be useful to compare with results from other countries characterized by similar intake. Still, further studies are also recommended in order to confirm these observations in other European or non-European countries.

5. Conclusions

1. Children, aged 10–12 years, with a higher food neophobia level may be characterized by lower vegetable intake than children with a lower neophobia level.
2. The association between food neophobia level and vegetable intake in the case of girls aged 10–12 years seems to be stronger than that in the case of boys.
3. In the case of children aged 10–12 years, in order to increase the vegetable intake, education must be conducted to achieve a reduction in the food neophobia level. However, further studies are also needed.

Author Contributions: D.Gu. made study conception and design; D.Gu., D.Gł., E.L. performed the research; D.Gł., analyzed the data; D.Gu., D.Gł., E.L., M.J.-Z. wrote the paper. All the authors read and approved the final manuscript.

References

1. Lim, S.S.; Vos, T.; Flaxman, A.D.; Danaei, G.; Shibuya, K.; Adair-Rohani, H.A.; AlMazroa, M.A.; Amann, M.; Anderson, R.; Andrews, K.G.; et al. A comparative risk assessment of burden of disease and injury attributable to 67 risk factors and risk factor clusters in 21 regions, 1990–2010: A systematic analysis for the Global Burden of Disease Study 2010. *Lancet* **2012**, *380*, 2224–2260. [CrossRef]
2. Increasing Fruit and Vegetable Consumption to Reduce the Risk of Noncommunicable Diseases Biological, Behavioural and Contextual Rationale. WHO, 2014. Available online: http://www.who.int/elena/titles/bbc/fruit_vegetables_ncds/en/ (accessed on 27 March 2017).
3. Lee, H.A.; Hwang, H.J.; Oh, S.Y.; Park, E.A.; Cho, S.J.; Kim, H.S.; Park, H. Which Diet-Related Behaviors in Childhood Influence a Healthier Dietary Pattern? From the Ewha Birth and Growth Cohort. *Nutrients* **2017**, *9*, 4. [CrossRef] [PubMed]
4. Galinski, G.; Lonnie, M.; Kowalkowska, J.; Wadolowska, L.; Czarnocinska, J.; Jezewska-Zychowicz, M.; Babicz-Zielinska, E. Self-Reported Dietary Restrictions and Dietary Patterns in Polish Girls: A Short Research Report (GEBaHealth Study). *Nutrients* **2016**, *8*, 796. [CrossRef] [PubMed]
5. Hall, J.N.; Moore, S.; Harper, S.B.; Lynch, J.W. Global variability in fruit and vegetable consumption. *Am. J. Prev. Med.* **2009**, *36*, 402–409. [CrossRef] [PubMed]
6. Borrmann, A.; Mensink, G.B.; KiGGS Study Group. Fruit and vegetable consumption by children and adolescents in Germany: Results of KiGGS wave 1. *Bundesgesundheitsblatt Gesundheitsforschung Gesundheitsschutz* **2015**, *58*, 1005–1014. (In German) [CrossRef] [PubMed]
7. Lock, K.; Pomerleau, J.; Causer, L.; McKee, M. Low fruit and vegetable consumption. In *Comparative Quantification of Health Risks. Global and Regional Burden of Disease Attribution to Selected Major Risk Factors*; Ezzati, M., Lopez, A.D., Rodgers, A., Murray, C.J.L., Eds.; Nonserial Publication; World Health Organization: Geneva, Switzerland; pp. 597–728.
8. Hebestreit, A.; Intemann, T.; Siani, A.; De Henauw, S.; Eiben, G.; Kourides, Y.A.; Kovacs, E.; Moreno, L.A.; Veidebaum, T.; Krogh, V.; et al. Dietary patterns of European children and their parents in association with family food environment: Results from the I. Family Study. *Nutrients* **2017**, *10*, 126. [CrossRef] [PubMed]
9. Rasmussen, M.; Krølner, R.; Klepp, K.-I.; Lytle, L.; Brug, J.; Bere, E.; Due, P. Determinants of fruit and vegetable consumption among children and adolescents: A review of the literature. Part I: Quantitative studies. *Int. J. Behav. Nutr. Phys. Act.* **2006**, *2*, 1–19.
10. Wardle, J.; Cooke, L. Genetic and environmental determinants of children's food preferences. *Br. J. Nutr.* **2008**, *99*, 15–21. [CrossRef] [PubMed]
11. Russell, C.G.; Worsley, A. A population-based study of preschoolers' food neophobia and its associations with food preferences. *J. Nutr. Educ. Behav.* **2008**, *40*, 11–19. [CrossRef] [PubMed]

12. Chu, Y.L.; Farmer, A.; Fung, C.; Kuhle, S.; Veugelers, P. Fruit and vegetable preferences and intake among children in Alberta. *Can. J. Diet. Pract. Res.* **2013**, *74*, 21–27. [CrossRef] [PubMed]
13. Pliner, P.; Hobden, K. Development of a scale to measure the trait of food neophobia in humans. *Appetite* **1992**, *19*, 105–120. [CrossRef]
14. Knaapila, A.; Tuorila, H.; Silventoinen, K.; Keskitalo, K.; Kallela, M.; Wessma, M.; Peltonen, L.; Cherkas, L.C.; Spector, T.D.; Perola, M. Food neophobia shows heritable variation in humans. *Physiol. Behav.* **2007**, *91*, 573–578. [CrossRef] [PubMed]
15. DeVellis, R.F. *Scale Development*; Sage Publications: Newbury Park, NJ, USA, 1991.
16. Tuorila, H.; Mustonen, S. Reluctant trying of an unfamiliar food induces negative affection for the food. *Appetite* **2010**, *43*, 418–421. [CrossRef] [PubMed]
17. Głąbska, D.; Guzek, D.; Sidor, P.; Włodarek, D. Vitamin D dietary intake questionnaire validation conducted among young Polish women. *Nutrients* **2016**, *5*, 36. [CrossRef] [PubMed]
18. Falciglia, G.A.; Couch, S.C.; Gribble, L.S.; Pabst, S.M.; Frank, R. Food neophobia in childhood affects dietary variety. *J. Am. Diet. Assoc.* **2000**, *100*, 1474–1481. [CrossRef]
19. Dovey, T.; Staples, P.; Gibson, E.; Halford, J. Food neophobia and 'picky/fussy' eating in children: A review. *Appetite* **2008**, *50*, 181–193. [CrossRef] [PubMed]
20. Ong, C.; Phuah, K.Y.; Salazar, E.; How, C.H. Managing the "picky eater" dilemma. *Singap. Med. J.* **2014**, *55*, 184–190. [CrossRef]
21. Mennella, J.A.; Nicklaus, S.; Jagolino, A.L.; Yourshaw, L.M. Variety is the spice of life: Strategies for promoting fruit and vegetable acceptance during infancy. *Physiol. Behav.* **2008**, *22*, 29–38. [CrossRef] [PubMed]
22. Lytle, L.A.; Seifert, S.; Greenstein, J.; McGovern, F. How do children's eating patterns and food choices change over time? Results from a cohort study. *Am. J. Health Promot.* **2000**, *14*, 222–228. [CrossRef] [PubMed]
23. Nicklaus, S.; Boggio, V.; Chabanet, C.; Issanchou, S. A prospective study of food variety seeking in childhood, adolescence and early adult life. *Appetite* **2005**, *44*, 289–297. [CrossRef] [PubMed]
24. Laureati, M.; Bergamaschi, V.; Pagliarini, E. School-based intervention with children. Peer-modeling, reward and repeated exposure reduce food neophobia and increase liking of fruits and vegetables. *Appetite* **2014**, *83*, 26–32. [CrossRef] [PubMed]
25. Nicklas, T.A.; Baranowski, T.; Baranowski, J.C.; Cullen, K.; Rittenberry, L.; Olvera, N. Family and child-care provider influences on preschool children's fruit, juice, and vegetable consumption. *Nutr. Rev.* **2001**, *59*, 224–235. [CrossRef] [PubMed]
26. Gillman, M.W.; Rifas-Shiman, S.L.; Frazier, A.L.; Rockett, H.R.; Camargo, C.A., Jr.; Field, A.E.; Berkey, C.S.; Colditz, G.A. Family dinner and diet quality among older children and adolescents. *Arch. Fam. Med.* **2000**, *9*, 235–240. [CrossRef] [PubMed]
27. Birch, L.L. Effects of peer models' food choices and eating behaviors on preschoolers' food preferences. *Child Dev.* **1980**, *51*, 489–496. [CrossRef]
28. Czarnocińska, J.; Anioła, J.; Grabowska, J.; Galiński, G.; Wądołowska, L. Food preferences, frequency and intake by schoolgirls. *Pol. J. Food Nutr. Sci.* **2009**, *59*, 251–254.
29. Babicz-Zielińska, E. Preference and consumption of vegetables and fruit among schoolchildren. *Pol. J. Food Nutr. Sci.* **1999**, *8*, 109–116.
30. Pérez-Rodrigo, C.; Ribas, L.; Serra-Majem, L.; Aranceta, J. Food preferences of Spanish children and young people: The enKid study. *Eur. J. Clin. Nutr.* **2003**, *57*, 45–48. [CrossRef] [PubMed]
31. Lafraire, J.; Rioux, C.; Giboreau, A.; Picard, D. Food rejections in children: Cognitive and social/environmental factors involved in food neophobiaand picky/fussy eating behavior. *Appetite* **2016**, *96*, 347–357. [CrossRef] [PubMed]
32. Coulthard, H.; Palfreyman, Z.; Morizet, D. Sensory evaluation of a novel vegetable in school age children. *Appetite* **2016**, *1*, 64–69. [CrossRef] [PubMed]
33. Cooke, L.J.; Wardle, J. Age and gender differences in children's food Preferences. *Br. J. Nutr.* **2005**, *93*, 741–746. [CrossRef] [PubMed]
34. Forestell, C.A.; Mennella, J.A. Early Determinants of Fruit and Vegetable Acceptance. *Pediatrics* **2007**, *120*, 1247–1254. [CrossRef] [PubMed]
35. Glendinning, J.I. Is the bitter rejection response always adaptive? *Physiol. Behav.* **1994**, *56*, 1217–1227. [CrossRef]

36. Galloway, A.; Lee, Y.; Birch, L.L. Predictors and consequences of food neophobia and pickiness in young girls. *J. Am. Diet. Assoc.* **2003**, *103*, 692–698. [CrossRef] [PubMed]
37. Hursti, U.; Sjödén, P. Food and general neophobia and their relationship with self-reported food choice: Familial resemblance in Swedish families with children of ages 7–17 years. *Appetite* **1997**, *29*, 89–103. [CrossRef] [PubMed]
38. Cooke, L.; Wardle, J.; Gibson, E. Relationship between parental report of food neophobia and everyday food consumption in 2–6-year-old children. *Appetite* **2003**, *41*, 205–206. [CrossRef]
39. Cooke, L.; Wardle, J.; Gibson, E.; Sapochnik, M.; Sheiham, A.; Lawson, M. Demographic, familial and trait predictors of fruit and vegetable consumption by pre-school children. *Public Health Nutr.* **2004**, *7*, 295–302. [CrossRef] [PubMed]
40. Cooke, L.; Carnell, S.; Wardle, J. Food neophobia and mealtime food consumption in 4–5 year old children. *Int. J. Behav. Nutr. Phys.* **2006**, *3*, 14. [CrossRef] [PubMed]
41. Wardle, J.; Carnell, S.; Cooke, L. Parental control over feeding and children's fruit and vegetable intake: How are they related? *J. Am. Diet. Assoc.* **2005**, *105*, 227–232. [CrossRef] [PubMed]
42. Coulthard, H.; Blissett, J. Fruit and vegetable consumption in children and their mothers. Moderating effects of child sensory sensitivity. *Appetite* **2009**, *52*, 410–415. [CrossRef] [PubMed]
43. Tsuji, M.; Nakamura, K.; Tamai, Y.; Wada, K.; Sahashi, Y.; Watanabe, K.; Ohtsuchi, S.; Ando, K.; Nagata, C. Relationship of intake of plant-based foods with 6-n-propylthiouracil sensitivity and food neophobia in Japanese preschool children. *Eur. J. Clin. Nutr.* **2012**, *66*, 47–52. [CrossRef] [PubMed]
44. Stein, L.J.; Nagai, H.; Nakagawa, M.; Beauchamp, G.K. Effects of repeated exposure and health-related information on hedonic evaluation and acceptance of a bitter beverage. *Appetite* **2003**, *40*, 119–129. [CrossRef]
45. Park, B.K.; Cho, M.S. Taste education reduces food neophobia and increases willingness to try novel foods in school children. *Nutr. Res. Pract.* **2016**, *10*, 221–228. [CrossRef] [PubMed]
46. Gibson, R.S. *Principles of Nutritional Assessment*, 2nd ed.; Oxford University Press: New York, NY, USA, 2005.
47. Nederhof, A.J. Methods of coping with social desirability bias: A review. *Eur. J. Soc. Psychol.* **1985**, *15*, 263–280. [CrossRef]
48. Data and Statistics—Food Supply—Statistics by Country. Available online: https://knoema.com/atlas/topics/Agriculture (accessed on 25 May 2017).

4

Food and Nutrients Intake in the School Lunch Program among School Children in Shanghai, China

Zhenru Huang, Runying Gao, Nadila Bawuerjiang, Yali Zhang, Xiaoxu Huang and Meiqin Cai *

School of Public Health, Shanghai Jiao Tong University,227 South Chongqing Rd, Huangpu Qu, Shanghai 200025, China; hzhenru@163.com (Z.H.); dly-slyj@hotmail.com (R.G.); nadirah@126.com (N.B.); abeney@126.com (Y.Z.); xiaoxuhuang0909@126.com (X.H.)

* Correspondence: caimeiqin@sjtu.edu.cn

Abstract: This study aimed to evaluate the intake of food and nutrients among primary, middle, and high schools students in Shanghai, and provide recommendations for possible amendments in new school lunch standards of Shanghai. Twenty schools were included in the school lunch menu survey. Of those, seven schools enrolled 5389 students and conducted physical measurement of plate waste and a questionnaire survey. The amount of food and nutrients was compared according to the new China National Dietary Guideline for School Children (2016) and Chinese Dietary Reference Intakes (2013). The provision of livestock and poultry meat in menus was almost 5–8 times the recommended amount. The amount of seafood was less than the recommended amount, and mostly came from half-processed food. The average percentage of energy from fat was more than 30% in students of all grades. The greatest amount of food wasted was vegetables with 53%, 42%, and 31%, respectively, among primary, middle and high school students. Intake of Vitamin A, Vitamin B_2, calcium, and iron was about 50% of the recommended proportion. Only 24.0% students were satisfied with the taste of school lunches. Higher proportions of livestock and poultry meat and low intake of vegetables have become integral problems in school lunch programs. Additionally, more attention needs to be paid to the serving size in primary schools with five age groups.

Keywords: students; school lunch; nutrient; intake; plate waste

---

1. Introduction

Children and adolescents are in a crucial period of body growth and maturation. Adequate nutrition during this period is of great importance. A number of studies has revealed that inappropriate nutrition in childhood is related to both the occurrence of diseases in youth [1] and the risks of developing obesity, cardiovascular diseases, and cancer in adulthood [2–4].

Lunch becomes a very important issue when it comes to school-aged children since a large number of students have lunch at school. The National School Lunch Program (NSLP) in the United States operates in more than 101,000 public and nonprofit private schools, and provides over 28 million low-cost or free lunches to children on a typical school day [5]. In Japan, more than 10 million schoolchildren in 32,400 schools participate in the lunch program [6]. China launched the first School Lunch Program in Hangzhou, Zhejiang Province in 1987 [7], and then expanded it to a number of cities. Shanghai, as a developed city in China, started the program in 1993, and now has more than 95% students having lunch at school [8], which is a total of 1.4 million students according to Shanghai Statistic Yearbook (2016) [9].

Since lunch is correlated to the health of young generations and involves so many students, it has drawn much attention worldwide. In developed countries, such as the US and Japan, they have called a legislative action to ensure well implemented school lunch programs. The U.S. signed the National School Lunch Act (NSLA) in 1946 and the Child Nutrition Act (CAN) in 1966, as well as subsequent amendments to the two acts that guide the program's administration [5]. Japan also introduced the School Lunch Act in 1954 and revised it in 2008 to change its aim to promote Shokuiku, which emphasizes food education. These acts clearly demonstrate the daily food and nutrient reference intake for each age group so that schools and companies that prepare lunches are able to provide adequate nutrition to students. China released the Amount of Nutritional Provision for School Lunch (ANPSL-1998) as the national standard for school lunches in 1998; there have been no amendments to date [10].

However, the health status and dietary structure of Chinese people have undergone tremendous changes within the last 20 years. Excessive intake of meat and insufficient consumption of dairy products and vegetables have emerged as concerns in Chinese dining habits [11]. Hence, it is very urgent and necessary to draw up an updated and feasible standard for the school lunch program, which requires on in-depth evaluation of the available data on the present status of school lunches. The former evaluation studies were all based on the ANPSL-1998, which might be inaccurate since China has published the new China National Dietary Guideline for School Children (2016) (CNDG-Children 2016) [12] and the Chinese Dietary Reference Intakes (2013) (DRIs-2013) [13]. To the best of our knowledge, this is the first study that applied the new guideline and DRIs to assess lunch intake in China. Additionally, unlike in the existing studies, we separated elementary, middle, and high school students into several sub-groups to obtain more information, as recommended by a recently published study by the NSLP in the US [14]. This is also the first time a comprehensive and regional-level investigation of school lunch program that involves multiple districts all over Shanghai has been conducted. As the study team of the new school lunch standardization commission in Shanghai, we aim to provide more evidence and scientific recommendations for updates.

Therefore, the objectives of this study were to evaluate the intake of food and nutrients among primary, middle and high schools students in Shanghai in reference to the CNDG-Children 2016 and the DRIs-2013 and to provide recommendations for possible amendments on new school lunch standards of Shanghai.

2. Methods

2.1. Sample Selection

Eight primary schools, five middle schools, and five high schools, two combined middle-high schools, making up a total of 20 schools, from seven districts of Shanghai, participated in the three-day lunch menu survey in 2015. Simultaneously, the intake survey and questionnaire survey were conducted among 5389 students from three primary schools (2936 students), three middle schools (1841 students), and one high school (612 students). The study population consisted of 2765 boys (51.3%) and 2624 girls (48.7%).

Signed informed consents were obtained from the students as well as their parents. No experiment and biological sample collection were conducted in this study. At no time were individual students associated with any particular lunch, and the questionnaire was anonymous without any personal identifying information, except for the students' grade and sex.

2.2. Data Collection

2.2.1. Menu Survey

Menu survey was a very common and easy way to assess the provision of school lunch [15,16]. Three-day lunch menus were obtained from 20 schools. Menus were analyzed with nutrient analysis software Fei Hua (2.a), Beijing Bowenshixun Technology Ltd., Beijing, China, which provided daily averages for staple food (including rice, noodles, and other cereal food), livestock and poultry meat, egg, seafood, bean products, and vegetables, as well as energy, protein, fat, carbohydrates, vitamins, and minerals. The oil, salt, and sugar used were also considered.

2.2.2. Intake Survey

In seven schools, menu survey was also applied. And plate waste measures were conducted over three days, using a previously validated physical measurement of aggregate selective plate waste [17,18]. Two randomly selected sample of school lunch trays were taken from each age group serving line before lunch. Meanwhile, the weights of food before and after cooking were recorded to calculate the raw/cooked ratio (Ration of r/c). Separate trash bins with plastic bags were prepared for each food category before lunch. The research team members waited at the designated spots and separated the leftovers into the corresponding trash bin when the students finished eating and brought their trays. The number of students who had lunch at school of every day was recorded.

Food Intake per Student (cooked) in grams for each food category was calculated as follows (1):

$$\text{Food Intake per student(cooked)} = \text{Sample Weight} - \frac{\text{Total Plate Waste}}{\text{Number of students}} \tag{1}$$

Since the nutrient analysis software and the reference standard both require raw food data, the Food Intake per Student (cooked) was transformed with the raw/cooked ratio (Ration of r/c) as shown in Formula (2) below.

$$\text{Food Intake per student(raw)} = \text{Food Intake per student(cooked)} \times \text{Ration of r/c} \tag{2}$$

Plate waste is defined as the quantity percentage of edible food served as part of the lunch but not consumed, as shown in Formula (3) below.

$$\%\text{Plate Waste} = \frac{\text{Total Plate waste/Number of students}}{\text{Sample weight}} \times 100 \tag{3}$$

Both menu and intake evaluation were based on the CNDG-Children 2016 for food category and the DRIs-2013 for nutrient assessment. To evaluate the lunch and nutrition intake, 40% of daily recommended intake in the CNDG-Children 2016 and the DRIs-2013 was used, as the CNDG 2016 distributes daily energy and nutrients into breakfast, lunch and dinner at the ratio 3:4:3 [19].

2.2.3. Questionnaire Survey

The aim of the questionnaire survey was to find out the reason for plate waste and the existing problems in the School Lunch Program.

Validity: Three nutrition and survey research experts were invited to evaluate the appropriateness of the survey questions and response options; then, face-to-face interviews were conducted with 36 students (three students from each grade level ranging from Grades 1–12) as a pilot. The students were asked to talk about the clarity of each question to ensure the targeted respondents understand what each question is asking as well as what each response means.

The questionnaire included the following information: (1) demographic background (i.e., age, sex); (2) knowledge and attitudes: basic knowledge of food and nutrients (including six questions, one point for each correct answer, six points in total), attitude towards healthy behaviors (including four behaviors, two points for very positive attitude, one point for positive attitude and zero point for neutral or negative attitude, eight points in total); and (3) opinions on food served at the school canteen (i.e., appearance, flavor, temperature, and portion size of the food served).

Reliability: Internal consistency reliability was calculated using Cronbach's alpha coefficient formula. Reliability of the questions related to knowledge, attitude and views on the school lunches were thus calculated to be 0.866, 0.807, and 0.792, respectively. This suggests that the reliability of this survey was adequate, since $\alpha \geq 0.7$ is generally considered to be the minimum for adequate internal consistency [20].

2.3. Data Analysis

Excel 2010 (Microsoft Corporation, Redmond, WA, USA) was used to record and calculate the food provided and intake. The nutrient analysis software Fei Hua (2.a) (Beijing Bowenshixun Technology Ltd., Beijing, China) was used to analyze nutrient contents. EpiData 3.1 (A comprehensive tool for validated entry and documentation of data. EpiData Association, Odense, Denmark) was used for double recording of questionnaire data. Data that presented abnormal distribution were analyzed using two independent samples via Wilcoxon rank sum test, while categorical variables were analyzed via chi-Square test using SPSS 21.0 (IBM SPSS Inc., Chicago, IL, USA). Differences found were determined to be statistically significant at $p \leq 0.05$.

3. Results

3.1. Evaluation of Food Provision

Amounts of staple food, livestock, and poultry meat in menus exceeded the recommended amount in all school grades; livestock and poultry meat were particularly high, almost 5–8 times the recommended amounts. On the contrary, the provision of seafood was insufficient. Additionally, we found the seafood supplied for lunch was mostly fish ball or other half-processed foods, instead of fresh products. Egg provision in the diet was higher than recommended for primary and middle school students. The amount of bean products and vegetables was generally adequate for all grades (see Table 1).

Table 1. Provision of food in the menus of twenty schools as compared to CNDG-Children 2016/g.

Category	Primary School		Middle School		High School	
	Recommended	Menu	Recommended	Menu	Recommended	Menu
Staple Food	**60–80**	99.6 ± 31.8	**90–100**	104.7 ± 42.7	**100–120**	154.3 ± 60.4
Livestock & Poultry Meat	**16**	123.4 ± 38.4	**20**	101.3 ± 44.9	**20–30**	135.4 ± 51.6
Egg	**10–16**	26.0 ± 27.8	**16–20**	22.8 ± 25.8	**20**	15.1 ± 20.6
Seafood	**16**	11.4 ± 23.7	**20**	28.3 ± 49.4	**20–30**	13.2 ± 24.5
Bean Product	**6**	9.0 ± 17.0	**6**	15.8 ± 25.5	**6–10**	32.2 ± 35.6
Vegetable	**120**	130.6 ± 60.8	**160–180**	189.2 ± 63.7	**180–200**	178.4 ± 84.5

Recommended amount is 40% of daily recommended intake in China National Dietary Guideline for School Children (2016) (CNDG-Children 2016).

Energy indicated in the menus was aligned with the recommendations. However, the proportion of fat in total energy exceeded the recommended percentage (20–30%). Protein was served excessively, at nearly twice the recommended amount, especially among primary school students. The percentage of energy from carbohydrate, which is supposed to be 50–65%, was found to be below the lower limit. As for the vitamins and minerals, Vitamin B_2 and calcium were insufficient. Vitamin A, Vitamin B_1, Vitamin C, iron, and zinc contents were consistent with the goals specified in the DRIs-2013 for students in all grades (see Table 2).

Table 2. Provision of energy and nutrients in 20 schools as compared to DRIs-2013/*n* (%).

Item	Primary School		Middle School		High School	
	DRIs	Menu	DRIs	Menu	DRIs	Menu
Energy (kcal)	621	696 ± 139 (112.0)	783	752 ± 229 (96.0)	844	1005 ± 179 (119.1)
Protein (g)	17.4	35.9 ± 7.5 (206.3)	23.4	32.0 ± 7.9 (136.8)	25.3	41.8 ± 10.0 (165.2)
Protein/%E	-	21 ± 4	-	18 ± 5	-	17 ± 4
Fat/%E	20–30	32 ± 10	20–30	39 ± 10	20–30	37 ± 12
Carbonhydrate/%E	50–65	47 ± 10	50–65	43 ± 7	50–65	46 ± 12
Vitamin A (μgRE)	199	204 ± 184 (102.5)	258	258 ± 173 (100)	272	221 ± 144 (81.3)
Vitamin B_1 (mg)	0.39	0.48 ± 0.21 (123.1)	0.5	0.49 ± 0.20 (98.0)	0.54	0.60 ± 0.21 (111.1)
Vitamin B_2 (mg)	0.39	0.33 ± 0.09 (84.6)	0.48	0.32 ± 0.08 (66.7)	0.51	0.37 ± 0.09 (72.5)
Vitamin C (mg)	26	39 ± 29 (150.0)	36	60 ± 34 (166.7)	38	54 ± 32 (142.1)
Calcium (mg)	390	140 ± 85 (35.9)	413	217 ± 196 (52.5)	375	226 ± 183 (60.3)
Iron (mg)	5.14	5.65 ± 1.77 (109.9)	6.28	6.91 ± 4.71 (110.0)	6.38	8.50 ± 4.71 (133.2)
Zinc (mg)	2.81	4.42 ± 1.65 (157.3)	3.66	4.28 ± 1.25 (116.9)	3.75	5.52 ± 1.52 (147.2)

DRIs are 40% of average of daily recommended intake in different age and sex group according to Chinese Dietary Reference Intakes (2013) (DRIs-2013). The value in brackets was the proportion that provision amount took up in the correspondent recommendation.

3.2. Evaluation of Food Intake and Plate Waste

The intake of staple food for grades 1–2 and middle school students was insufficient (with plate waste ranging from 15–24%), but was adequate for grades 3–5 and high school students (with 16–21% of plate waste). All students consumed livestock and poultry meat in amounts exceeding the recommended amount. Egg intake was in accordance with the recommended amounts, except among high school students. Seafood intake was in a severe shortage for primary school and high school students since their provision was also insufficient. Bean product consumption was deficient among primary school students, but reasonable among middle and high school students. Vegetable consumption was the lowest and the accompanying plate waste levels ranked the highest, with 53%, 42%, and 31%, of waste among primary, middle, and high school students, respectively. Livestock and poultry meat, and egg followed as the second ranking plate waste among all food categories (see Table 3). Additionally, students of lower grades in primary school seemed to waste more food than students of higher grades ($p < 0.05$). Girls tended to waste more food and nutrients than boys ($p < 0.05$).

Table 3. Actual food intake and plate waste percentage in seven schools among different age groups and sexes/g (%).

Stage		Staple Food	Livestock & Poultry Meat	Egg	Seafood	Bean Product	Vegetable
Primary School	Recommended	60–80	16	10–16	16	6	120
	Menu	79.5	141.6	24.9	0.4	5.0	101.6
	Grades 1–2	52.9 (34%)	73.7 (46%)	10.5 (50%)	0.2 (50%)	2.4 (50%)	38.9 (57%)
	Grades 3–5	63.1 (21%)	75.0 (45%)	14.8 (30%)	0.2 (50%)	3.2 (33%)	45.1 (50%)
	Average Intake	58.8 (27%)	74.5 (46%)	13.0 (38%)	0.2 (50%)	2.9 (40%)	42.5 (53%)
Middle School	Recommended	90–100	20	16–20	20	6	160–180
	Menu	93.4	119.4	34.9	27.9	14.9	176.7
	Grades 6–7 (Male)	74.5 (11%)	106.3 (14%)	16.2 (29%)	25.8 (12%)	10.5 (20%)	118.2 (35%)
	Grades 6–7 (Female)	64.4 (23%)	96.7 (22%)	14.1 (38%)	21.7 (26%)	7.9 (40%)	104.1 (43%)
	Grades 8–9 (Male)	81.0 (3%)	95.1 (23%)	16.3 (28%)	25.6 (13%)	9.0 (32%)	105.3 (42%)
	Grades 8–9 (Female)	61.5 (26%)	82.1 (34%)	15.2 (33%)	24.9 (15%)	8.8 (33%)	87.8 (52%)
	Average Intake	70.9 (15%)	96.7 (22%)	15.5 (32%)	24.6 (16%)	9.2 (30%)	105.9 (42%)
High School	Recommended	100–120	20–30	20	20–30	6–10	180–200
	Menu	140.4	164.3	18.4	2.0	23.0	198.1
	Grades 10–12 (Male)	149.0 (1%)	161.0 (0%)	17.6 (24%)	2.0 (0%)	18.6 (18%)	154.2 (27%)
	Grades 10–12 (Female)	103.0 (31%)	141.1 (12%)	13.4 (42%)	1.3 (35%)	14.4 (37%)	139.4 (34%)
	Average Intake	126.7 (16%)	151.3 (6%)	15.5 (33%)	1.6 (20%)	16.6 (27%)	147.0 (31%)

Energy intake for students in Grades 1–9 was under the recommended amount. The intakes of protein and fat for all students were excessive, while the carbohydrate intake was deficient. Primary school students were facing a lack of vitamins in their diet, including Vitamin B_1, Vitamin B_2, and Vitamin C. Calcium intake was very low for all students. Iron intake was low except for boys in high school. Zinc intake was matched with the recommended amount. In summary, Vitamin A, Vitamin B_2, calcium, and iron were the most deficient micronutrients in school lunches, which corresponded to about 50% of the recommendation (see Table 4).

Table 4. Actual intake and proportion to the recommended amounts of energy and nutrients in seven schools among different age groups and sexes/*n* (%).

Stage		Energy kcal	Protein g	Fat %E	Carbonhydrate %E	Vitamin A μgRE	Vitamin B_1 mg	Vitamin B_2 mg	Vitamin C mg	Calcium mg	Iron mg	Zinc mg
Primary School	Recommended	662	19	20–30	50–65	212	0.42	0.42	28	416	5.5	3.0
	Menu	638 (96.4)	35 (188.2)	35	42	156 (73.6)	0.38 (91.3)	0.32 (76.9)	28 (100.0)	95 (22.8)	4.7 (85.4)	4.3 (143.3)
	Grades 1–2	409 (61.8)	20 (107.5)	37	43	58 (27.4)	0.19 (45.7)	0.19 (45.7)	10 (35.7)	48 (11.5)	2.9 (52.2)	2.5 (83.3)
	Grades 3–5	480 (72.5)	22 (118.3)	38	43	79 (37.3)	0.25 (60.1)	0.21 (50.5)	12 (42.9)	60 (14.4)	3.1 (56.6)	2.8 (93.3)
	Average Intake	451 (68.1)	21 (112.9)	37	43	70 (33.0)	0.23 (55.3)	0.20 (48.1)	11 (39.3)	55 (13.2)	3.0 (54.7)	2.7 (90.0)
Middle School	Recommended	835	25	20–30	50–65	275	0.53	0.51	38	440	6.7	3.9
	Menu	665 (79.6)	32 (128.0)	38	43	232 (84.4)	0.59 (111.3)	0.30 (58.8)	55 (144.7)	168 (38.2)	5.1 (76.1)	3.8 (97.4)
	Grades 6–7 (Male)	612 (73.3)	29 (116.0)	42	39	148 (53.8)	0.63 (118.9)	0.25 (49.0)	35 (92.1)	117 (26.6)	4.0 (59.6)	3.2 (82.1)
	Grades 6–7 (Female)	542 (64.9)	26 (104.0)	43	38	127 (46.2)	0.60 (113.2)	0.23 (45.1)	30 (78.9)	104 (23.6)	3.5 (52.8)	2.9 (74.4)
	Grades 8–9 (Male)	599 (71.7)	28 (112.0)	40	41	131 (47.6)	0.58 (109.4)	0.24 (47.1)	32 (84.2)	105 (23.9)	3.8 (56.7)	3.2 (82.1)
	Grades 8–9 (Female)	499 (59.8)	24 (96.0)	42	39	112 (40.7)	0.48 (90.6)	0.20 (39.2)	26 (68.4)	89 (20.2)	3.2 (48.1)	2.6 (66.7)
	Average Intake	570 (68.3)	27 (108.0)	42	39	132 (48.0)	0.58 (109.4)	0.23 (45.1)	31 (81.6)	106 (24.1)	3.7 (55.2)	3.0 (76.9)
High School	Recommended	900	27	20–30	50–65	290	0.58	0.54	40	400	6.8	4.0
	Menu	924 (102.7)	46 (170.4)	35	46	242 (83.4)	0.71 (121.9)	0.40 (74.1)	61 (152.5)	180 (45.0)	7.5 (110.3)	5.4 (135.0)
	Grades 10–12 (Male)	910 (101.1)	45 (166.7)	30	51	190 (65.5)	0.70 (120.7)	0.39 (72.2)	45 (112.5)	146 (36.5)	6.9 (101.5)	5.3 (132.5)
	Grades 10–12 (Female)	697 (77.4)	36 (133.3)	33	46	158 (54.5)	0.55 (94.8)	0.31 (57.4)	40 (100.0)	112 (28.0)	5.0 (73.5)	4.1 (102.5)
	Average Intake	807 (89.7)	40 (148.1)	32	49	175 (60.3)	0.62 (106.9)	0.35 (64.8)	43 (107.5)	129 (32.3)	6.0 (88.2)	4.7 (117.5)

The value in brackets was the proportion that actual intake took up in the correspondent recommendation.

3.3. Analysis for Possible Reasons for Plate Waste

A total of 5937 students from seven schools were administered questionnaires, of which 5389 (90.8%) valid responses were included in this study.

Results from the questionnaire showed that the percentage of students who often or always had leftovers was 56.3%. The main reason for plate waste among primary school students was food being too much (43.3%) and unpalatable food (43.4%). However, the main reason for plate waste in 54.5% of the middle school and 61.9% of the high school students was unpalatable food.

As for knowledge about nutrition, students from primary, middle, and high schools scored 4.44 ± 1.50, 4.69 ± 1.21 and 4.92 ± 0.98, respectively, with accuracy over 70%. However, their scores towards healthy behaviors were relatively low, at 5.80 ± 2.10, 4.25 ± 2.46, and 3.15 ± 2.18, for primary, middle, and high school students, respectively.

Students rated the food temperature and portion size as satisfactory; however, they were not satisfied with food appearance and flavor. Only 24% of the students marked the overall food taste as good (see Table 5).

Table 5. Students' opinion on school lunches/n (%).

Rank	Good	Neutral	Bad
Appearance	1067 (19.8%)	2689 (49.9%)	1633 (30.3%)
Flavor	1515 (28.1%)	2705 (50.2%)	1169 (21.7%)
Temperature	2716 (50.4%)	2177 (40.4%)	496 (9.2%)
Adequate in Portion Size	2792 (51.8%)	1918 (35.6%)	679 (12.6%)
Overall Food Taste	1293 (24.0%)	2905 (53.9%)	1191 (22.1%)

4. Discussion

The latest report on nutrition status and chronic diseases of Chinese people issued in 2015 revealed that the wasting percentage of Chinese adolescents aged 6–17 years was 9%, while the overweight and obesity percentages were 9.6% and 6.4%, respectively [21]. Diet-related problems including anorexia and obesity have been increasing among school children [6]. School lunch, as one of the important meals in a day, also provides direct access to nutrition for students.

Nevertheless, problems continue to exist in the School Lunch Program. In the present study, we evaluated the provision and actual intake, as well as the students' opinion on school lunches to uncover the existing problems and come up with feasible recommendations when amending the new school lunch standards of Shanghai. In particular, the provision of livestock and poultry meat was too excessive while seafood was in a severe shortage. This study highlighted the fact that excessive provision of animal protein in school lunch diets may be associated with a greater intake of fat. This high-level of fat content in school lunches is a common issue worldwide. To decrease children's access to lunches with a high fat content, the US Department of Agriculture implemented School Meals Initiative for Healthy Children in 1995 [22]. However, this program did not show favorable results, since the three School Nutrition Dietary Assessment Studies showed that the average percentages of energy from total fat were 38% (school year 1991–1992), 33–34% (school year 1998–1999) and 33.8% (school year 2004–2005), respectively [23–25]. The higher-fat provision in school lunch should be given more attention as obesity has become a global public health threat [26].

The actual food intake was also unsatisfying. The plate waste of livestock and poultry meat, eggs and vegetables was higher than other food category. The provision of livestock and poultry meat, as well as eggs, far exceeded the recommended amounts, and this may be the reason for high plate waste. However, the situation for vegetables was different. The vegetable provision was within the recommended range, but accounted for the highest plate waste. Having further investigated, we found that vegetables were prepared in a large cauldron, in a manner that resulted in overcooking. Additionally, the time between cooking and consumption was about 1.5–2 h, and individual lunch sets were covered with a plastic covering to prevent contamination. This may have resulted in the vegetables gaining an unpleasant color and unpalatable flavor, leading to increased plate waste.

In fact, vegetables were reported to be the food items that are wasted the most, and this is very common all over the world [18,27]. A study involving students from grades 3–8 in four schools in the U.S. showed the waste percentage of vegetables was up to 58.9% [28]. Another study conducted in Beijing, China also indicated that vegetables were the dominant wasted food with 42% of plate waste [29], comparable with the present study ranging from 31–53%.

Due to high plate waste of vegetables and other foods, intake for energy and a majority of nutrients did not meet the recommended targets in this study. The reason for higher intake of fat and protein was the unreasonable high fat content of lunches. Intake of micronutrients, such as Vitamin A, Vitamin B_2 and iron, was also less than the recommended level, which might be a consequence of high plate waste, especially for vegetables. However, we should notice that, for most Chinese people, they are used to eat more at dinner rather than lunch. Hence, the distribution of breakfast, lunch and dinner at the ratio 3:4:3 might not be the occasion and whether the nutrient intake over a full day is adequate remains unknown. Calcium insufficiency was also found in this study. As people usually drink milk in the morning or at night, it is difficult to judge the intake of calcium at lunch. However, the insufficiency of calcium intake has always been a problem among Chinese students because of low-milk dietary habits of Chinese people [21].

A number of factors could influence food intake, causing the unreasonable nutrient intake among students. Previous studies have concluded that students' knowledge, attitude, and eating behaviors [29,30], as well as characteristics of the food itself (including the appearance, flavor, and temperature) [31], were the main influencing factors leading to plate waste. It was inspiring that the students achieved about 70% accuracy when answering nutrition-related questions. However, their attitudes toward healthy behaviors were not very positive. Therefore, future nutrition education should focus more on how to encourage students to turn their good nutrition knowledge into actions. In terms of the characteristics of food, the results revealed a low satisfaction in the appearance of food (19.8%) and flavor (28.1%), which might be a result of comprehensive factors, such as cooking skills of the kitchen staff, food quality, food preparation equipment and storage and so on. Furthermore, 50.4% students were satisfied with the food temperature, showing that the supply chain worked quite successfully.

Plate waste may also be due to serving size. We found that younger students wasted more food than the older ones in primary school. This must be addressed since the lunch patterns and serving sizes for food were similar within school level (primary, middle, and high school). For example, a primary school may contain five grades of different age students, but their serving sizes are the same. In addition, the recommendations for different age groups do not correspond with the actual real-life situation. DRIs-2013 for school children and CNDG-Children 2016 determined the recommendations at three age levels, i.e., 7–10 years, 11–13 years, and 14–17 years. However, the primary, middle, and high schools in Shanghai include students aged from 7–11 years, 12–15 years, and 16–18 years old, respectively. Apparently, the age group in DRIs-2013 and CNDG-Children is different from the actual situation. It should be mentioned that ANPSL-1998 successfully matched the age groups with actual school stage and separated recommendations for two age groups for primary school (i.e., students aged 6–8 years and 9–11 years). However, the recommendation for students older than 15 years is absent in ANPSL-1998. Hence, some gaps between the present recommendations and the actual situation were found. Whether the younger students in primary school need less energy, nutrients, or smaller portion sizes remains unknown. This is in accordance with the opinion of Niaki et al. from the U.S. [14]. Another study from Portugal and Denmark also suggested that portion sizes need to be reconsidered in School Lunch Program [32,33].

The physical measurement of plate waste was recommended and commonly used in dietary surveys in China [17]. Its advantages of providing detailed and accurate plate waste information were also demonstrated in a report to the U.S. Congress [18]. It overcomes the need to rely on students' memory or lack of ability to accurately estimate portion sizes, which are common limitations of 24 h recall investigations [34]. However, the measurement of plate waste in this study was an average estimation based on total plate waste across food items rather than the individual plate waste. We did not take into account any differences in individual behaviors. Measurement of individual plate waste is quite costly and time-consuming, especially for samples over 50–100 persons [35]. Hence, visual estimation and digital photography methods have been applied in some plate waste studies [36–38]. Digital photography was proven to be a more accurate method to estimate plate waste since it can be standardized and offers a way to enhance the reliability and validity of recording dietary intake [36,38]. The digital photography method is worth further development, although it is not used widely in China yet.

This study was conducted in Shanghai so it has limitations to generalize to other cities or at the national level. However, some findings, such as excessive provision of livestock and poultry meat, low intake of vegetables and low satisfaction about school lunches from students, were very common across China.

5. Conclusions

Based the above, the recommendations for the new school lunch standards of Shanghai are as follows: (1) emphasize the provision of less livestock and poultry meat, and more fresh seafood instead of half-processed products; (2) recommend mixed-vegetable dishes. Leafy vegetables could be cooked with other food categories, such as bean products and mushrooms to improve the flavor of vegetables. More importantly, multi-component interventions should be encouraged, which was proven to be an effective way to increase the consumption of vegetables in many countries [6,39,40]; (3) recommend yogurt at lunch or milk at breakfast but this is not compulsory according to Chinese dietary habits; and (4) supplement the recommendations for students aged 15–18 years to cover the missing points in the old standard (ANPSL-1998), while separating the recommendations for primary school students as in the old standard.

Acknowledgments: The authors would like to thank the Shanghai Association Student Nutrition and Health Promotion for funding (Grant #SXYJ-2015) and confirm that the financial supporters had no role in the design and implementation of the study, including data collection, analysis, and interpretation. Additionally, we would like to thank all of the participants who participated in the study. We are also grateful to the teachers and other staff from the schools and companies that prepared lunch in support of our field investigation.

Author Contributions: Z.H., R.G., N.B., Y.Z. and X.H. conceived, designed the study and collected the data in the field; Z.H. and R.G. analyzed the data; Z.H. wrote the first draft of the paper. All the authors participated in the revising of this article. M.C. was the corresponding author and provided professional guidance during the entire study. All authors provided assistance in the completion of the manuscript.

References

1. Papandreou, D.; Makedou, K.; Zormpa, A.; Karampola, M.; Ioannou, A.; Hitoglou-Makedou, A. Are Dietary Intakes Related to Obesity in Children? *Maced. J. Med. Sci.* **2016**, *4*, 194–199. [CrossRef] [PubMed]
2. Liang, Y.; Hou, D.; Zhao, X.; Wang, L.; Hu, Y.; Liu, J.; Cheng, H.; Yang, P.; Shan, X.; Yan, Y.; et al. Childhood obesity affects adult metabolic syndrome and diabetes. *Endocrine* **2015**, *50*, 87–92. [CrossRef] [PubMed]
3. Petkeviciene, J.; Klumbiene, J.; Kriaucioniene, V.; Raskiliene, A.; Sakute, E.; Ceponiene, I. Anthropometric measurements in childhood and prediction of cardiovascular risk factors in adulthood: Kaunas cardiovascular risk cohort study. *BMC Public Health* **2015**, *15*, 218. [CrossRef] [PubMed]
4. Wiseman, M. The second World Cancer Research Fund/American Institute for Cancer Research expert report. Food, nutrition, physical activity, and the prevention of cancer: A global perspective. *Proc. Nutr. Soc.* **2008**, *67*, 253–256. [CrossRef] [PubMed]
5. Ralston, K.; Newman, C.; Clauson, A.; Guthrie, J.; Buzby, J.C. *The National School Lunch Program: Background, Trends, and Issues*; Economic Research Report Number 61; U.S. Department of Agriculture: Washington, DC, USA, 2008; p. 2.

6. Tanaka, N.; Miyoshi, M. School lunch program for health promotion among children in Japan. *Asia Pac. J. Clin. Nutr.* **2012**, *21*, 155–158. [PubMed]
7. Hu, C.K. The current situation and future development perspective of School Lunch Program in China. *Food Nutr. China* **2008**, *2*, 4–6. (In Chinese).
8. Guo, P.; Yang, M.Y.; Chen, D.M. The analysis of school lunch industries in Shanghai. *Chin. J. Sch. Health* **2004**, *25*, 376–377. (In Chinese).
9. Shanghai Bureau of Statistics. Shanghai Statistic Yearbook. 2016. Available online: http://www.stats-sh.gov.cn/tjnj/nj16.htm?d1=2016tjnj/C2003.htm (accessed on 17 February 2017).
10. Ministry of Health People's Republic of China. *Amount of Nutritional Provision for School Lunch*; WS/T 100-1998; Ministry of Health People's Republic of China: Beijing, China, 1998; pp. 78–82.
11. Zhang, B.; Zhai, F.Y.; Du, S.F.; Popkin, B.M. The China Health and Nutrition Survey, 1989–2011. *Obes. Rev.* **2014**, *15* (Suppl. 1), 2–7. [CrossRef] [PubMed]
12. Chinese Nutrition Society. *China National Dietary Guideline for School Children (2016)*, 1st ed.; People's Medical Publishing House: Beijing, China, 2016; p. 49. (In Chinese)
13. Chinese Nutrition Society. *Chinese Dietary Reference Intakes (2013)*, 1st ed.; Science Press: Beijing, China, 2014; pp. 649–660. (In Chinese)
14. Niaki, S.F.; Moore, C.E.; Chen, T.A.; Weber Cullen, K. Younger Elementary School Students Waste More School Lunch Foods than Older Elementary School Students. *J. Acad. Nutr. Diet.* **2017**, *117*, 95–101. [CrossRef] [PubMed]
15. Smith, S.L.; Cunningham-Sabo, L. Food choice, plate waste and nutrient intake of elementary-and middle-school students participating in the US National School Lunch Program. *Public Health Nutr.* **2014**, *17*, 1255–1263. [CrossRef] [PubMed]
16. Condon, E.M.; Crepinsek, M.K.; Fox, M.K. School Meals: Types of Foods Offered to and Consumed by Children at Lunch and Breakfast. *J. Am. Diet. Assoc.* **2009**, *109*, S67–S78. [CrossRef] [PubMed]
17. Sun, C.H.; Ling, W.H.; Huang, G.W. *Nutrition and Food Hygiene*, 7th ed.; People's Medical Publishing House: Beijing, China, 2012; p. 201. (In Chinese)
18. Buzby, J.C.; Guthrie, J.F. *Plate Waste in School Nutrition Programs: Report to Congress*; E-FAN-02-009; Economic Research Service, U.S. Department of Agriculture: Washington, DC, USA, 2002.
19. Chinese Nutrition Society. *China National Dietary Guideline (2016)*, 1st ed.; People's Medical Publishing House: Beijing, China, 2016; p. 309. (In Chinese)
20. Bland, J.M.; Altman, D.G. Statistics notes: Cronbach's alpha. *BMJ* **1997**, *314*, 572. [CrossRef] [PubMed]
21. National Health and Family Planning Commission of the People's Republic of China. Report on Nutrition Status and Chronic Diseases of Chinese People. 2015. Available online: http://www.nhfpc.gov.cn/xcs/s3574/201506/6b4c0f873c174ace9f57f11fd4f6f8d9.shtml (accessed on 17 February 2017).
22. Office of the Federal Register, National Archives and Records Administration. *National School Lunch Program and School Breakfast Program: School Meals Initiative for Healthy Children*; Office of the Federal Register: Washington, DC, USA, 1995; pp. 31188–31222.
23. Crepinsek, M.K.; Gordon, A.R.; McKinney, P.M.; Condon, E.M.; Wilson, A. Meals offered and served in US public schools: Do they meet nutrient standards? *J. Am. Diet. Assoc.* **2009**, *109* (Suppl. 2), S31–S43. [CrossRef] [PubMed]
24. Clark, M.A.; Fox, M.K. Nutritional quality of the diets of US public school children and the role of the school meal programs. *J. Am. Diet. Assoc.* **2009**, *109* (Suppl. 2), S44–S56. [CrossRef] [PubMed]
25. Fox, M.K. School nutrition dietary assessment study-II. *Math. Policy Res. Rep.* **2001**, *67* (Suppl. 1), 67–69.
26. NCD Risk Factor Collaboration (NCD-RisC). Trends in adult body-mass index in 200 countries from 1975 to 2014: A pooled analysis of 1698 population-based measurement studies with 19.2 million participants. *Lancet* **2016**, *387*, 1377–1396.
27. Byker, C.J.; Farris, A.R.; Marcenelle, M.; Davis, G.C.; Serrano, E.L. Food Waste in a School Nutrition Program After Implementation of New Lunch Program Guidelines. *J. Nutr. Educ. Behav.* **2014**, *46*, 406–411. [CrossRef] [PubMed]
28. Cohen, J.F.; Richardson, S.; Parker, E.; Catalano, P.J.; Rimm, E.B. Impact of the New U.S. Department of Agriculture School Meal Standards on Food Selection, Consumption, and Waste. *Am. J. Prev. Med.* **2014**, *46*, 388–394. [CrossRef] [PubMed]

29. Liu, Y.; Cheng, S.; Liu, X.; Cao, X.; Xue, L.; Liu, G. Plate Waste in School Lunch Programs in Beijing, China. *Sustainability* **2016**, *8*, 1288. [CrossRef]
30. Baik, J.Y.; Lee, H. Habitual plate-waste of 6-to 9-year-olds may not be associated with lower nutritional needs or taste acuity, but undesirable dietary factors. *Nutr. Res.* **2009**, *29*, 831–838. [CrossRef] [PubMed]
31. Marlette, M.A.; Templeton, S.B.; Panemangalore, M. Food Type, Food Preparation, and Competitive Food Purchases Impact School Lunch Plate Waste by Sixth-Grade Students. *J. Am. Diet. Assoc.* **2005**, *105*, 1779–1782. [CrossRef] [PubMed]
32. Thorsen, A.V.; Lassen, A.D.; Andersen, E.W.; Christensen, L.M.; Biltoft-Jensen, A.; Andersen, R.; Damsgaard, C.T.; Michaelsen, K.F.; Tetens, I. Plate waste and intake of school lunch based on the new Nordic diet and on packed lunches: A randomised controlled trial in 8-to 11-year-old. *J. Nutr. Sci.* **2015**, *4*, e20. [CrossRef] [PubMed]
33. Dinis, D.; Martins, M.L.; Rocha, A. Plate Waste as an Indicator of Portions Inadequacy at School Lunch. *Int. Sch. Sci. Res. Innov.* **2013**, *7*, 477–480.
34. Warren, J.M.; Henry, C.J.; Livingstone, M.B.; Lightowler, H.J.; Bradshaw, S.M.; Perwaiz, S. How well do children aged 5–7 years recall food eaten at school lunch? *Public Health Nutr.* **2003**, *6*, 41–47. [CrossRef] [PubMed]
35. Comstock, E.M.; St Pierre, R.G.; Mackiernan, Y.D. Measuring individual plate waste in school lunches. Visual estimation and children's ratings vs. actual weighing of plate waste. *J. Am. Diet. Assoc.* **1981**, *79*, 290–296. [PubMed]
36. Swanson, M. Digital photography as a tool to measure school cafeteria consumption. *J. Sch. Health* **2008**, *78*, 432–437. [CrossRef] [PubMed]
37. Nicklas, T.A.; O'Neil, C.E.; Stuff, J.; Goodell, L.S.; Liu, Y.; Martin, C.K. Validity and Feasibility of a Digital Diet Estimation Method for Use with Preschool Children: A Pilot Study. *J. Nutr. Educ. Behav.* **2012**, *44*, 618–623. [CrossRef] [PubMed]
38. Martins, M.L.; Cunha, L.M.; Rodrigues, S.S.P.; Rocha, A. Determination of plate waste in primary school lunches by weighing and visual estimation methods: A validation study. *Waste Manag.* **2014**, *34*, 1362–1368. [CrossRef] [PubMed]
39. Thomson, C.A.; Ravia, J. A systematic review of behavioral interventions to promote intake of fruit and vegetables. *J. Am. Diet. Assoc.* **2011**, *111*, 1523–1535. [CrossRef] [PubMed]
40. Blanchette, L.; Brug, J. Determinants of fruit and vegetable consumption among 6–12-year-old children and effective interventions to increase consumption. *J. Hum. Nutr. Diet.* **2005**, *18*, 431–443. [CrossRef] [PubMed]

5

Associations between Physical Activity and Food Intake among Children and Adolescents: Results of KiGGS Wave 2

Kristin Manz *, Gert B. M. Mensink, Jonas D. Finger, Marjolein Haftenberger, Anna-Kristin Brettschneider, Clarissa Lage Barbosa, Susanne Krug and Anja Schienkiewitz

Department of Epidemiology and Health Monitoring, Robert Koch Institute, 13353 Berlin, Germany; MensinkG@rki.de (G.B.M.M.); FingerJ@rki.de (J.D.F.); HaftenbergerM@rki.de (M.H.); BrettschneiderA@rki.de (A.-K.B.); Lage-BarbosaC@rki.de (C.L.B.); KrugS@rki.de (S.K.); SchienkiewitzA@rki.de (A.S.)

* Correspondence: ManzK@rki.de

Abstract: A balanced diet and sufficient physical activity are essential for the healthy growth of children and adolescents and for obesity prevention. Data from the second wave of the population-based German Health Interview and Examination Survey for Children and Adolescents (KiGGS Wave 2; 2014–2017) were used to analyse the association between food intake and physical activity among 6- to 17-year-old children and adolescents (n = 9842). Physical exercise (PE) and recommended daily physical activity (RDPA) were assessed with self-administered questionnaires and food intake by a semi-quantitative food frequency questionnaire. Multivariable logistic regression was used to analyse the association between food group intake (dependent variable) and level of PE or RDPA. High levels of physical activity (PE or RDPA) were associated with higher consumption of juice, water, milk, dairy products, fruits, and vegetables among both boys and girls, and among boys with a higher intake of bread, potatoes/pasta/rice, meat, and cereals. Higher PE levels were also less likely to be associated with a high soft drink intake. High levels of RDPA were associated with high intake of energy-dense foods among boys, which was not observed for PE. This study indicates that school-aged children and adolescents with higher levels of physical activity consume more beneficial foods and beverages compared to those with lower physical activity levels.

Keywords: Physical activity; exercise; food intake; diet; children; adolescents; KiGGS

---

1. Introduction

A balanced diet and sufficient physical activity are essential for a healthy growth and development of children and adolescents and are important determinants of health throughout the life course. Unbalanced dietary patterns (with high amounts of highly processed and energy dense foods) are associated with unfavourable cardiometabolic risk factors (e.g., blood pressure, blood glucose, insulin levels, and lipid profile) among adolescents [1,2]. Higher levels of physical activity are associated with better physical, psychological, and cognitive health of children and adolescents [3], whereas a predominantly sedentary lifestyle is associated with less favourable levels of cardiometabolic risk factors [4]. In addition to genetic predisposition [5], dietary behaviour and physical activity are important determinants of obesity [6,7].

The prevalence of childhood obesity has significantly increased in recent years and is, therefore, a priority for health promotion and prevention policy and action [8]. Current data from KiGGS wave 2 (2014–2017) show that 15% of the 3- to 17-year-old children and adolescents in Germany are overweight; almost 6% are obese [9]. Compared to the KiGGS baseline survey (2003–2006), the prevalence of overweight and obesity has not increased further in the last ten years among children and adolescents, but remains at a high level [9].

There are only a few studies that have comprehensively analysed the relation between the two key components of obesity development, dietary behaviour, and physical activity in children and adolescents. In two studies, one conducted among high school students in the USA and the other among 12-year-old children from France, a higher level of physical activity is associated with a higher intake of fruits and vegetables [10,11]. The international study ISCOLE among 9- to 12-year-old children from 12 countries showed that achieving a higher number of specific physical activity recommendations (for sedentary behaviour, physical activity, and sleep duration) is associated with a more preferable dietary pattern [12]. A review of several studies investigating obesogenic behaviours using cluster analyses indicated that diet, physical activity, and sedentary behaviour cluster in both unhealthy and healthy ways and that cluster patterns differ by sex, age, and socioeconomic status [6].

Most existing studies investigating the relation between physical activity and dietary behaviour cover just a small age-range of childhood and do not indicate how the intake of single food items differ by the level of physical activity. Indicators of the current physical activity levels, as well as consumption of particular food items of children and adolescents have been described for Germany [13,14]. However, the interrelationship between these two behavioural aspects has not yet been analysed.

The aim of this study is to analyse whether children and adolescents aged 6 to 17 years with higher levels of physical activity differ in their food intake compared to those with lower levels of physical activity.

2. Materials and Methods

2.1. Study Design and Study Population

KiGGS (German Health Interview and Examination Survey for Children and Adolescents) is part of the Federal Health Monitoring System of the Robert Koch Institute and consists of regularly conducted representative cross-sectional surveys among children and adolescents aged between 0 and 17 years living in Germany. KiGGS Wave 2 was conducted between 2014 and 2017. The design and methodology of KiGGS Wave 2 have been described in detail elsewhere [15,16]. In brief, the study sample was drawn from the German resident population aged 0 to 17 years using a two-stage cluster sampling approach. Firstly, 167 sample points were randomly selected proportional to the population densities in the federal states and community sizes within the Federal Republic of Germany. Secondly, within each sample point age-stratified samples of individuals were randomly selected from the local population registries. In total, 15,023 children and adolescents (7538 girls; 7,485 boys) participated in the cross-sectional survey of KiGGS Wave 2.

KiGGS Wave 2 was conducted in accordance with the Declaration of Helsinki, and the protocol was approved by the Federal Commissioner for Data Protection and Freedom of Information and by the ethics committee of the Hannover Medical School (Number 2275–2014). A written informed consent was obtained by parents and all participants aged 14 years and above before data collection.

2.2. Data Collection and Aggregation

In KiGGS, parents (or legal guardians) of the 3- to 10-year-olds completed self-administered questionnaires which provided information on their children's health and health behaviour (e.g., food intake and physical activity). Similar questionnaires were filled in by 11- to 17-year-olds themselves.

2.3. Food Intake

KiGGS Wave 2 included a self-administered semi-quantitative food frequency questionnaire (FFQ) to assess the consumption of selected food items [17]. The FFQ starts with a short written introduction about the questionnaire. Participants are instructed how to report the frequency and number of standard portions which were consumed during the last four weeks. An illustration is provided as an example to report two slices of bread that were eaten twice a day during the past four weeks. A further illustration shows how to make corrections in case this is necessary. Finally, a telephone number was provided for further questions about the completion of the questionnaire. The 11- to 17-year-old participants or parents of 3- to 10-year-old participants were asked about the food items they or their children had consumed 'during the last four weeks'. The questionnaire contained 48 food items for younger participants and 53 food items (including alcoholic beverages) for those aged 11 years and above. First, the consumption frequency of each food item was assessed with the question: 'How often did your child/did you eat/drink food/drink X?' and in most cases, examples of the particular food items were given. Answer categories were: 'never', 'once per month', '2–3 times per month', '1–2 times per week', '3–4 times per week', '5–6 times per week', 'daily', '2 times per day', '3 times per day', '4–5 times per day', 'more than five times per day'. Second, portion size information was obtained by questions following the pattern: 'If your child/you eat/drink food/drink X, how much does your child/do you usually eat/drink?' To support portion size estimation, pictures were included as a reference for predefined portion sizes. In each case, five answering categories were given, which varied depending on the food item. These were, for instance, '$\frac{1}{2}$ a glass (or less)', '1 glass', '2 glasses', '3 glasses', and '4 glasses (or more)'. For some food items, a specific aspect of the food consumption was inquired, such as the dilution ratio of juice and water.

For the presented analyses, the information on food consumption frequencies was transformed into the number of occasions of consumption of each food over a four-week period (28 days). The portions were converted into grams or millilitres. For each food item, the estimated amount consumed per day was obtained by multiplying the converted food consumption frequency and the portion amount, and dividing this by 28. The following food groups were used for the analyses, partly constructed by summarising the amounts of multiple food items (in parenthesis): Soft drinks (sugar-sweetened soft drinks; reduced calorie soft drinks), juices (fruit juices; vegetable juices), water, milk, dairy products (cream cheese; cheese; quark, yoghurt or soured milk), fast food (hamburger or doner kebab; grilled sausages; French fries; pizza), fruits (fresh fruits; processed fruits), vegetables (raw vegetables; legumes; cooked vegetables), bread (whole-grain bread or rolls; brown or mixed bread or rolls; white bread or rolls), potatoes, noodles & rice (cooked potatoes; fried potatoes; noodles; rice), meat (poultry; red meat; meat portion in hamburger or doner kebab; grilled sausages; sausage; ham), breakfast cereals (corn flakes; muesli), savoury snacks (potato crisps; salty snacks or crackers), confectionery (cakes, tartes or sweet pastries; biscuits; chocolate; sweets; ice cream; sweet spreads). Based on the consumed amounts of these food groups, participants were ranked into quintiles. Quintiles were calculated separately for boys and girls in the age groups 6–10, 11–13 and 14–17 years in order to account for gender- and age-related differences in energy and nutrient requirements. For each food group, the top two quintiles (40%) were assigned to the category 'high intake'. A table with the threshold values for the category 'high intake' can be found in the Supplemental Table S1.

2.4. Recommended Daily Physical Activity (RDPA) and Physical Exercise (PE)

In KiGGS Wave 2, RDPA and PE information was also obtained using self-administered questionnaires. The indicator RDPA describes the amount of days per week with physical activity (light to vigorous intensity) of at least 60 min. To assess RDPA, participants were asked 'How many days of a normal week are you/is your child physically active for at least 60 min on a single day?' The eight answer categories ranged from 'Seven days' to 'None'. The answers were assigned to the categories 'low' (one hour/day on less than 3 days/week), 'medium' (one hour/day on 3 to 5 days/week) and 'high' (one 1 hour/day on 6 to 7 days/week). The instrument was initially used to verify if participants met the 'at least 60 min daily physical activity' criteria recommended by the World Health Organization [18] and was adapted from Prochaska and colleagues [19] A validation study showed moderate test-retest reliability with a Kappa coefficient of 0.54 and a significant Spearman correlation coefficient of 0.24 for validity when compared with objectively measured physical activity by accelerometers [20]. The indicator PE should include sports activities like running or playing soccer. To obtain information on PE, participants were asked whether they participate in physical exercises, adding that this referred to all kinds of sports regardless if it was within a sports club or not. Physical education at school should not be included. The question could be answered with 'Yes' or 'No'. Participants who answered 'Yes' were consecutively asked how many minutes or hours they usually participate in physical exercises per week. The data on PE was used to assign the persons to categories 'low' (less than one hour of sport/week), 'medium' (1–3 h/week) and 'high' (more than 3 h/week).

2.5. *Socioeconomic Status (SES)*

In the KiGGS study, an index is used to measure parental socioeconomic status (SES), which is based on information about the parents' education, their occupational status and income [21,22]. A detailed description of the construction of the socioeconomic variables and the SES index can be found elsewhere [22]. Based on the SES index, individuals were categorized into 'low', 'medium' and 'high' SES.

2.6. *Body Mass Index (BMI)*

In the physical examination component, standardized measurements of body height and weight were obtained [9]. The body mass index (BMI) was calculated from body weight divided by the square of body height. BMI percentiles were modelled as a function of age (BMI-for-age) and transformed to a standard normal distribution (BMI-for-age *z*-score).

2.7. *Data Analysis*

Since preschool children have a considerably different physical activity and food consumption pattern from older children, 3- to 5-year-olds were not included in the present analysis. The current analysis was, therefore, restricted to 11,014 participants aged 6 to 17 years (5582 girls and 5432 boys).

Food consumption information was completely set to missing for some cases in the original dataset ($n = 38$). This was done if the frequency answers contained more than 20 missing values or if the calculated total intake was implausibly high (total daily amount of beverages exceeded 15 litres, of solid foods exceeded 10 kg or if there was a combination of the amount of beverages exceeding 4 L and solid foods exceeding 6 kg). In the current analysis, participants with missing information on at least one of the aggregated food intake variables were excluded from the current analysis ($n = 1172$, 10.6%). The sample for multivariable regression analyses among boys comprises 4472 participants for PE and 4557 participants for RDPA, after excluding participants with missing information on PE, RDPA or SES. Among girls, the sample for the multivariable regression comprises 5016 for PE and 5073 participants for RDPA.

Statistical analyses were conducted using Stata SE 15 (StataCorp. 2017. Stata Statistical Software: Release 15. StataCorp LLC, College Station, TX, USA). All analyses were performed with survey design procedures to adjust for the clustered sampling design. A weighting factor was applied to correct deviations within the sample from the German population with regard to age, gender, federal state (as of 31.12.2015), nationality (as of 21.12.2014), and the parents' level of education (Mikrozensus 2013). Multivariable logistic regression was used to analyse if medium and high versus low RDPA and PE were associated with food intake variables. Odds ratios (OR) were reported to describe the odds of having a high intake of a food depending on the variables PE and RDPA. The associations were stepwise adjusted for age (model 1) and parental SES (model 2). In a sensitivity analysis, BMI-for-age *z*-scores were added to model 2. The criterion for statistical significance was set at $p < 0.05$.

3. Results

Demographic characteristics and physical activity behaviour of the study sample stratified by sex, age, and SES are shown in Table 1. PE was low among 25.7%, medium among 36.7% and high among 37.6% of the participants, while RDPA was low among 25.2%, medium among 47.8% and high among

27.0% of the participants. Boys more often had a high level of PE and RDPA than girls. The proportion of boys and girls with a high PE level was higher among older age groups, whereas the proportion with a high RDPA level was lower among older age groups. The proportion of boys and girls with a high PE level increased with increasing SES, while there were no statistically significant differences in the frequency of high RDPA levels by SES. However, the proportion of participants with low RDPA significantly decreased with increasing SES.

3.1. Binary Associations

A higher PE level was significantly associated with a high intake of water, dairy products, fruits, and vegetables in boys and girls, and a high intake of juice and breakfast cereals in boys (Table 2). A medium or high PE level was less often associated with a high soft drink intake than a low PE level among boys and girls. Furthermore, a low PE level was more often associated with a higher meat intake for girls compared to medium or high PE level, while a low PE level was associated with a high intake of savoury snacks for both genders.

Higher RDPA was significantly associated with a high intake of fruits and vegetables among boys and girls. Furthermore, among boys, higher levels of RDPA were associated with a high intake of water, milk, dairy products, bread, potatoes/pasta/noodles, breakfast cereals, and confectionery (Table 2). Girls with a low RDPA level more often had a high intake of soft drinks, savoury snacks, and confectionery than girls with a medium or high RDPA level.

3.2. Multivariable Analyses

Almost all significant associations in the binary analyses for PE remained significant in the logistic regression analyses after adjustment for age and SES (model 2; Table 3). Exceptions were the associations of PE with water and with meat among girls. Furthermore, the association of PE and a high intake of breakfast cereals and savoury snacks among girls became significant after adjusting for age, but did not remain significant after further adjustment for SES.

For boys, a high compared to a low level of PE was less likely associated with a high soft drink intake (OR 0.7), but was more likely associated with a high intake of juice (OR 1.3), water (OR 1.3), dairy products (OR 1.5), fruits (OR 1.9), vegetables (OR 1.7), and breakfast cereals (OR 1.5) (Table 3). For girls, a high compared to a low level of PE was less likely associated with a high intake of soft drinks (OR 0.7), and more likely associated a high intake of dairy products (OR 1.2), fruits (OR 1.6), and vegetables (OR 1.5).

Many binary associations of RDPA with a certain food group intake remained significant in the multivariable analyses (Table 4). Among boys, the non-significant association observed for a high intake of juice and meat with higher levels of RDPA became significant after adjustment for age and SES. For girls, the significant binary association between RDPA and high soft drink intake did not remain significant after adjusting for age and SES, whereas the associations between RDPA and high intake of juice, water, milk, and dairy products became significant.

For boys, a high compared to a low RDPA was more likely associated with a high intake of juice (OR 1.3), water (OR 1.4), milk (OR 1.7), dairy products (OR 1.4), fruits (OR 2.1), vegetables (OR 1.5) bread (OR 1.5), potatoes/pasta/rice (OR 1.4), meat (OR 1.3), breakfast cereals (OR 1.3), and confectionery (OR 1.6) for boys (Table 4). For girls, a high compared to a low RDPA was more likely associated with a high intake of water (OR 1.3), milk (OR 1.3), dairy products (OR 1.4), fruits (OR 1.9), and vegetables (OR 1.5). A medium compared to a low RDPA was less likely associated with a high intake of savoury snacks (OR 0.8) and confectionery (OR 0.8), and more likely associated with a high intake of juice (OR 1.3) for girls.

The inclusion of BMI-for-age z-scores into model 2 did not alter the relation between PE nor RDPA and food intake (data not shown).

Table 1. Demographic characteristics for categories of physical activity behaviour of the study sample ($N = 9842$).

		Total	Sex		Age (Years)			Socioeconomic Status [a]		
			Boys	Girls	6–10	11–13	14–17	Low	Medium	High
	n	% 95% CI	% 95% CI	% 95% CI	% 95% CI	% 95% CI	% 95% CI	% 95% CI	% 95% CI	% 95% CI
n		100.0 9842	47.2 4646	52.8 5196	32.0 3146	35.2 3464	32.8 3232	12.2 1184	62.3 6065	25.5 2480
Physical exercise [b]										
Low	2295	25.7 24.4–27.0	22.1 20.4–23.8	29.2 27.4–31.1	23.5 21.1–26.0	23.1 21.1–25.2	29.9 27.7–32.1	44.2 40.4–48.1	24.0 22.6–25.6	12.9 11.3–14.7
Medium	3639	36.7 35.3–38.1	32.5 30.7–34.3	40.7 38.8–42.8	48.3 45.7–50.8	36.4 34.1–38.8	27.3 25.5–29.2	30.4 27.1–34.0	37.6 36.0–39.4	40.0 38.0–42.2
High	3654	37.6 36.2–39.1	45.4 43.2–47.7	30.1 28.3–31.9	28.3 26.3–30.4	40.5 38.0–43.1	42.9 40.8-45.0	25.3 22.5–28.5	38.3 36.5–40.1	47.0 44.5–49.6
Recommended daily physical activity [c]										
Low	2305	25.2 23.9–26.6	20.3 18.5–22.2	30.1 28.3–31.9	17.1 15.4–18.9	22.8 20.9–24.9	34.2 32.1–36.4	34.1 30.3–38.2	24.1 22.7–25.7	19.7 17.9–21.6
Medium	4786	47.8 46.4–49.2	48.8 46.9–50.6	46.9 44.9–49.0	44.9 42.5–47.3	50.0 47.6–52.5	48.4 46.1–50.6	40.3 36.4–44.2	48.8 47.0–50.5	52.4 50.0–54.8
High	2639	27.0 25.6–28.4	31.0 29.2–32.9	23.0 21.3–24.9	38.0 35.6–40.6	27.1 24.8–29.6	17.4 15.8–19.2	25.6 22.5–29.1	27.1 25.6–28.7	27.9 26.1–29.9

[a] 113 missing; [b] 254 missing; low: < 1 h/week, medium: 1–3 h/week, high: >3 h/week; [c] 112 missing; low: <3 days/week 1 h/day, medium: 3–5 days/week 1 h/day, high: 6–7 days/week 1 h/day; CI—confidence interval.

Table 2. Percentage with high intake of specific foods among 6- to 17-year-old children and adolescents in total and stratified by physical activity variables (binary associations).

		Total	Physical Exercise [a]				Recommended Daily Physical Activity [b]			
			Low	Medium	High	*P* *	Low	Medium	High	*P* *
High Intake		%	%	%	%		%	%	%	
Soft drinks	boys	39.7	48.2	36.3	37.2	<0.001	42.4	37.4	40.5	0.128
	girls	38.0	47.3	33.2	33.9	<0.001	42.0	35.3	36.0	0.008
	total	38.8	47.7	34.6	35.8	<0.001	42.2	36.3	38.6	0.003
Juice	boys	34.5	31.1	33.8	37.3	0.012	31.5	34.9	36.2	0.210
	girls	35.5	32.4	36.0	36.0	0.223	33.2	37.1	35.2	0.231
	total	35.0	31.9	35.0	36.8	0.014	32.5	36.0	35.8	0.092
Water	boys	39.7	36.8	37.0	42.1	0.016	35.9	39.2	42.8	0.045
	girls	33.5	33.7	31.1	36.5	0.042	32.2	32.9	36.7	0.118
	total	36.5	35.0	33.7	39.8	<0.001	33.7	36.1	40.2	<0.001
Milk	boys	25.6	25.5	24.7	27.1	0.496	21.2	25.7	28.3	0.015
	girls	29.9	30.9	27.8	32.1	0.124	30.8	29.6	29.4	0.776
	total	27.8	28.6	26.4	29.1	0.170	27.0	27.6	28.7	0.557
Dairy products	boys	39.0	33.2	38.6	42.5	0.001	33.8	39.7	41.1	0.013
	girls	39.3	36.8	38.6	43.1	0.021	36.0	40.1	41.9	0.057
	total	39.1	35.3	38.6	42.7	<0.001	35.1	39.9	41.5	<0.001
Fast food	boys	40.0	36.6	39.0	41.0	0.220	39.8	40.1	39.2	0.928
	girls	41.4	43.6	40.4	39.8	0.219	41.3	42.0	39.6	0.614
	total	40.7	40.7	39.8	40.5	0.852	40.7	41.0	39.4	0.628
Fruits	boys	36.0	27.4	33.5	41.9	<0.001	24.3	37.7	41.3	<0.001
	girls	37.1	33.5	35.0	43.9	<0.001	30.6	38.5	41.7	<0.001
	total	36.5	30.9	34.4	42.7	<0.001	28.1	38.1	41.5	<0.001
Vegetables	boys	38.4	31.0	35.6	44.1	<0.001	32.1	38.9	41.9	0.001
	girls	40.1	35.3	38.7	47.6	<0.001	34.7	42.0	43.8	<0.001
	total	39.3	33.5	37.4	45.5	<0.001	33.7	40.5	42.7	<0.001
Bread	boys	37.4	39.3	34.7	37.2	0.168	33.5	36.6	40.9	0.016
	girls	38.8	39.7	38.5	37.5	0.689	36.9	37.9	41.5	0.180
	total	38.1	39.5	36.8	37.3	0.295	35.5	37.2	41.1	0.008

Table 2. *Cont.*

		Total	Physical Exercise [a]				Recommended Daily Physical Activity [b]			
			Low	Medium	High	P *	Low	Medium	High	P *
High Intake		%	%	%	%		%	%	%	
Potatoes/pasta/rice	boys	38.5	36.7	37.2	39.7	0.417	35.6	36.8	42.6	0.013
	girls	39.2	40.5	38.4	38.6	0.596	37.7	40.6	37.5	0.309
	total	38.8	38.9	37.9	39.2	0.663	36.9	38.7	40.4	0.174
Meat	boys	39.8	37.6	38.9	41.1	0.361	37.7	38.6	42.3	0.172
	girls	41.3	45.4	38.9	40.0	0.013	42.2	40.0	42.3	0.438
	total	40.6	42.1	38.9	40.7	0.162	40.4	39.3	42.3	0.159
Breakfast cereals	boys	36.8	31.2	34.0	41.9	<0.001	32.2	38.1	37.7	0.042
	girls	39.3	36.4	39.2	41.6	0.113	37.3	39.3	42.4	0.104
	total	38.0	34.2	37.0	41.8	<0.001	35.3	38.7	39.7	0.020
Savoury snacks	boys	41.0	43.3	39.9	40.1	0.417	40.8	40.9	40.8	0.999
	girls	41.2	44.5	40.0	39.1	0.080	45.0	38.4	41.4	0.011
	total	41.1	44.0	40.0	39.7	0.033	43.3	39.7	41.1	0.098
Confectionery	boys	35.2	31.4	34.2	37.0	0.109	30.7	34.4	39.0	0.009
	girls	40.6	43.9	39.6	40.1	0.143	44.3	37.5	42.8	0.002
	total	37.9	38.6	37.2	38.2	0.719	38.9	35.9	40.6	0.011

[a] $n = 9488$; boys: $n = 4472$, girls: $n = 5016$; low: <1 h/week, medium: 1–3 h/week, high: >3 h/week; [b] $n = 9630$, boys: $n = 4557$, girls: $n = 5073$; low: <3 days/week 1 h/day, medium: 3–5 days/week 1 h/day, high: 6–7 days/week 1 h/day; * P-values of test for differences between groups (chi-square).

Table 3. Results of logistic regression analyses between food intake and physical exercise [a].

High intake of Food Group		Boys (n = 4472) Physical Exercise Level		Girls (n = 5016) Physical Exercise Level	
		Medium	High	Medium	High
		OR (95% CI)	OR (95% CI)	OR (95% CI)	OR (95% CI)
Soft drinks	Model [1]	**0.6 (0.5–0.8)**	**0.6 (0.5–0.8)**	**0.6 (0.5–0.7)**	**0.6 (0.5–0.7)**
	Model [2]	**0.7 (0.6–0.9)**	**0.7 (0.6–0.9)**	**0.7 (0.5–0.8)**	**0.7 (0.6–0.8)**
Juice	Model [1]	1.2 (1.0–1.4)	**1.3 (1.1–1.6)**	1.2 (1.0–1.6)	1.2 (1.0–1.5)
	Model [2]	1.2 (0.9–1.4)	**1.3 (1.0–1.5)**	1.2 (1.0–1.6)	1.2 (1.0–1.5)
Water	Model [1]	1.0 (0.8–1.2)	**1.2 (1.0–1.5)**	0.9 (0.7–1.1)	1.1 (0.9–1.4)
	Model [2]	1.1 (0.9–1.3)	**1.3 (1.1–1.6)**	0.9 (0.8–1.1)	1.2 (1.0–1.5)
Milk	Model [1]	1.0 (0.8–1.3)	1.0 (0.8–1.4)	1.0 (0.8–1.2)	1.1 (0.9–1.3)
	Model [2]	1.0 (0.8–1.3)	1.0 (0.8–1.4)	1.0 (0.8–1.3)	1.1 (0.9–1.4)
Dairy products	Model [1]	**1.3 (1.0–1.6)**	**1.5 (1.2–1.8)**	1.1 (0.9–1.3)	**1.3 (1.1–1.6)**
	Model [2]	**1.3 (1.0–1.7)**	**1.5 (1.2–1.9)**	1.0 (0.9–1.3)	**1.2 (1.0–1.5)**
Fast food	Model [1]	1.1 (0.9–1.4)	1.2 (1.0–1.5)	0.9 (0.7–1.0)	0.9 (0.7–1.1)
	Model [2]	1.2 (0.9–1.5)	1.2 (1.0–1.5)	1.0 (0.8–1.1)	0.9 (0.8–1.2)
Fruits	Model [1]	1.3 (1.0–1.7)	**2.0 (1.5–2.5)**	1.1 (0.9–1.4)	**1.6 (1.3–1.9)**
	Model [2]	1.2 (1.0–1.6)	**1.9 (1.5–2.4)**	1.1 (0.9–1.4)	**1.6 (1.3–1.9)**
Vegetables	Model [1]	1.2 (1.0–1.6)	**1.7 (1.4–2.2)**	1.2 (1.0–1.4)	**1.7 (1.4–2.0)**
	Model [2]	1.2 (0.9–1.5)	**1.7 (1.3–2.1)**	1.0 (0.8–1.3)	**1.5 (1.2–1.8)**
Bread	Model [1]	0.9 (0.7–1.1)	0.9 (0.7–1.1)	1.0 (0.8–1.2)	0.9 (0.7–1.1)
	Model [2]	0.9 (0.7–1.1)	0.9 (0.8–1.1)	1.0 (0.8–1.2)	0.9 (0.8–1.2)
Potatoes/pasta/rice	Model [1]	1.1 (0.8–1.4)	1.1 (0.9–1.4)	0.9 (0.8–1.1)	0.9 (0.8–1.1)
	Model [2]	1.1 (0.8–1.3)	1.1 (0.9–1.4)	1.0 (0.8–1.1)	0.9 (0.8–1.2)
Meat	Model [1]	1.1 (0.9–1.4)	1.1 (0.9–1.4)	**0.8 (0.7–1.0)**	**0.8 (0.7–1.0)**
	Model [2]	1.1 (0.9–1.5)	1.2 (1.0–1.5)	0.8 (0.7–1.0)	0.9 (0.7–1.1)
Breakfast cereals	Model [1]	1.2 (0.9–1.5)	**1.6 (1.2–2.0)**	1.1 (0.9–1.4)	**1.2 (1.0–1.6)**
	Model [2]	1.1 (0.9–1.4)	**1.5 (1.2–1.8)**	1.1 (0.9–1.3)	1.2 (1.0–1.5)
Savoury snacks	Model [1]	0.9 (0.7–1.1)	0.9 (0.7–1.1)	0.8 (0.7–1.0)	**0.8 (0.6–1.0)**
	Model [2]	1.0 (0.7–1.2)	1.0 (0.8–1.2)	0.9 (0.7–1.1)	0.9 (0.7–1.1)
Confectionery	Model [1]	1.2 (0.9–1.5)	1.2 (1.0–1.6)	0.8 (0.7–1.0)	0.9 (0.7–1.0)
	Model [2]	1.2 (0.9–1.5)	1.3 (1.0–1.6)	0.9 (0.7–1.1)	0.9 (0.7–1.1)

[1] Model adjusted for age; [2] Model adjusted for age and socioeconomic status; [a] low: <1 h/week (reference group), medium: 1–3 h/week, high: >3 h/week; OR—odds ratio; CI—confidence interval; bold: The odds ratio is significantly different from 1 (reference is low PE with $p < 0.05$).

Table 4. Results of logistic regression analyses between food intake and recommended daily physical activity [a].

High intake of Food Group		**Boys (n = 4557) Daily Physical Activity Level**		**Girls (n = 5073) Daily Physical Activity Level**	
		Medium	High	Medium	High
		OR (95% CI)	OR (95% CI)	OR (95% CI)	OR (95% CI)
Soft drinks	Model [1]	0.8 (0.7–1.0)	1.0 (0.8–1.2)	**0.8 (0.6–1.0)**	0.8 (0.7–1.1)
	Model [2]	0.9 (0.7–1.1)	1.0 (0.8–1.3)	0.8 (0.7–1.0)	0.9 (0.7–1.1)
Juice	Model [1]	1.2 (0.9–1.5)	**1.3 (1.0–1.6)**	**1.3 (1.0–1.5)**	1.2 (1.0–1.6)
	Model [2]	1.2 (0.9–1.5)	**1.3 (1.0–1.6)**	**1.3 (1.1–1.6)**	1.3 (1.0–1.6)
Water	Model [1]	1.2 (0.9–1.4)	**1.4 (1.1–1.8)**	1.0 (0.9–1.2)	**1.3 (1.0–1.6)**
	Model [2]	1.2 (1.0–1.5)	**1.4 (1.1–1.8)**	1.1 (0.9–1.3)	**1.3 (1.0–1.6)**
Milk	Model [1]	**1.3 (1.0–1.7)**	**1.6 (1.2–2.2)**	1.1 (0.9–1.4)	**1.3 (1.0–1.7)**
	Model [2]	**1.3 (1.0–1.7)**	**1.7 (1.3–2.2)**	1.1 (0.9–1.4)	**1.3 (1.0–1.7)**
Dairy products	Model [1]	**1.3 (1.1–1.6)**	**1.4 (1.1–1.8)**	**1.2 (1.0–1.5)**	**1.4 (1.1–1.7)**
	Model [2]	**1.3 (1.1–1.6)**	**1.4 (1.1–1.8)**	1.2 (1.0–1.5)	**1.4 (1.1–1.7)**
Fast food	Model [1]	1.0 (0.8–1.3)	1.0 (0.8–1.3)	1.0 (0.9–1.3)	0.9 (0.8–1.2)
	Model [2]	1.0 (0.8–1.3)	1.0 (0.8–1.3)	1.1 (0.9–1.3)	1.0 (0.8–1.2)
Fruits	Model [1]	**1.9 (1.5–2.3)**	**2.1 (1.7–2.7)**	**1.5 (1.3–1.9)**	**1.9 (1.6–2.4)**
	Model [2]	**1.8 (1.5–2.3)**	**2.1 (1.6–2.7)**	**1.5 (1.3–1.8)**	**1.9 (1.6–2.3)**
Vegetables	Model [1]	**1.4 (1.1–1.7)**	**1.6 (1.2–2.0)**	**1.4 (1.2–1.7)**	**1.6 (1.2–2.0)**
	Model [2]	**1.3 (1.1–1.6)**	**1.5 (1.2–2.0)**	**1.3 (1.1–1.6)**	**1.5 (1.2–1.9)**
Bread	Model [1]	1.2 (1.0–1.4)	**1.5 (1.2–1.8)**	1.1 (0.9–1.3)	1.2 (1.0–1.6)
	Model [2]	1.2 (1.0–1.5)	**1.5 (1.2–1.9)**	1.1 (0.9–1.3)	1.3 (1.0–1.6)
Potatoes/pasta/rice	Model [1]	1.1 (0.8–1.3)	**1.4 (1.1–1.8)**	1.2 (1.0–1.4)	1.1 (0.9–1.3)
	Model [2]	1.1 (0.8–1.3)	**1.4 (1.1–1.8)**	1.2 (1.0–1.5)	1.1 (0.9–1.3)
Meat	Model [1]	1.0 (0.8–1.3)	1.3 (1.0–1.6)	1.0 (0.8–1.1)	1.1 (0.9–1.4)
	Model [2]	1.1 (0.9–1.3)	**1.3 (1.0–1.6)**	1.0 (0.8–1.2)	1.1 (0.9–1.4)
Breakfast cereals	Model [1]	**1.3 (1.1–1.6)**	**1.4 (1.1–1.7)**	1.1 (0.9–1.3)	1.2 (1.0–1.5)
	Model [2]	**1.3 (1.0–1.6)**	**1.3 (1.1–1.6)**	1.1 (0.9–1.3)	1.2 (1.0–1.5)
Savoury snacks	Model [1]	1.0 (0.8–1.2)	1.0 (0.8–1.3)	**0.8 (0.6–0.9)**	0.9 (0.7–1.1)
	Model [2]	1.1 (0.9–1.3)	1.1 (0.9–1.4)	**0.8 (0.7–1.0)**	0.9 (0.7–1.1)
Confectionery	Model [1]	1.2 (0.9–1.5)	**1.6 (1.2–2.0)**	**0.8 (0.6–0.9)**	0.9 (0.8-1.1)
	Model [2]	1.2 (0.9–1.5)	**1.6 (1.2–2.0)**	**0.8 (0.6–0.9)**	1.0 (0.8–1.2)

[1] Model adjusted for age; [2] Model adjusted for age and socioeconomic status; [a] low: <3 days/week 1 h/day (reference group), medium: 3–5 days/week 1 h/day, high: 6–7 days/week 1 h/day; OR—odds ratio; CI—confidence interval; bold: The odds ratio is significantly different from 1 (reference is low RDPA with $p < 0.05$).

4. Discussion

Adequate levels of physical activity and a balanced diet are important requirements for an optimal physiological and cognitive development, as well as for the maintenance of good physical conditions and health in general. A good balance between physical activity and diet may also help to prevent or reduce the occurrence of obesity [23]. For a holistic prevention approach, it is important to understand and take into account that these health behaviours may interact with each other. The aim of the current study was, therefore, to analyse differences in intake of various food groups between low, medium and high physical activity behaviour groups among children and adolescents. To our knowledge, this study is the first study to investigate the associations between two different aspects of physical activity behaviour and 14 different food groups based on representative data from children and adolescents living in Germany. These analyses among boys and girls aged 6 to 17 years indicate that higher physical activity levels are more often associated with a high intake of predominantly preferable foods (with some exceptions) and a less frequent high intake of some less beneficial foods. For example, boys and girls with a high RDPA level were twice as likely to consume fruits in high amounts and had 50% higher odds to consume vegetables in high amounts than those with a lower RDPA. Furthermore, the odds ratio of a high soft drink intake was 30% lower in children and adolescents with a high compared to a low PE level.

The more often observed high intake of several food groups among children and adolescents with higher physical activity levels (PE and RDPA), some of which are dairy products, fruits, and vegetables, may partly be explained by a higher energy requirement due to a higher physical activity. A derivation of accurate estimates of the energy intake is not possible due to the relatively short food frequency questionnaire used in KiGGS Wave 2. Nevertheless, a high RDPA level was more often associated with a high intake for many food groups for boys, which may suggest a higher energy intake for this group. Among girls, high intakes of some food groups, i.e., for water, fruits, and vegetables, were associated with higher RDPA levels, although these are not energy-dense foods. Overall, this suggests that differences in energy needs may not explain all observed differences in food intake. The observed association of high intake of water and higher physical activity levels may be related to higher transpiration losses during enhanced physical activity. The authors of a review summarised that the relation between energy expenditure caused by physical activity and energy intake in children and adolescents are still inconclusive due to a lack of data [24]. However, it was observed that nutritional adaptation occurs as a response to physical activity, not only to compensate for the expended energy [24,25]. These adaptations may be changes in food choices as well as in appetite sensation, depending on duration, intensity, and type of physical activity [26,27]. Differences in duration, intensity and type of physical activity between boys and girls might also explain why, in this present analysis, more food groups were associated with physical activity in boys compared to girls. The higher levels of RDPA and PE among boys than girls [13] might have a stronger impact on their food choices. Furthermore, our results confirm that different types of physical activity are differently associated with a high consumption of food items: RDPA was more often associated with a high intake of individual foods compared to PE. Various reasons may lead to engagement in more PE or RDPA. These include body weight loss or maintenance, to gain muscle power, to improve body fitness, or physical skills as well as social aspects [28]. These purposes may differ between genders as well as for RDPA and PE, and could partly explain the observed differences in associations with food intake.

Studies comparing the intake of different food groups and physical activity in children and adolescents are rare. The observed higher fruit and vegetable consumption in children with higher physical activity is in line with studies among school-aged children in the USA and France [10,11]. In a representative sample of adolescents attending grade 9 to 12 in the USA, a higher fruit, vegetable, and soft drink consumption was associated with higher daily physical activity [10]. Regarding the soft drink intake, our study showed contradictory results: a lower soft drink intake was associated with a high PE level. There was no significant association observed between a high soft drink intake and RDPA. A study among 12-year-olds from France showed that the consumption of fruits, vegetables, and fruit juice was positively associated with organised physical activity [11]. In our study, in addition to the observed association with fruit and vegetable intake, fruit juice was also positively associated with PE and RDPA in boys and with RDPA in girls.

Most studies regarding physical activity and food intake in children summarise the assessed food intake into the categories 'healthy dietary pattern' and 'unhealthy dietary pattern'. If we apply these categories to the food groups presented in our study, a high intake of water, fruits, and vegetables would be considered as components of a healthy dietary behaviour, whereas a high intake of soft drinks, fast food, savoury snacks, and confectionery would be unhealthy [29]. From this perspective, the current results suggest that a high PE level is more likely associated with a healthy food pattern, reflected by high intakes of fruit and vegetables and low intakes of soft drinks. High RDPA also seems to be associated with more beneficial intakes of fruits, vegetables, and drinking water. Additionally, high RDPA seems to be associated with higher intakes of energy-dense food groups and less beneficial food groups, like confectionery and meat, among boys. Among girls, higher RDPA was associated with a lower intake of savoury snacks and confectionery. The positive association between PE and a healthy food intake might be explained by a higher overall health consciousness which influences multiple health behaviours [30,31]. For younger children, the motivation of the parents and family to live a healthy lifestyle will be relevant rather than the individual preference [32].

The authors of a review about the clustering of physical activity, sedentary behaviour and diet in children and adolescents concluded that these behaviours show inconsistent clustering patterns, sometimes corresponding with healthy behaviours and sometimes not [6]. Two studies found a consistency in preferable physical activity and dietary behaviour which confirms our results. However, in a cluster analysis conducted with children and adolescents aged 11 to 17 years living in Germany no cluster with high scores in physical activity and healthy diet was observed [33].

Data of the International Study of Childhood Obesity, Lifestyle and the Environment (ISCOLE) were used to examine if meeting recommendations related to physical activity, screen-time and sleep (≥60 min/day moderate-to-vigorous physical activity; ≤2 h/day screen time; 9 to 11 h/night sleep duration) were associated with dietary patterns among 9- to 11-year-old children from 12 different countries [12]. Results showed that a healthier diet was observed when more recommendations were met, which confirm partly a positive relation between sufficient physical activity and a healthy diet.

A strength of the study is that it is based on a large nationwide and representative sample of young persons living in Germany. In addition, the information on two different aspects of physical activity, as well as on the intake of many food groups, allows a broad analysis of the association between physical activity and food intake among children and adolescents. Our analyses have some limitations that should be considered. The assessment of physical activity and food intake was based on self-reports which is subject to recall and social desirability bias [34,35]. This may lead to overreporting of healthy behaviours (e.g., physical activity, intake of fruits, and vegetables) and an underreporting of unhealthy behaviours (e.g., intake of soft drinks, snacks, and sweets). The use of objective methods, such as activity monitors, may help to reduce such bias for physical activity. However, bias might still be present, since the measurement of specific physical activities by activity monitors is only possible in combination with a self-reported diary, and the consciousness of activity being measured may also alter actual behaviour [36]. In a free-living population setting, it is hardly possible to objectively measure dietary intake. The food frequency instrument used in this survey is not comprehensive and detailed enough to give a complete and precise overview of food consumption and energy intake. In addition, the specific information on food consumption and physical activity behaviour is gathered from parents for the younger children (up to the age of 11 years) and from those above 11 years themselves, which could have biased the results. Although this is inevitable because young children cannot give reliable information on major parts of the requested items, parents may also not have a complete overview of what their children eat (especially out of home) and how physically active they are. So for the different age groups the level of misreporting could be different. However, we constructed age-specific quintiles for the reported food intakes, so persons are ranked according to reported consumption relative to those within their age group. This may at least reduce in some extent the possible bias introduced by the responder. Furthermore, the association between physical activity and food intake may be confounded by other variables, which we have not considered for adjustment. We adjusted for age and SES because these dimensions could bias the association between physical activity and food intake. In a sensitivity analysis, we additionally adjusted for BMI-for-age z-scores. This, however, had no substantial impact on the regression results (data not shown). Due to the cross-sectional nature of the data, causal inferences cannot be derived. Finally, around 10% of the participants were excluded because of missing values in the analysed items which might have biased the results. These excluded participants were more often boys, younger children, and participants with lower SES.

5. Conclusions

The analysis of the association between RDPA and PE with food intake among school-aged children and adolescents indicates that higher levels of RDPA and PE are associated with more beneficial intakes of particular food items, such as a high fruit and vegetable intake and a lower soft drink intake. RDPA is additionally more often associated with high intakes of some energy-dense foods among boys, but not among girls. Detailed information on activity patterns and food intake can make a considerable contribution to focused primary prevention strategies which promote a healthy lifestyle of children and adolescents.

Author Contributions: K.M. conducted the present analysis and drafted the manuscript. K.M., J.D.F., A.S. and G.B.M.M. conceptualised the present study and statistical analyses. K.M. and J.D.F. conducted the statistical analyses. A.S., A.K.-B., K.M., J.D.F. and G.B.M.M. were involved in the design and conduct of KiGGS Wave 2. G.B.M.M. was responsible for the construction and conversion of the food frequency questionnaire. All authors contributed to the writing, interpretation of findings, reviewed, edited and approved the final manuscript.

Acknowledgments: First: we would like to thank the participants and their parents as well as everyone at the 167 study sites who provided us with space and active support on site. KiGGS Wave 2 could not have been conducted without the dedication of numerous colleagues at the Robert Koch Institute. We would especially like to thank the study teams for their excellent work and their exceptional commitment during the three-year data collection phase.

References

1. Cunha, C.M.; Costa, P.R.F.; de Oliveira, L.P.M.; Queiroz, V.A.O.; Pitangueira, J.C.D.; Oliveira, A.M. Dietary patterns and cardiometabolic risk factors among adolescents: Systematic review and meta-analysis. *Br. J. Nutr.* **2018**, *119*, 859–879. [CrossRef]
2. Rocha, N.P.; Milagres, L.C.; Longo, G.Z.; Ribeiro, A.Q.; Novaes, J.F. Association between dietary pattern and cardiometabolic risk in children and adolescents: A systematic review. *J. Pediatr.* **2017**, *93*, 214–222. [CrossRef]
3. Poitras, V.J.; Gray, C.E.; Borghese, M.M.; Carson, V.; Chaput, J.P.; Janssen, I.; Katzmarzyk, P.T.; Pate, R.R.; Connor Gorber, S.; Kho, M.E.; et al. Systematic review of the relationships between objectively measured physical activity and health indicators in school-aged children and youth. *Appl. Physiol. Nutr. Metab.* **2016**, *41*, S197–S239. [CrossRef]
4. Carson, V.; Hunter, S.; Kuzik, N.; Gray, C.E.; Poitras, V.J.; Chaput, J.P.; Saunders, T.J.; Katzmarzyk, P.T.; Okely, A.D.; Connor Gorber, S.; et al. Systematic review of sedentary behaviour and health indicators in school-aged children and youth: An update. *Appl. Physiol. Nutr. Metab.* **2016**, *41*, S240–S265. [CrossRef]
5. Hebebrand, J.; Bammann, K.; Hinney, A. Genetic determinants of obesity. Current issues. *Bundesgesundheitsblatt Gesundheitsforschung Gesundheitsschutz* **2010**, *53*, 674–680. [CrossRef] [PubMed]

6. Leech, R.M.; McNaughton, S.A.; Timperio, A. The clustering of diet, physical activity and sedentary behavior in children and adolescents: A review. *Int. J. Behav. Nutr. Phys. Act.* **2014**, *11*, 4. [CrossRef] [PubMed]
7. Fisberg, M.; Maximino, P.; Kain, J.; Kovalskys, I. Obesogenic environment - intervention opportunities. *J. Pediatr.* **2016**, *92*, S30–S39. [CrossRef] [PubMed]
8. Commission on Ending Childhood Obesity. *Report of the Commission on Ending Childhood Obesity*; World Health Organization: Geneva, Switzerland, 2016.
9. Schienkiewitz, A.; Brettschneider, A.K.; Damerow, S.; Schaffrath Rosario, A. Overweight and obesity among children and adolescents in Germany. Results of the cross-sectional KiGGS Wave 2 study and trends. *J. Health Monit.* **2018**, *3*.
10. Lowry, R.; Michael, S.; Demissie, Z.; Kann, L.; Galuska, D.A. Associations of Physical Activity and Sedentary Behaviors with Dietary Behaviors among US High School Students. *J. Obes.* **2015**, *2015*, 876524. [CrossRef]
11. Platat, C.; Perrin, A.E.; Oujaa, M.; Wagner, A.; Haan, M.C.; Schlienger, J.L.; Simon, C. Diet and physical activity profiles in French preadolescents. *Br. J. Nutr.* **2006**, *96*, 501–507.
12. Thivel, D.; Tremblay, M.S.; Katzmarzyk, P.T.; Fogelholm, M.; Hu, G.; Maher, C.; Maia, J.; Olds, T.; Sarmiento, O.L.; Standage, M.; et al. Associations between meeting combinations of 24-hour movement recommendations and dietary patterns of children: A 12-country study. *Prev. Med.* **2019**, *118*, 159–165. [CrossRef]
13. Krug, S.; Finger, J.D.; Lange, C.; Richter, A.; Mensink, G.B. Sports and dietary behaviour among children and adolescents in Germany. Results of the cross-sectional KiGGS Wave 2 study and trends. *J. Health Monit.* **2018**, *3*. [CrossRef]
14. Finger, J.D.; Varnaccia, G.; Borrmann, A.; Lange, C.; Mensink, G.B. Physical activity among children and adolescents in Germany. Results of the cross-sectional KiGGS Wave 2 study and trends. *J. Health Monit.* **2018**, *3*.
15. Mauz, E.; Gößwald, A.; Kamtsiuris, P.; Hoffmann, R.; Lange, M.; von Schenck, U.; Allen, J.; Butschalowsky, H.; Frank, L.; Hölling, H.; et al. Neue Daten für Taten. Die Datenerhebung zur KiGGS Welle 2 ist beendet. *J. Health Monit.* **2017**, *2*.
16. Hoffmann, R.; Lange, M.; Butschalowsky, H.; Houben, R.; Schmich, P.; Allen, J.; Kuhnert, R.; Schaffrath Rosario, A.; Gößwald, A. Querschnitterhebung von KiGGS Welle 2 – Teilnehmendengewinnung, Response und Repräsentativität. *J. Health Monit.* **2018**, *3*.
17. Haftenberger, M.; Heuer, T.; Heidemann, C.; Kube, F.; Krems, C.; Mensink, G.B. Relative validation of a food frequency questionnaire for national health and nutrition monitoring. *Nutr. J.* **2010**, *9*, 36. [CrossRef]
18. World Health Organization. *Global Recommendations on Physical Activity for Health*; World Health Organization: Geneva, Switzerland, 2010.
19. Prochaska, J.J.; Sallis, J.F.; Long, B. A physical activity screening measure for use with adolescents in primary care. *Arch. Pediatr. Adolesc. Med.* **2001**, *155*, 554–559. [CrossRef]
20. Jekauc, D.; Wagner, M.O.; Kahlert, D.; Woll, A. Reliability and validity of MoMo-Physical-Activity-Questionnaire for Adolescents (MoMo-AFB). *Diagnostica* **2013**, *59*, 100–111. [CrossRef]
21. Lampert, T.; Müters, S.; Stolzenberg, H.; Kroll, L.E. Messung des sozioökonomischen Status in der KiGGS-Studie Erste Folgebefragung (KiGGS Welle 1). *Bundesgesundheitsblatt Gesundheitsforschung Gesundheitsschutz* **2014**, *57*, 762–770. [CrossRef]
22. Lampert, T.; Hoebel, J.; Kuntz, B.; Müters, S.; Kroll, L.E. Socioeconomic status and subjective social status measurement in KiGGS Wave 2. *J. Health Monit.* **2018**, *3*.
23. Sahoo, K.; Sahoo, B.; Choudhury, A.K.; Sofi, N.Y.; Kumar, R.; Bhadoria, A.S. Childhood obesity: Causes and consequences. *J. Family Med. Prim. Care* **2015**, *4*, 187–192. [CrossRef]
24. Thivel, D.; Aucouturier, J.; Doucet, E.; Saunders, T.J.; Chaput, J.P. Daily energy balance in children and adolescents. Does energy expenditure predict subsequent energy intake? *Appetite* **2013**, *60*, 58–64. [CrossRef]
25. King, N.A.; Horner, K.; Hills, A.P.; Byrne, N.M.; Wood, R.E.; Bryant, E.; Caudwell, P.; Finlayson, G.; Gibbons, C.; Hopkins, M.; et al. Exercise, appetite and weight management: Understanding the compensatory responses in eating behaviour and how they contribute to variability in exercise-induced weight loss. *Br. J. Sports Med.* **2012**, *46*, 315–322. [CrossRef]
26. Thivel, D.; Blundell, J.E.; Duche, P.; Morio, B. Acute exercise and subsequent nutritional adaptations: What about obese youths? *Sports Med. (Auckland, N.Z.)* **2012**, *42*, 607–613. [CrossRef]

27. Thivel, D.; Chaput, J.P. Are post-exercise appetite sensations and energy intake coupled in children and adolescents? *Sports Med. (Auckland, N.Z.)* **2014**, *44*, 735–741. [CrossRef]
28. Allender, S.; Cowburn, G.; Foster, C. Understanding participation in sport and physical activity among children and adults: A review of qualitative studies. *Health Educ. Res.* **2006**, *21*, 826–835. [CrossRef]
29. Moreno, L.A.; Rodriguez, G. Dietary risk factors for development of childhood obesity. *Curr. Opin. Clin. Nutr. Metab. Care* **2007**, *10*, 336–341. [CrossRef]
30. Birkenhead, K.L.; Slater, G. A Review of Factors Influencing Athletes' Food Choices. *Sports Med. (Auckland, N.Z.)* **2015**, *45*, 1511–1522. [CrossRef]
31. Elder, S.J.; Roberts, S.B. The effects of exercise on food intake and body fatness: A summary of published studies. *Nut. Rev.* **2007**, *65*, 1–19. [CrossRef]
32. Birch, L.L.; Davison, K.K. Family environmental factors influencing the developing behavioral controls of food intake and childhood overweight. *Pediatr. Clin. North Am.* **2001**, *48*, 893–907. [CrossRef]
33. Spengler, S.; Mess, F.; Mewes, N.; Mensink, G.B.; Woll, A. A cluster-analytic approach towards multidimensional health-related behaviors in adolescents: The MoMo-Study. *BMC Public Health* **2012**, *12*, 1128. [CrossRef]
34. Sallis, J.F.; Saelens, B.E. Assessment of physical activity by self-report: Status, limitations, and future directions. *Res. Q. Exerc. Sport* **2000**, *71*, S1–S14. [CrossRef]
35. Macdiarmid, J.; Blundell, J. Assessing dietary intake: Who, what and why of under-reporting. *Nutr. Res. Rev.* **1998**, *11*, 231–253. [CrossRef]
36. Baumann, S.; Gross, S.; Voigt, L.; Ullrich, A.; Weymar, F.; Schwaneberg, T.; Dorr, M.; Meyer, C.; John, U.; Ulbricht, S. Pitfalls in accelerometer-based measurement of physical activity: The presence of reactivity in an adult population. *Scand. J. Med. Sci. Sports* **2018**, *28*, 1056–1063. [CrossRef]

6

Design, Development and Construct Validation of the Children's Dietary Inflammatory Index

Samira Khan [1,2], Michael D. Wirth [1,2,3,4], Andrew Ortaglia [3], Christian R. Alvarado [1,3], Nitin Shivappa [1,2,3], Thomas G. Hurley [1,2] and James R. Hebert [1,2,3,*]

1 Statewide Cancer Prevention and Control Program (CPCP), Arnold School of Public Health, University of South Carolina, 915 Greene Street, Columbia, SC 29208, USA; khans@mailbox.sc.edu (S.K.); wirthm@mailbox.sc.edu (M.D.W.); alvarac@email.sc.edu (C.R.A.); shivappa@mailbox.sc.edu (N.S.); thurley@mailbox.sc.edu (T.G.H.)

2 Connecting Health Innovations, LLC, Columbia, SC 29201, USA; skhan@chi-llc.net (S.K.); mwirth@chi-llc.net (M.D.W.); nshivappa@chi-llc.net (N.S.); thurley@chi-llc.net (T.G.H.)

3 Epidemiology and Biostatistics, Arnold School of Public Health, University of South Carolina, 915 Greene Street, Columbia, SC 29208, USA; ORTAGLIA@mailbox.sc.edu

4 College of Nursing, University of South Carolina, Columbia, SC 29208, USA

* Correspondence: jhebert@mailbox.sc.edu or jhebert@chi-llc.net

Abstract: Objective: To design and validate a literature-derived, population-based Children's Dietary Inflammatory Index (C-DII)^{TM}. Design: The C-DII was developed based on a review of literature through 2010. Dietary data obtained from children in 16 different countries were used to create a reference database for computing C-DII scores based on consumption of macronutrients, vitamins, minerals, and whole foods. Construct validation was performed using quantile regression to assess the association between C-reactive protein (CRP) concentrations and C-DII scores. Data Sources: All data used for construct validation were obtained from children between six and 14 years of age ($n = 3300$) who participated in the U.S. National Health and Nutrition Examination Survey (NHANES) (2005–2010). Results: The C-DII was successfully validated with blood CRP concentrations in this heterogeneous sample of 3300 children from NHANES (52% male; 29% African American, 25% Mexican American; mean age 11 years). The final model was adjusted for sex, age, race, asthma, body mass index (BMI), and infections. Children in level 3 (i.e., quartiles 3 and 4 combined) of the C-DII (i.e., children with the most pro-inflammatory diets) had a CRP value 0.097 mg/dL higher than that in level 1 (i.e., quartile 1) for CRP values at the 75th percentile of CRP using quantile regression ($p < 0.05$). Conclusion: The C-DII predicted blood CRP concentrations among children 6–14 years in the NHANES. Further construct validation with CRP and other inflammatory markers is required to deepen understanding of the relationship between the C-DII and markers of inflammation in children.

Keywords: diet; inflammation; children's-dietary inflammatory index

---

1. Introduction

Inflammation is regulated in the body through a variety of processes that involve intercellular signaling via well-characterized cytokine and chemokine messengers [1–4]. An acute inflammatory response is necessary for normal physiologic functioning, including response to infectious disease agents [5–9]. This acute inflammatory response is characterized by an increase in vascular permeability and blood flow accompanied by the accumulation of inflammatory mediators, fluid, and leukocytes. Acute inflammatory responses are time-limited and require negative feedback signaling between pro-inflammatory cytokines that turn on the response and anti-inflammatory cytokines that signal acute inflammatory responses to cease [10,11]. Because of the unique nutritional needs of children, and because it is imperative to deal with enteric and other infections, to which children are especially vulnerable, much of the initial focus of the field of immunology was on children and childhood nutrition [9,12].

In contrast to acute inflammation, chronic systematic inflammation results when negative feedback does not occur (or is either incomplete or inefficient) [10,13]. The chronic phase is characterized by a specific cellular immune response along with specific humoral responses [14,15]. In addition to its role in regulating acute inflammatory responses, diet also has been implicated in regulating chronic inflammation [16,17].

The Dietary Inflammatory Index (DII®) was developed to classify human dietary patterns on a continuous scale from anti-inflammatory to pro-inflammatory [18]. Although the original DII could predict changes in C-reactive protein (CRP) levels, a newer version of the DII was developed that reflected an update in the review of peer-reviewed articles by adding those published from 2007 to 2010 and a refined scoring algorithm [19]. Subsequently, the new DII has been construct validated in nine studies against inflammatory biomarkers in different populations and under varying conditions [20–26].

In the process of publishing the new DII, we observed that the relationship between total caloric intake and DII score is highly idiosyncratic across populations, and by body size. For example, in most populations, DII scores decrease with increasing caloric intake [27–29]. This observation led, in part, to development of the Energy Density-DII (E-DII) and then to the Children's Dietary Inflammatory Index (C-DII™). In addition, the world standard database used for the DII includes data on dietary parameters only from adults, and not all the parameters that comprise the DII (e.g., alcohol intake) are appropriate to include when evaluating children's dietary intake. With these limitations in mind, we set out to create a "world" standard database of food parameters that could be used to calculate C-DII scores among children. At the same time, it was understood that construct validation of the C-DII was necessary. Therefore, we also sought to conduct a construct validation to test the relationship between C-DII scores and levels of an inflammatory biomarker, CRP. We hypothesized that children with more pro-inflammatory diets (i.e., higher C-DII scores) will have higher values of CRP compared to children with lower C-DII scores.

This paper describes the development of the C-DII and the relationship between C-DII scores and blood concentrations of CRP in a nationally representative sample of children.

2. Methods

2.1. C-DII™ Development

To develop the C-DII, methods similar to those used to develop the current version of the DII were employed [19]. First, the "inflammatory effect scores", which were derived from an extensive literature search to develop the DII, were still applicable and therefore used for the development of the C-DII. The Dietary Inflammatory Index (DII®) was developed to classify human dietary patterns on a continuous scale from anti-inflammatory to pro-inflammatory [18]. Although the original DII could predict changes in CRP levels, a newer version of the DII was developed that reflected an update in the review of peer-reviewed articles by adding those published from 2007 to 2010 and a refined scoring algorithm [19]. Subsequently, the new DII has been construct validated in nine studies against inflammatory biomarkers in different populations and under varying conditions [20–26]. This work entailed a literature review of 1943 articles that was conducted to identify food parameters which are associated with six inflammatory biomarkers: Interleukin-1beta (IL-1β), interleukin-4 (IL-4), interleukin-6 (IL-6), interleukin-10 (IL-10), tumor necrosis factor-alpha (TNF-α), and CRP. By contrast with the constrained list of the six inflammatory biomarkers, the list of dietary parameters was open. For each article reviewed, a score was assigned for each food parameter based on its effect on inflammation. A '+1' was assigned if the effect of the parameter was pro-inflammatory, a '−1' was assigned if the effect of the parameter was anti-inflammatory; and '0' was assigned if the effect of the parameter was neutral. Each food parameter for which a finding existed was assigned a score for each article separately [19]. Published articles were weighted by study design, with highest weight assigned to experimental studies in humans and the lowest weight assigned to cell culture experiments. Based on the weights, pro- or anti-inflammatory fractions were calculated for each food parameter. Next, the overall inflammatory effect score specific to each food parameter was calculated by subtracting the anti-inflammatory fraction from pro-inflammatory fraction [19].

The food parameters used to calculate C-DII scores are: vitamin A, thiamine, riboflavin, niacin, vitamin B6, folic acid, vitamin B12, vitamin D, vitamin C, vitamin E, beta carotene, energy, carbohydrates, fiber, total fat, saturated fat, mono-unsaturated fatty acid (MUFA), poly-unsaturated fatty acid (PUFA), cholesterol, protein, alcohol, iron (Fe), magnesium (Mg), selenium (Se), and zinc (Zn).

Developing a Composite Database Representing a Diversity of Children's Diets

Dietary intakes from a wide range of diverse populations from different countries representing six continents were used to construct a composite database for the C-DII. The methodology used was virtually identical to that employed for developing the DII for adults. Data collection began in August 2016 and ended in May 2017. Using the National Library of Medicine database (Medline), we identified 35 different published papers with sample size over 200 with children's diet data collected using either a food frequency questionnaire (FFQ) or diet recalls. Overall, data were collected from 16 different countries representing diverse diets from six different continents.

Dietary data for creating a global database were collected from three different sources: (1) datasets (n = 11) received directly from the study principal investigators (from collaborations during DII development); (2) from published articles (n = 3); (3) National Health and Nutrition Examination (NHANES) Survey reports (n = 2). We sent emails to the authors of the 35 published articles with sample size >200 to obtain consent to use data. After three attempts to obtain consent to use data, we finalized a list of the articles from which we could extract dietary data for the global database. The decision was based on the availability of macro and micronutrients presented in the tables in the articles for children age 6–14 years.

The world database used for the C-DII contains dietary information from the following countries (and sources): (i) USA—the NHANES data set 2005–2011 [30]; (ii) Australia—mean values were taken from the National Nutrition Survey report of 1999 [31]; (iii) Japan—means were taken from the National Nutrition Survey Report [32]; (iv) Korea—mean values were taken from the Korean National Health and Nutrition Examination Survey (KNHANES); (v) Spain, (vi) Belgium, (vii) Greece, (viii) Germany, (ix) France, (x) Italy, (xi) Sweden, and (xii) Austria—means were taken from the Healthy Lifestyle in Europe by Nutrition in Adolescence (HELENA) study [33]; (xiii) Venezuela—means were taken from an article published by Bernal et al. [34]; (xiv); United Arab Emirates—means were taken from an article published by Ali et al. [35]; and (xvi) Chile—means were taken from an article published by Liberona et al. [36].

Missing food parameters for countries included in the database were left blank, and the overall mean and standard deviation were calculated using only data from the datasets that had information on that specific food parameter. For example, the mean and standard deviation for vitamin A were calculated using 13 countries because South Africa, Venezuela, and Chile did not have information on that food parameter. Some sources of data provided mean intake values separately for males and females or for different age groups within the range of 6–14 years; in such cases, the values were averaged. For example, the data from the United Emirates, gathered from the article by Ali et al. [35], had children separated by sex, and by age group: 6–8, 9–13, and 14–18 years. In this case, the values were averaged first between age groups for each sex, and then averaged between males and females. The list of 25 food parameters and the information regarding each country (present or missing for each food parameter) is presented in Supplementary Table S1.

Individual estimates of consumption were standardized to a global database of children's dietary intake, in a manner analogous to methods used to compute adult DII scores. As children's diet differs from the adult diet, one difference between the DII and the C-DII is that the C-DII identified only 25 food parameters, compared to the 45 used in scoring of the adult DII.

2.2. Calculation of the Children's Dietary Inflammatory Index

Calculation of the C-DII is based on the dietary intake data that are related to the regionally representative world database. These values become multipliers to express an individual child's exposure relative to the 'standard global mean' as a Z-score. This is done by subtracting the 'standard mean' from the reported amount and dividing this value by the global standard deviation. This Z-score is then converted to a proportion to avoid 'right skewing'. A symmetrical distribution was achieved with values centered on 0 (null) and bounded between −1 (maximally anti-inflammatory) and +1 (maximally pro-inflammatory), by doubling each proportion and then subtracting '1'. This centered proportion score is then multiplied by the 'overall food parameter-specific inflammatory effect score'. In the final step, 'food parameter-specific DII scores' are added to create the 'overall C-DII score' for an individual child. This approach eliminates the problem of non-comparability of units because the Z-scores and centered proportion scores are independent of the units of measurement [19]. This technique is the same as that used previously in the development of the DII [19]. Additionally, the C-DII, just like recent developments in the DII, can be calculated per 1000 calories consumed to take into account differing amounts of energy consumption between people.

2.3. Validation Study: NHANES Study Population

The NHANES survey examines a nationally representative sample of about 10,000 persons each year, and it employees a complex, multistage probability sampling design and generates weights to create a nationally representative dataset of the US population. More detailed information about the NHANES methods and protocols can be found on the Centers for Disease Control and Prevention (CDC)—National Center for Health Statistics website [37].

The proposed study population was restricted to children age 6–14 years (primary inclusion criterion) from the NHANES dataset (2005–2010) who had complete dietary data, demographics, and blood results, including CRP. There were 3445 children with CRP information and 145 were removed due to missing information. The final sample for analysis included data from 3300 children.

2.4. Dietary Assessment

NHANES 24-h dietary recall data were used to calculate C-DII scores. These data were collected through in-person interviews conducted by trained dietary interviewers fluent in English and Spanish. These staff members and the USDA's Food Survey Research Group were responsible for the dietary data collection, maintenance of the databases, and data processing. The food parameters from the NHANES data set included carbohydrates, protein, fat, fiber, fatty acids, vitamins (A, B1, B2, B6, B12, C, D, E), iron, magnesium, zinc, selenium, folic acid and beta carotene. To account for total energy intake, the C-DII was calculated per 1000 calories of food consumed.

2.5. CRP Data

The blood samples for CRP determination were processed, stored and analyzed at the University of Washington, Seattle, WA, using Behring Nephelometer for quantitative CRP determination (NHANES 2009–2010 data documentation, 2011). The blood specimens for children aged 3 years and older were collected in a mobile examination clinic by using regular or serum-separator vacutainers, and specimens were kept frozen at <-20 °C if testing was not done within 24 h of specimen collection. The serum or plasma was separated from the cells within 60 min of collection; recommended sample volume for assay is 1.0 mL. Specimens are stored in glass or plastic vials and kept tightly sealed. The lower detection limit for CRP was 0.02 ng/mL.

2.6. Study Population and Covariates

Study covariates included demographic characteristics, such as age, sex, race, body mass index (BMI kg/m^2), ethnicity, self-reported asthma, and infection at the time of data collection. Subjects with missing information on any of these variables were removed from the analysis.

2.7. Statistical Analyses

The statistical software SAS 9.4® (SAS Institute, Cary, NC, USA) and R 3.4.3® (The R Foundation, Vienna, Austria) were used for analyses. For descriptive analysis, we report continuous variables with means and standard deviation (SD) and categorical variables using frequencies and percentage across C-DII quartiles. Chi Square tests were performed for descriptive statistics of categorical covariates across C-DII quartiles, and Analysis of Variance (ANOVAs) were used for the continuous covariates (See Table 1 for a list of covariates).

Table 1. Participants' characteristics across quartiles of the children's dietary inflammatory index (C-DII) among 3300 children. NHANES, 2005–2012.

	C-DII Quartiles				
	1st	2nd	3rd	4th	
Participant Characteristics	(−3.99, −0.04)	(−0.05, 1.14)	(1.14, 2.07)	(2.08, 4.39)	*p*-value [a]
Age (years)					<0.0001
	10.0 ± 3.0	11.0 ± 3.0	11.0 ± 3.0	11.0 ± 3.0	
Sex					0.29
Male	411 (48.52)	430 (51.62)	413 (49.64)	409 (51.9)	
Female	436 (51.48)	403 (48.38)	419 (50.36)	379 (48.1)	
Race					<0.0001
Non-Hispanic Black	180 (21.25)	212 (25.45)	223 (26.8)	229 (29.06)	
Non-Hispanic White	224 (26.45)	228 (27.37)	229 (27.52)	251 (31.85)	
Mexican American	323 (38.13)	267 (32.05)	262 (31.49)	198 (25.13)	
Other	120 (14.17)	126 (15.13)	118 (14.18)	110 (13.96)	
Body mass index (tertiles) [b,c,d]					0.19
I	705 (83.43)	682 (82.17)	671 (81.04)	640 (81.42)	
II	82 (9.7)	103 (12.41)	101 (12.2)	84 (10.69)	
III	58 (6.69)	45 (5.42)	56 (6.76)	62 (7.89)	
Asthma [e]					0.01
Yes	128 (15.11)	134 (16.13)	145 (17.45)	155 (19.7)	
No	719 (84.89)	697 (83.87)	686 (82.55)	632 (80.3)	
Infection [e]					0.06
Yes	252 (27.39)	237 (25.76)	225 (24.46)	206 (22.39)	
No	571 (24.72)	579 (25.06)	595 (25.76)	565 (24.46)	

[a] *p* Value for Chi-square test; [b] BMI (kg/m^2): Category I Under or Normal weight (i.e., <25 kg/m^2); [c] BMI (kg/m^2): Category II Overweight (i.e., ≥25 kg/m^2 and <30 kg/m^2); [d] BMI (kg/m^2): Category III Obese (i.e., ≥30 kg/m^2); [e] Asthma and Infection are self-reported; Column percentages may not equal 100% due to rounding. Stratum total may not equal column totals due to missing data. For categorical covariates, frequencies (%) were presented, and chi-square tests were used to derive *p*-values. For continuous covariates, means and standard deviations were presented, and ANOVAs were used to derive *p*-values.

The C-DII scores were expressed as quartiles, and CRP weighted percentiles were used for analysis (see Table 2 for percentile details). For this analysis, we combined quartiles 3 and 4 of the C-DII because the ranges in values for these quartiles were somewhat narrow and, together, represented the most pro-inflammatory diets. Also, combining these two quartiles provided a larger sample size for the comparison of interest, therefore, providing more statistical power. For these analyses, C-DII scores were expressed as three levels, with 1 = quartile 1 (anti-inflammatory); 2 = quartile 2 (neutral); and 3 = quartiles 3 + 4 (most pro-inflammatory). For all comparative analyses, C-DII quartile 1 was used as the reference. Categorizing the C-DII initially into quartiles was done because the DII is typically analyzed using quartiles, and C-DII follows strategies and methodologies used to assess and validate the DII [22,24].

Table 2. The quantile regression coefficients for children's dietary inflammatory index treated categorically with 3 levels (level 1 is the reference level) adjusted for sex, age, race, asthma, BMI and infection, NHANES, 2005–2012 *.

	Weighted CRP Levels											
	25th Percentile			50th Percentile			75th Percentile			90th Percentile		
	Est.	SE	95% CI	Est.	SE	95% CI	Est.	SE	95% CI	Est.	SE	95% CI
C-DII Level												
2 (Quartile 2)	0.014	0.009	(−0.004, 0.032)	† 0.045	0.020	(0.005, 0.085)	† 0.113	0.055	(0.005, 0.221)	0.233	0.192	(−0.144, 0.609)
3 (Quartiles 3 + 4)	0.017	0.009	(−0.001, 0.035)	† 0.054	0.023	(0.009, 0.099)	† 0.097	0.041	(0.016, 0.177)	0.157	0.142	(−0.122, 0.436)

CRP, C-reactive protein. * Tabulated data are: The quantile regression coefficients (Est.), standard errors (SE) and 95% confidence intervals (CI). † Indicates a significant value (at $\alpha = 0.05$).

Quantile regression was used to assess the association between C-DII levels and weighted CRP, treated as the dependent variable, across adjusted CRP percentiles (25th, 50th, 75th and 90th) after controlling for sex, age, race, asthma, BMI, and infections. "R" version 3.43 was used for the quantile regression analysis, with the survey package extended to accommodate quantile regression, accounting for the NHANES complex survey design using standard errors calculated via replicate weights [38].

Quantile regression has the advantage of allowing the examination of relationships across the entire CRP distribution, allowing for a comprehensive evaluation of the association between C-DII and CRP. Quantile regression coefficients are interpreted similarly to mean regression coefficients except that a quantile regression coefficient indicates the change in the value at the modeled percentile, not the mean, of the dependent variable. For example, consider a categorical predictor such as C-DII classified by quartile, with the lowest C-DII quartile being the reference level. A coefficient estimate of 0.1 mg/L for the second quartile of C-DII in the quantile regression model for the 90th percentile would indicate that the 90th percentile of CRP is estimated to be 0.1 mg/L greater for children in the second C-DII quartile as compared to children in the first C-DII quartile after controlling for other covariates in the model (See Figure 1 for a depiction).

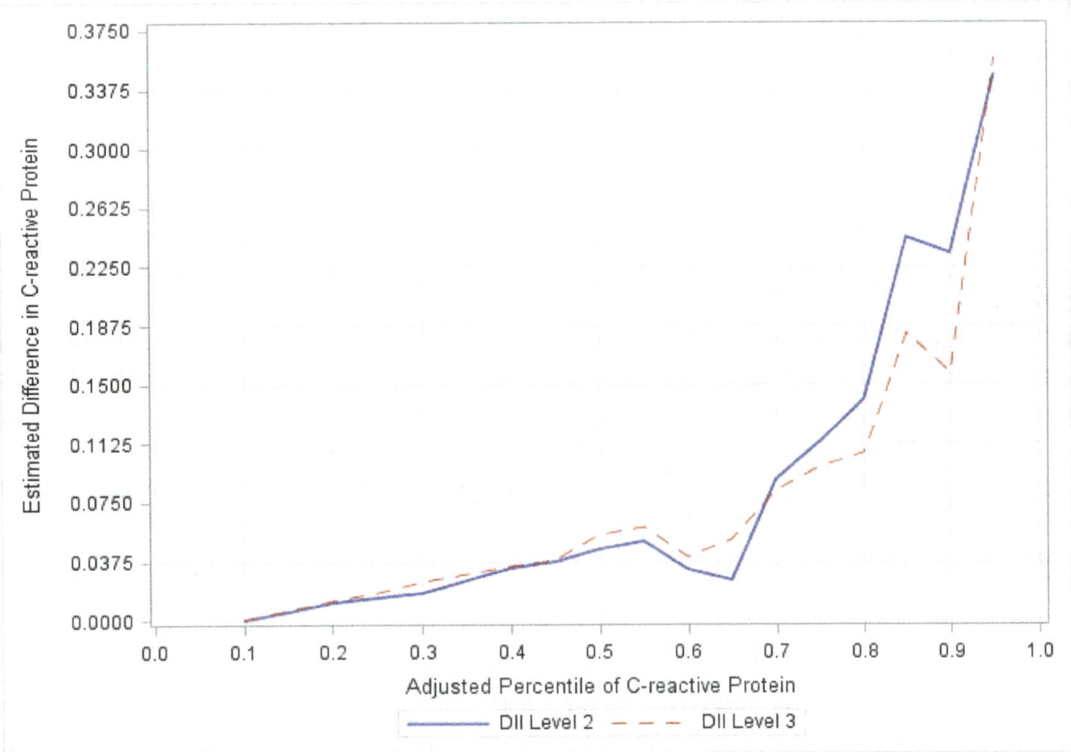

Figure 1. Plot of regression coefficients (C-DII and CRP). The magnitude of the differences in CRP increases at the upper percentiles up to the 85th percentile. CRP for children in C-DII group 2 as compared to C-DII group 1 at the 85th percentile is over 5 times the difference in CRP at the median, NHANES, 2005–2012.To reinforce the validity of our study, a logistic regression was performed using dichotomized CRP as the dependent variable (designated as high risk if CRP $\geq$ 0.50 mg/L or low risk <0.50 mg/dL) using a median cut-point. The odds of a CRP value $\geq$ 0.50 mg/L were obtained for those in C-DII level 3 compared to level 1, controlling for sex, age, race, asthma, BMI, and infections.

3. Results

Characteristics of children from the NHANES database (2005–2010 two-year cycles) whose data were used to validate C-DII scores are presented in Table 1. Weighted mean CRP value (n = 3193) was 0.84 mg/dL (standard error (SE) = 0.03). C-DII mean score was +0.99 (SE = 0.05), with values ranging from a maximally anti-inflammatory value of −3.98 to a maximally pro-inflammatory value of +4.39. Participants in quartile 1 had the least inflammatory scores (−3.98 to −0.04) and children in upper quartiles 3 and 4 had the most pro-inflammatory diet (2.07 to 4.39). The majority (≈82%) of the children in all quartiles were normal weight. More children in upper quartiles 3 and 4 reported asthma (17.4% and 19.7%, respectively) ($p < 0.01$) compared to lower quartiles (15.1% and 16.1%).

Significant differences in CRP were observed at the adjusted 50th and 75th percentiles for both groups, that is levels 2 (quartile 2) and 3 (quartiles 3 + 4 combined). Differences in CRP for children in C-DII level 2 as compared to C-DII level 1 were 0.045 and 0.113 mg/dL at the 50th and 75th percentiles, respectively. Similarly, differences in CRP for children in C-DII level 3 as compared to C-DII level 1 were 0.054 and 0.097 mg/dL at the 50th and 75th percentiles, respectively (see Table 2). The estimates for the association of C-DII on the adjusted 25th, 50th, 75th and 90th percentile CRP values are shown in Table 2.

For both C-DII levels 2 and 3, the magnitude of the estimated impact of C-DII tended to increase with increasing CRP percentiles. The magnitude of the differences in CRP between C-DII level 3 and 1 increase up to the 85th percentile. The estimated difference in CRP for children in C-DII level 2, as compared to C-DII level 3, at the 85th percentile is over 5 times the difference in CRP at the median (see Figure 1). The regression coefficients at the 90th percentile did not reach the nominal cut-point for statistical significance because the standard errors also increased, which tends to occur at the upper tail of the distribution.

Based on the logistic regression results, children in C-DII levels 2 and 3 had increased odds of having a CRP value above 0.50 mg/L. Specifically, children in C-DII level 2 (which equates to quartile 2) had 22% increased odds (95% confidence intervals (CI) = 0.94–1.59) of a CRP value above 0.50 mg/L compared to children in C-DII level 1. However, this did not achieve statistical significance. Children in C-DII level 3 (which equates to C-DII quartiles 3 and 4) had statistically significant 38% increased odds of an elevated CRP compared to children in C-DII level 1 (odds ratio (OR) = 1.38, 95% CI = 1.11–1.71, data not tabulated).

We also conducted sensitivity analyses, limiting the data set to observations for children without asthma and without an infection (as suggested by the reviewer) (Supplementary Table S2). This deletion of 1239 observations, or about 40% of the previous unweighted sample size, reduced the sample size from 3112 to 1873. There was no change in the direction of any regression coefficient. The only noteworthy difference between analyses is that the coefficient for the 90th percentile for CDII quartile 3 became statistically significant. Due to the significant reduction in the total number of observations, the appropriateness of the NHANES supplied survey weights becomes questionable.

4. Discussion

Results from this study showed that: (1) We were able to construct a global reference database for C-DII analogous to what we had done for the DII; and (2) Results from the construct validation indicated that the resulting C-DII scores were associated with CRP values among children 6 to 14 years of age in the NHANES data set. Analyses were performed to examine the association between three levels of the C-DII and the complete distribution of CRP using quantile regression. The major finding from these analyses is that CRP levels differ across the levels of the C-DII and the association of the C-DII is not constant across the CRP distribution. Specifically, we found that in level 2 of the C-DII there was significant increase in levels of CRP at the 50th, 55th, 70th, 75th, 80th, and 85th percentiles. This also is consistent with previous studies that have shown that quantile regression allows for the examination of outcomes at multiple levels, and is not influenced by outliers or skewness of the dependent variable [39]. Results in level 3 of the C-DII, representing the 3rd and 4th C-DII quartiles were more strongly in support of our hypothesis. Increased levels of the C-DII are associated with an increase in levels of CRP which is a risk factor for obesity and chronic disease.

Obesity is a pro-inflammatory state and childhood obesity is strongly associated with chronic inflammation and is on the rise [40–42]. It is known that obese children often become obese adults [43] and are more likely to suffer from insulin resistance [44], high blood pressure, unhealthy levels of serum lipids, and increased cardiovascular disease (CVD) risk [45]. This obesity epidemic is the result of specific changes in our environment and health-related behaviors [46,47]. High-calorie, inexpensive foods have become widely available and are heavily advertised [47,48]. Therefore, it is important to develop tools that can help monitor children's diet to tackle childhood obesity and its important correlate, inflammation.

Diet plays an essential role in the regulation of chronic inflammation [18,49–51]. Western diets rich in red meat, high-fat, sugar, dairy products, and refined grains have been associated with higher levels of CRP and other inflammatory markers [52,53]. Several studies have investigated individual food items such as meat or individual nutrients, such as vitamin C, and have observed associations with inflammation [54–59]. However, it is important to note that nutrients and individual foods are rarely consumed alone in a diet. Therefore, a nutrient or individual food effect may not be independent of the effect of other nutrients in the diet. Until recently, no dietary index was developed to predict inflammatory potential of whole diet; i.e., not just individual items or nutrients. Few research studies have investigated the effects of dietary indices such as the Healthy Eating Index (HEI), and Mediterranean Diet scores [60,61]. Therefore, there was a need to develop a comprehensive tool that can help children and their parents make healthier food choices that, in turn, can help reduce the risk of chronic diseases by directly influencing inflammation and preventing, or at least greatly limiting, weight gain.

The DII was developed and validated against inflammatory markers in adult populations and has been associated with a range of outcomes including cancer, metabolic syndrome, and asthma [19,62–65]. An important component of the DII calculation is the standardization of food parameter intake estimates to a "global" database of intake for the food parameters [19]. Furthermore, in developing the DII we identified eleven food consumption data sets from different parts of the world to represent a range of dietary intakes, which was used as the 'reference' database [19]. However, DII use among younger individuals (e.g., 6–14 year olds) is limited because of the "global" database used for this index. There are several barriers that prevent use of the current DII among children. The "global" standard database includes only adult dietary intakes and not all of the food parameters that comprise the DII (e.g., alcohol) may be appropriate for children dietary intake. Furthermore, we could not obtain data on garlic from any dataset we collected for the global database. Therefore, we developed C-DII, which can provide guidance for improving diets among children, and in combating obesity. Childhood obesity has been on the rise in the US, and obese children are more likely to become obese adults who experience risk factors associated with chronic disease risk [40–43,45]. Therefore, it is imperative that we create tools to monitor dietary patterns that can contribute to fluctuations in inflammation levels in the body resulting in obesity and chronic diseases [50,66]. To address this need, we developed the C-DII, which is based on the scoring algorithm of the DII.

A necessary step in the process was to identify dietary data collected in children from around the world. A total of 16 such data sets were obtained that included the US NHANES [30], the Korean NHANES [67], HELENA study (in ten European cities in Greece, Germany, Belgium, France, Hungary, Italy, Sweden, Austria, and Spain) [33], and a dataset from South Africa [68] that helped create the "world" database for C-DII.

The C-DII represents an innovative tool for evaluating the inflammatory potential of children's diet and it can be applied to any child population in which dietary information of sufficient quality has been gathered. The C-DII is not limited to data from 24-h recalls but can be used with a wide range of dietary data from various sources, including children-appropriate food frequency questionnaires (FFQ). The C-DII can be used to establish intervention strategies regarding an individual child's dietary goals to reduce inflammation and the risk of various health conditions [19].

This study has several strengths. It is the first study to develop and validate an index to explore the inflammatory potential of children's diet based on a global database. Second, it provided a unique opportunity to assess the inflammatory potential of diet in relation to CRP in a nationally representative sample. Third, it was possible to control for several confounding factors such as age, sex, race, BMI, and infection, and asthma.

Despite its strengths, there were several limitations to this study including a relative paucity of robust and reliable data on child nutrition. Regular public health surveillance of child nutrition occurs infrequently around the world, and few research studies have collected children dietary data, so to find reliable sources for these data was challenging, and not all datasets provided 100% complete dietary data. Additionally, we were limited by the availability of dietary data (i.e., a single 24-h dietary recall) in the NHANES.

5. Conclusions

Results indicate that the C-DII predicts CRP among children aged 6 to 14 years, and it appears that the C-DII is more strongly predictive of CRP among the higher levels CRP compared to lower levels of CRP. The C-DII can be used as a means for informing primary prevention and for educating physicians and other providers, parents and children on the importance of a healthy diet to reduce chronic disease rates and to enhance feelings of well-being and to improve quality of life. Further construct validation is required to deepen the understanding of the relationship between the C-DII and markers of inflammation in children. Additionally, more research should be focused on the role of diet in inflammation-related conditions in children.

Author Contributions: N.S., M.D.W. and S.K. were involved in the design of the C-DII, analyzed the data and collaborated with J.R.H. in writing the original draft of the paper. C.R.A. provided data management and critical input in revising drafts of the paper. T.G.H. was involved in the design of the C-DII, provided data management expertise, and helped in writing the paper. A.O. was involved in analyzing the data, provided high-level statistical expertise and had input in writing the paper. J.R.H. devised the initial dietary inflammatory index concept, guided the design of all phases of developing the C-DII and took the lead in writing the paper.

Acknowledgments: The authors wish to thank Seul Ki Choi, who helped with the KNHANES data, and Jumpei Kodama, who helped with the Japanese NHANES data.

References

1. Neumann, P.A.; Koch, S.; Hilgarth, R.S.; Perez-Chanona, E.; Denning, P.; Jobin, C.; Nusrat, A. Gut commensal bacteria and regional Wnt gene expression in the proximal versus distal colon. *Am. J. Pathol.* **2014**, *184*, 592–599. [CrossRef] [PubMed]
2. Shehzad, A.; Ha, T.; Subhan, F.; Lee, Y.S. New mechanisms and the anti-inflammatory role of curcumin in obesity and obesity-related metabolic diseases. *Eur. J. Nutr.* **2011**, *50*, 151–161. [CrossRef] [PubMed]
3. Maihöfner, C.; Charalambous, M.P.; Bhambra, U.; Lightfoot, T.; Geisslinger, G.; Gooderham, N.J. Expression of cyclooxygenase-2 parallels expression of interleukin-1beta, interleukin-6 and NF-kappaB in human colorectal cancer. *Carcinogenesis* **2003**, *24*, 665–671. [CrossRef] [PubMed]
4. McCullough, L.E.; Miller, E.E.; Calderwood, L.E.; Shivappa, N.; Steck, S.E.; Forman, M.R.; Mendez, M.A.; Maguire, R.; Fuemmeler, B.F.; Kollins, S.H.; et al. Maternal inflammatory diet and adverse pregnancy outcomes: Circulating cytokines and genomic imprinting as potential regulators? *Epigenetics* **2017**, *12*, 688–697. [CrossRef] [PubMed]
5. Chandra, R.K. Immunodeficiency in undernutrition and overnutrition. *Nutr. Rev.* **1981**, *39*, 225–231. [CrossRef] [PubMed]

6. Chandra, R.K.; Tejpar, S. Diet and immunocompetence. *Int. J. Immunopharmacol.* **1983**, *5*, 175–180. [CrossRef]
7. Chandra, R.K. Nutrition, immunity, and infection: Present knowledge and future directions. *Lancet* **1983**, *1*, 688–691. [PubMed]
8. Kortman, G.A.; Mulder, M.L.; Richters, T.J.; Shanmugam, N.K.; Trebicka, E.; Boekhorst, J.; Timmerman, H.M.; Roelofs, R.; Wiegerinck, E.T.; Laarakkers, C.M.; et al. Low dietary iron intake restrains the intestinal inflammatory response and pathology of enteric infection by food-borne bacterial pathogens. *Eur. J. Immunol.* **2015**, *45*, 2553–2567. [CrossRef] [PubMed]
9. Jones, K.D.; Thitiri, J.; Ngari, M.; Berkley, J.A. ; Childhood malnutrition: Toward an understanding of infections, inflammation, and antimicrobials. *Food Nutr. Bull.* **2014**, *35*, S64–S70. [CrossRef] [PubMed]
10. Elenkov, I.J.; Iezzoni, D.G.; Daly, A.; Harris, A.G.; Chrousos, G.P. Cytokine dysregulation, inflammation and well-being. *Neuroimmunomodulation* **2005**, *12*, 255–269. [CrossRef] [PubMed]
11. Kiecolt-Glaser, J.K.; Derry, H.M.; Fagundes, C.P. Inflammation: Depression fans the flames and feasts on the heat. *Am. J. Psychiatry* **2015**, *172*, 1075–1091. [CrossRef] [PubMed]
12. Hebert, J.R. Growth monitoring: The "G" in GOBI FFF. In *Child Health and Survival: The UNICEF GOBI FFF Program*; Cash, R., Keusch, G.T., Lamstein, J., Eds.; Croom Helm: London, UK, 1987; pp. 11–20.
13. Mathe, E.; Nguyen, G.H.; Funamizu, N.; He, P.; Moake, M.; Croce, C.M.; Hussain, S.P. Inflammation regulates microRNA expression in cooperation with p53 and nitric oxide. *Int. J. Cancer* **2012**, *131*, 760–765. [CrossRef] [PubMed]
14. Larsen, J.M. The immune response to *Prevotella bacteria* in chronic inflammatory disease. *Immunology* **2017**, *151*, 363–374. [CrossRef] [PubMed]
15. Kagnoff, M.F. Immunology of the intestinal tract. *Gastroenterology* **1993**, *105*, 1275–1280. [CrossRef]
16. Saita, E.; Kondo, K.; Momiyama, Y. Anti-inflammatory diet for atherosclerosis and coronary artery disease: Antioxidant foods. *Clin. Med. Insights Cardiol.* **2014**, *8*, 61–65. [CrossRef] [PubMed]
17. Ramallal, R.; Toledo, E.; Martinez, J.A.; Shivappa, N.; Hébert, J.R.; Martínez-González, M.A.; Ruiz-Canela, M. Inflammatory potential of diet, weight gain, and incidence of overweight/obesity: The SUN cohort. *Obesity* **2017**, *25*, 997–1005. [CrossRef] [PubMed]
18. Cavicchia, P.P.; Steck, S.E.; Hurley, T.G.; Hussey, J.R.; Ma, Y.; Ockene, I.S.; Hébert, J.R. A new dietary inflammatory index predicts interval changes in high-sensitivity c-reactive protein. *J. Nutr.* **2009**, *139*, 2365–2372. [CrossRef] [PubMed]
19. Shivappa, N.; Steck, S.E.; Hurley, T.G.; Hussey, J.R.; Hébert, J.R. Designing and developing a literature-derived population-based dietary inflammatory index. *Public Health Nutr.* **2014**, *17*, 1689–1696. [CrossRef] [PubMed]
20. Shivappa, N.; Steck, S.E.; Hurley, T.G.; Hussey, J.R.; Ma, Y.; Ockene, I.S.; Tabung, F.; Hébert, J.R. A population-based dietary inflammatory index predicts levels of c-reactive protein (CRP) in the SEASONS Study. *Public Health Nutr.* **2014**, *17*, 1825–1833. [CrossRef] [PubMed]
21. Shivappa, N.; Hebert, J.R.; Rietzschel, E.R.; De Buyzere, M.L.; Langlois, M.; Debruyne, E.; Marcos, A.; Huybrechts, I. Associations between dietary inflammatory index and inflammatory markers in the Asklepios Study. *Br. J. Nutr.* **2015**, *113*, 665–671. [CrossRef] [PubMed]
22. Shivappa, N.; Wirth, M.D.; Hurley, T.G.; Hébert, J.R. Association between the Dietary Inflammatory Index (DII) and telomere length and C-reactive protein from the National Health and Nutrition Examination Survey-1999-2002. *Mol. Nutr. Food Res.* **2016**, *61*, 1600630. [CrossRef] [PubMed]
23. Tabung, F.K.; Steck, S.E.; Zhang, J.; Ma, Y.; Liese, A.D.; Agalliu, I.; Hingle, M.; Hou, L.; Hurley, T.G.; Jiao, L.; et al. Construct validation of the dietary inflammatory index among postmenopausal women. *Ann. Epidemiol.* **2015**, *25*, 398–405. [CrossRef] [PubMed]
24. Wirth, M.D.; Shivappa, N.; Davis, L.; Hurley, T.G.; Ortaglia, A.; Drayton, R.; Blair, S.N.; Hébert, J.R. Construct validation of the Dietary Inflammatory Index among African Americans. *J. Nutr. Health Aging* **2017**, *21*, 487–491. [CrossRef] [PubMed]
25. Vahid, F.; Shivappa, N.; Hekmatdoost, A.; Hebert, J.R.; Davoodi, S.H.; Sadeghi, M. Association between Maternal Dietary Inflammatory Index (DII) and Abortion in Iranian Women and Validation of DII with Serum Concentration of Inflammatory Factors: Case-Control Study. *Appl. Physiol. Nutr. Metab.* **2017**, *42*, 511–516. [CrossRef] [PubMed]

26. Boden, S.; Wennberg, M.; Van Guelpen, B.; Johansson, I.; Lindahl, B.; Andersson, J.; Shivappa, N.; Hebert, J.R.; Nilsson, L.M. Dietary inflammatory index and risk of first myocardial infarction; a prospective population-based study. *Nutr. J.* **2017**, *16*, 21. [CrossRef] [PubMed]
27. Ge, I.; Rudolph, A.; Shivappa, N.; Flesch-Janys, D.; Hébert, J.R.; Chang-Claude, J. Dietary inflammation potential and postmenopausal breast cancer risk in a German case-control study. *Breast* **2015**, *24*, 491–496. [CrossRef] [PubMed]
28. Peres, L.C.; Bandera, E.V.; Qin, B.; Guertin, K.A.; Shivappa, N.; Hebert, J.R.; Abbott, S.E.; Alberg, A.J.; Barnholtz-Sloan, J.; Bondy, M.; et al. Dietary Inflammatory Index and Risk of Epithelial Ovarian Cancer in African American Women. *Int. J. Cancer* **2017**, *140*, 535–543. [CrossRef] [PubMed]
29. Harmon, B.E.; Wirth, M.D.; Boushey, C.J.; Wilkens, L.R.; Draluck, E.; Shivappa, N.; Steck, S.E.; Hofseth, L.; Haiman, C.A.; Le Marchand, L.; et al. The Dietary Inflammatory Index Is Associated with Colorectal Cancer Risk in the Multiethnic Cohort. *J. Nutr.* **2017**, *147*, 430–438. [CrossRef] [PubMed]
30. *2005–2011 National Health and Nutrition Examination Survey (NHANES)*; Centers for Disease Control and Prevention, US Department of Health and Human Services: Hyattsville, MD, USA, 2011.
31. Commonwealth Scientific Industrial Research Organisation (CSIRO). *2007 Australian National Children's Nutrition and Physical Activity Survey: Main Findings*; Australian Bureau of Statistics, Australian Government Publishing Service: Canberra, Australia, 2008.
32. Ministry of Health, Labour and Welfare, Tokyo, Japan. National Health and Nutrition Survey, Continuous through Sept 2017. Available online: http://www.mhlw.go.jp/bunya/kenkou/kenkou_eiyou_chousa.html (accessed on 26 July 2018).
33. Shivappa, N.; Hebert, J.R.; Marcos, A.; Diaz, L.E.; Gomez, S.; Nova, E.; Michels, N.; Arouca, A.; González-Gil, E.; Frederic, G.; et al. Association between dietary inflammatory index and inflammatory markers in the HELENA study. *Mol. Nutr. Food Res.* **2017**, *61*, 1600707. [CrossRef] [PubMed]
34. Bernal, J.; Lorenzana, A. Dietary diversity and associated factors among beneficiaries of 77 child care centers: Central Regional, Venezuela. *Arch. Latinoam. Nutr.* **2003**, *53*, 52–58.
35. Ali, H.; Ng, S.; Zaghloul, S.; Harrison, G.G.; Qazaq, H.S.; El Sadig, M.; Yeatts, K. ; High proportion of 6 to 18-year-old children and adolescents in the United Arab Emirates are not meeting dietary recommendations. *Nutr. Res.* **2013**, *33*, 447–456. [CrossRef] [PubMed]
36. Liberona, Y.; Castillo, O.; Engler, V.; Villarroel, L.; Rozowski, J. Nutritional profile of schoolchildren from different socio-economic levels in Santiago, Chile. *Public Health Nutr.* **2010**, *14*, 142–149. [CrossRef] [PubMed]
37. US Centers for Disease Control and Prevention (CDC), National Center for Health Statistics. National Health and Nutrition Examination Survey. Atlanta, GA, USA. Available online: https://www.cdc.gov/nchs/nhanes/index.htm (accessed on 26 July 2018).
38. Lumley, T. *Complex. Surveys: A Guide to Analysis Using R*; John Wiley & Sons: Hoboken, NJ, USA, 2010.
39. Bottai, M.; Frongillo, E.A.; Sui, X.; O'Neill, J.R.; McKeown, R.E.; Burns, T.L.; Liese, A.D.; Blair, S.N.; Pate, R.R. Use of Quantile Regression to Investigate the Longitudinal Association between Physical Activity and Body Mass Index. *Obesity* **2014**, *22*, E149–E156. [CrossRef] [PubMed]
40. Ogden, C.L.; Carroll, M.D.; Curtin, L.R.; McDowell, M.A.; Tabak, C.J.; Flegal, K.M. Prevalence of overweight and obesity in the United States, 1999–2004. *JAMA* **2006**, *295*, 1549–1555. [CrossRef] [PubMed]
41. Ogden, C.L.; Carroll, M.D.; Curtin, L.R.; Lamb, M.M.; Flegal, K.M. Prevalence of high body mass index in US children and adolescents, 2007–2008. *JAMA* **2010**, *303*, 242–249. [CrossRef] [PubMed]
42. Ogden, C.L.; Carroll, M.D.; Kit, B.K.; Flegal, K.M. Prevalence of Childhood and Adult Obesity in the United States, 2011–2012. *JAMA* **2014**, *311*, 806–814. [CrossRef] [PubMed]
43. Freedman, D.S.; Khan, L.K.; Serdula, M.K.; Dietz, W.H.; Srinivasan, S.R. The relation of childhood BMI to adult adiposity: The Bogalusa Heart Study. *Pediatrics* **2005**, *115*, 22–27. [CrossRef] [PubMed]
44. Nathan, B.M.; Moran, A. Metabolic complications of obesity in childhood and adolescence: More than just diabetes. *Curr. Opin. Endocrinol.* **2008**, *15*, 21–29. [CrossRef] [PubMed]
45. Sen, S.; Rifas-Shiman, S.L.; Shivappa, N.; Wirth, M.D.; Hebert, J.R.; Gold, D.R.; Gillman, M.W.; Oken, E. Associations of prenatal and early life dietary inflammatory potential with childhood adiposity and cardiometabolic risk in Project Viva. *Pediatr. Obes.* **2018**, *13*, 292–300. [CrossRef] [PubMed]
46. Nielsen, S.J.; Siega-Riz, A.M.; Popkin, B.M. Trends in energy intake in U.S. between 1977 and 1996: Similar shifts seen across age groups. *Obes. Res.* **2002**, *10*, 370–378. [CrossRef] [PubMed]

47. Nielsen, S.J.; Popkin, B.M. Patterns and trends in food portion sizes, 1977–1998. *JAMA* **2003**, *289*, 450–453. [CrossRef] [PubMed]
48. Nielsen, S.J.; Popkin, B.M. Changes in beverage intake between 1977 and 2001. *Am. J. Prev. Med.* **2004**, *27*, 205–210. [CrossRef] [PubMed]
49. Cui, X.; Jin, Y.; Singh, U.P.; Chumanevich, A.A.; Harmon, B.; Cavicchia, P.; Hofseth, A.B.; Kotakadi, V.; Poudyal, D.; Stroud, B.; et al. Suppression of DNA damage in human peripheral blood lymphocytes by a juice concentrate: A randomized, double-blind, placebo-controlled trial. *Mol. Nutr. Food Res.* **2012**, *56*, 666–670. [CrossRef] [PubMed]
50. Giugliano, D.; Ceriello, A.; Esposito, K. The effects of diet on inflammation: Emphasis on the metabolic syndrome. *J. Am. Coll. Cardiol.* **2006**, *48*, 677–685. [CrossRef] [PubMed]
51. Porrata-Maury, C.; Hernandez-Triana, M.; Rodriguez-Sotero, E.; Vilá-Dacosta-Calheiros, R.; Hernández-Hernández, H.; Mirabal-Sosa, M.; Campa-Huergo, C.; Pianesi, M. Medium- and short-term interventions with ma-pi 2 macrobiotic diet in type 2 diabetic adults of Bauta, Havana. *J. Nutr. Metab.* **2012**, *2012*, 856342. [CrossRef] [PubMed]
52. Hickling, S.; Hung, J.; Knuiman, M.; Divitini, M.; Beilby, J. Are the associations between diet and C-reactive protein independent of obesity? *Prev. Med.* **2008**, *47*, 71–76. [CrossRef] [PubMed]
53. Lopez-Garcia, E.; Schulze, M.B.; Manson, J.E.; Meigs, J.B.; Albert, C.M.; Rifai, N.; Willett, W.C.; Hu, F.B. Consumption of (*n*-3) fatty acids is related to plasma biomarkers of inflammation and endothelial activation in women. *J. Nutr.* **2004**, *134*, 1806–1811. [CrossRef] [PubMed]
54. Bertran, N.; Camps, J.; Fernandez-Ballart, J.; Arija, V.; Ferre, N.; Tous, M.; Simo, D.; Murphy, M.M.; Vilella, E.; Joven, J. Diet and lifestyle are associated with serum C-reactive protein concentrations in a population-based study. *J. Lab. Clin. Med.* **2005**, *145*, 41–46. [CrossRef] [PubMed]
55. Esmaillzadeh, A.; Kimiagar, M.; Mehrabi, Y.; Azadbakht, L.; Hu, F.B.; Willett, W.C. Fruit and vegetable intakes, C-reactive protein, and the metabolic syndrome. *Am. J. Clin. Nutr.* **2006**, *84*, 1489–1497. [CrossRef] [PubMed]
56. King, D.E.; Mainous, A.G., III; Geesey, M.E.; Woolson, R.F. Dietary magnesium and C-reactive protein levels. *J. Am. Coll. Nutr.* **2005**, *24*, 166–171. [CrossRef] [PubMed]
57. Ma, Y.; Griffith, J.A.; Chasan-Taber, L.; Olendzki, B.C.; Jackson, E.; Sanek, E.J., III; Li, W.; Pagoto, S.L.; Hafner, A.R.; Ockene, I.S. Association between dietary fiber and serum C-reactive protein. *Am. J. Clin. Nutr.* **2006**, *83*, 760–766. [CrossRef] [PubMed]
58. Viscogliosi, G.; Cipriani, E.; Liguori, M.L.; Marigliano, B.; Saliola, M.; Ettorre, E.; Andreozzi, P. Mediterranean dietary pattern adherence: Associations with prediabetes, metabolic syndrome, and related microinflammation. *Metab. Syndr. Relat. Disord.* **2013**, *11*, 210–216. [CrossRef] [PubMed]
59. Wannamethee, S.G.; Lowe, G.D.; Rumley, A.; Bruckdorfer, K.R.; Whincup, P.H. Associations of vitamin C status, fruit and vegetable intakes, and markers of inflammation and hemostasis. *Am. J. Clin. Nutr.* **2006**, *83*, 567–574. [CrossRef] [PubMed]
60. Boynton, A.; Neuhouser, M.L.; Wener, M.H.; Wood, B.; Sorensen, B.; Chen-Levy, Z.; Kirk, E.A.; Yasui, Y.; Lacroix, K.; McTiernan, A. Associations between healthy eating patterns and immune function or inflammation in overweight or obese postmenopausal women. *Am. J. Clin. Nutr.* **2007**, *86*, 1445–1455. [CrossRef] [PubMed]
61. Serrano-Martinez, M.; Palacios, M.; Martinez-Losa, E.; Lezaun, R.; Maravi, C.; Prado, M.; Martínez, J.A.; Martinez-Gonzalez, M.A. A Mediterranean dietary style influences TNF-alpha and VCAM-1 coronary blood levels in unstable angina patients. *Eur. J. Nutr.* **2005**, *44*, 348–354. [CrossRef] [PubMed]
62. Wirth, M.D.; Burch, J.; Shivappa, N.; Violanti, J.M.; Burchfiel, C.M.; Fekedulegn, D.; Andrew, M.E.; Hartley, T.A.; Miller, D.B.; Mnatsakanova, A.; et al. Association of a dietary inflammatory index with inflammatory indices and metabolic syndrome among police officers. *J. Occup. Environ. Med.* **2014**, *56*, 986–989. [CrossRef] [PubMed]
63. Shivappa, N.; Bosetti, C.; Zucchetto, A.; Serraino, D.; La Vecchia, C.; Hébert, J.R. Dietary inflammatory index and risk of pancreatic cancer in an Italian case-control study. *Br. J. Nutr.* **2015**, *113*, 292–298. [CrossRef] [PubMed]

64. Hebert, J.R.; Shivappa, N.; Tabung, F.K.; Steck, S.E.; Wirth, M.D.; Hurley, T.G. On the use of the dietary inflammatory index in relation to low-grade inflammation and markers of glucose metabolism in the Cohort study on Diabetes and Atherosclerosis Maastricht (CODAM) and the Hoorn study. *Am. J. Clin. Nutr.* **2014**, *99*, 1520. [CrossRef] [PubMed]
65. Wood, L.G.; Shivappa, N.; Berthon, B.S.; Gibson, P.G.; Hebert, J.R. Dietary inflammatory index is related to asthma risk, lung function and systemic inflammation in asthma. *Clin. Exp. Allergy* **2015**, *45*, 177–183. [CrossRef] [PubMed]
66. Saneei, P.; Hashemipour, M.; Kelishadi, R.; Esmaillzadeh, A. The Dietary Approaches to Stop Hypertension (DASH) diet affects inflammation in childhood metabolic syndrome: A randomized cross-over clinical trial. *Ann. Nutr. Metab.* **2014**, *64*, 20–27. [CrossRef] [PubMed]
67. Shim, Y.J.P.H. Reanalysis of 2007 Korean National Health and Nutrition Examination Survey (2007 KNHANES) Results by CAN-Pro 3.0 Nutrient Database. *Korean J. Nutr.* **2009**, *42*, 577–595. [CrossRef]
68. Oldewage-Theron, W.; Kruger, R. The association between diet quality and subclinical inflammation among children aged 6–18 years in the Eastern Cape, South Africa. *Public Health Nutr.* **2017**, *20*, 102–111. [CrossRef] [PubMed]

7

Weight Status is Related with Gender and Sleep Duration but not with Dietary Habits and Physical Activity in Primary School Italian Children

Alice Rosi [1], Maria Vittoria Calestani [1], Liborio Parrino [2], Giulia Milioli [2], Luigi Palla [3], Elio Volta [4], Furio Brighenti [1] and Francesca Scazzina [1,*]

1 Human Nutrition Unit, Department of Food and Drug, University of Parma, 43125 Parma, Italy; alice.rosi.g@gmail.com (A.R.); vittoria.calestani@hotmail.com (M.V.C.); furio.brighenti@unipr.it (F.B.)
2 Sleep Disorders Center, Department of Medicine and Surgery, University of Parma, 43126 Parma, Italy; liborio.parrino@unipr.it (L.P.); giulia.milioli@gmail.com (G.M.)
3 Department of Medical Statistics, Faculty of Epidemiology and Population Health, London School of Hygiene and Tropical Medicine, London WC1E 7HT, UK; luigi.palla@lshtm.ac.uk
4 Giocampus Steering Committee, 43124 Parma, Italy; voltaelio@giocampus.it
* Correspondence: francesca.scazzina@unipr.it

Abstract: The prevalence of overweight and obesity in children has risen greatly worldwide. Diet and poor physical activity are the two risk factors usually examined, but epidemiological evidence exists suggesting a link between sleep duration and overweight/obesity in children. The aim of this study was to describe the relationship among body mass index (BMI), diet quality, physical activity level, and sleep duration in 690 children attending the 5th grade in primary schools (9–11 years old) in the city of Parma (Italy) involved in the Giocampus educational program. This was achieved through (i) measuring anthropometric data to compute body mass index; (ii) administering a food questionnaire to evaluate adherence to the Mediterranean Diet (KIDMED score); and (iii) administering a lifestyle questionnaire to classify children physical activity level (PAL), sleep duration, and school achievement. A highly significant negative association was found between BMI and sleep hours. Moreover, there was a significant positive association between PAL and KIDMED scores. No evidence was found of association between BMI and PAL, nor between BMI and KIDMED score. Data from this study established that BMI is correlated to gender and sleep duration, defining sleep habits as one of the factors linked to overweight and obesity.

Keywords: Mediterranean diet; KIDMED; sleep; physical activity; children; school; BMI; lifestyle; Giocampus

---

1. Introduction

The incidence of overweight and obesity is increasing in all age groups worldwide. In Italy, overweight or obesity prevalence in children reach 35% in some regions, an extremely high level considering that obesity is high risk exposure for future health conditions [1,2]. In particular, overweight/obesity during childhood and adolescence is associated to a higher risk of developing chronic diseases during adulthood, such as several types of cancer, cardiovascular diseases, and metabolic syndrome [3]. The main determinants of overweight and obesity during childhood are an excessive energy intake, the lack of physical activity, and an inadequate sleep duration [4]. In the last few years, the time spent by children in outdoor activities or sports has considerably decreased, while time spent in screen activities, such as watching TV, playing videogames, or using electronic devices in their spare time has increased [5]. Even dietary habits have radically changed in recent years.

The consumption of high energy density and processed foods has risen significantly at the expense of fruit, vegetables, legumes, and whole cereals, the latter being those food groups the Mediterranean diet is based upon [6]. This fact is even more alarming as a high adherence to the Mediterranean diet has been related to a lower risk of developing chronic diseases and mortality in adults [7]. Different studies have also shown that a short sleep duration is often related to a non-balanced food intake and to unhealthy lifestyle habits, such as a reduction of physical activity [8–10]. Nevertheless, only a few studies have analyzed the relationship among dietary habits, physical activity, and sleep duration in school-aged children [11].

For all these reasons, it is paramount to create a surveillance system for monitoring the actual incidence of overweight and obesity in children and for defining the relative contribution of lifestyle habits (dietary, physical activity and sleep related). Moreover, it is important to educate children about a healthy lifestyle, explaining the importance of a balanced diet, regular physical activity, and adequate sleep duration [12]. In this framework, schools seem to be the optimal context for promoting programs aimed at improving lifestyle habits in children [13].

In the state primary schools in the city of Parma (Italy), an educational school program named "Giocampus" has been created for improving the wellbeing of future generations through healthy eating education and promotion of physical activity. An integrated "learning through playing" approach for delivering nutritional education has been successful in improving children's knowledge about healthy foods and a healthy lifestyle [14]. Professionally guided programs of physical education may also lead to significant progress in the development of conditional and coordinative abilities [15].

The aim of this study was to describe the relationship among body mass index (BMI), adherence to the Mediterranean diet (MD), physical activity level (PAL), and sleep duration in school-aged children attending the Giocampus program.

2. Materials and Methods

2.1. Participants and Study Design

The study was carried out during the 2015–2016 school years in the city of Parma (North Italy), in primary schools participating to the Giocampus program. All the students enrolled in the fifth grade (9–11 years old) were asked to participate in this observational study, through letters sent to the schools. Before acceptance, school principals, teachers, and parents were fully informed about the study protocol and the methods of assessment.

Data for each child were collected on the same day during school hours by two trained researchers through (i) measuring anthropometric data; (ii) administering a diet questionnaire aimed at defining the adherence to the MD; and (iii) administering a lifestyle questionnaire allowing classification of children PAL, sleep duration, and school achievement. The two questionnaires were administered directly to children.

The study was performed according to the Declaration of Helsinki and was approved by the Ethical Committee of the University of Parma (n5348-15/02/16).

2.2. Anthropometric Measurements

Anthropometric measurements were collected in the morning, during the physical activity class, ensuring privacy for each child, and following the WHO guidelines [16]. Body weight was measured to the nearest 100 g by using an electronic scale (MQ919, Maniquick, Niederkassel, Germany) with the child wearing only T-shirt and shorts, and was then corrected according to a simplified method validated within the Italian national surveillance system Okkio alla SALUTE [17]. Height was measured to the nearest 100 mm using a portable stadiometer (Leicester Tanita HR 001, Tanita, IL, USA). BMI was calculated as weight in kilograms divided by the square of the height in meters. Weight status was defined through the International Obesity Task Force gender- and age-related cut-offs for children BMI [18].

2.3. Dietary Habits

Adherence to the MD was assessed through the Mediterranean Diet Quality Index for children and adolescents (KIDMED) [19]. The KIDMED questionnaire comprises 16 dichotomous yes/no questions related to 12 positive and 4 negative dietary habits. Based on their correspondence with the principles of the MD, questions with a positive connotation were scored +1 point and questions with a negative connotation -1 point. A total KIDMED score ranging from 0 to 12 points was calculated for each child. The adherence to the MD was considered low, medium, or high if the KIDMED score was ≤ 3, between 4 and 7, and ≥ 8, respectively.

2.4. Physical Activity Level

According to the Italian national survey on children lifestyle [20], the PAL of children was defined by asking children about four types of activity they may be practicing during a usual week: transport-related activity, leisure time, screen-related activity, and sport. For each question, children chose one out of four possible answers, to which a score between 1 (sedentary habit) and 4 (high physical activity) was assigned. The mean score of the questions corresponded to the final activity level of the child, in keeping with the PAQ-C questionnaire [21]. Based on their final score, children were classified into one of four PAL categories as sedentary, low active, active, and very active [22,23].

2.5. Sleep Behaviors

Sleep habits were explored in terms of sleep duration and sleep pattern by asking about the wake up time in the morning and the time children went to sleep, for both weekdays and weekend days. Total sleep time was calculated in hours as the difference between bedtime and wake up time for weekdays and weekend days, and as the average weighted duration using the equation: (weekday time $\times$ 5 + weekend day time $\times$ 2)/7.

On the basis of the National Sleep Foundation recommendations for school-age children [24], sleep duration was classified as low if less than 9 h per night, recommended if between 9 and 11 h per night or high if more than 11 h per night.

In addition, sleep pattern was defined using the median value of the total week average sleep-wake schedule and classified as early bed/early rise (EE) (before 22:04 and before 07:38), early bed/late rise (EL) (before 22:04 and after 07:38), late bed/early rise (LE) (after 22:04 and before 07:38), or late bed/late rise (LL) (after 22:04 and after 07:38) [25,26].

2.6. School Achievement

School performance was assessed by asking the average grade (across subjects) of the current school year as a number, since in Italy school grades could range between 0 (very poor) and 10 (outstanding). In addition, child response was classified in three categories: mostly 10 and 9 (excellent-very good level), mostly 8 and 7 (good-very satisfactory level), and mostly 6 or less (satisfactory-poor level).

2.7. Statistical Analysis

All data were analyzed using descriptive statistics. Continuous variables were expressed as mean $\pm$ standard deviation (SD) of the total samples and by gender groups, BMI groups, or adherence to the MD groups. Categorical variables are presented as absolute frequencies and percentages of the total in the sample of respondents and by BMI groups or adherence to the MD groups.

The Kolmogorov–Smirnov test was applied to assess the normality of data distribution. The Student t-test was used to compare continuous variables between gender or BMI groups, while one-way ANOVA with Bonferroni post hoc test was used to compare among adherence to the MD groups, once the equality of variance was assessed by using the Levene's test. A Pearson chi-square test was performed to compare categorical variables between genders, BMI groups, and adherence to the MD groups.

The statistical analysis was completed through the Statistical Package for the Social Sciences (SPSS®, version 24.0, IBM, Chicago, IL, USA), with the significance set at $p < 0.05$.

3. Results

From a total of 1062 potentially eligible children, written consent to participate from parents was collected for 711 students (response rate 67%). In addition, 21 pupils did not give their verbal consent to participate or were absent during the assessment day. A total of 690 children, 357 females (52%) and 333 males (48%), with a mean age of 10.8 ± 0.4 years old, correctly completed all study requests. Children characteristics for the total sample and by gender are presented in Table 1.

Table 1. Participant characteristics (total sample and by gender).

Characteristic	Total Sample (n = 690)	Female (n = 357)	Male (n = 333)	p Value
Age (years)	10.8 ± 0.4	10.8 ± 0.3	10.8 ± 0.4	0.175
Weight (kg)	39.6 ± 8.7	39.2 ± 8.6	40.1 ± 8.8	0.152
Height (cm)	144.7 ± 6.8	145.0 ± 7.2	144.5 ± 6.5	0.357
BMI (kg/cm^2)	18.8 ± 3.2	18.5 ± 3.1	19.1 ± 3.3	0.019
KIDMED Score	6.5 ± 2.2	6.7 ± 2.1	6.4 ± 2.3	0.034
Physical Activity Level				<0.001
Low	92 (13.3)	57 (8.3)	35 (5.1)	
Medium	129 (18.7)	82 (11.9)	47 (6.8)	
High	372 (53.9)	177 (25.7)	195 (28.3)	
Very high	97 (14.1)	41 (5.9)	56 (8.1)	
Sleep Duration				
Total Sleep (hh)	9.5 ± 0.8	9.6 ± 0.7	9.4 ± 0.8	0.010
Week days (hh)	9.3 ± 0.8	9.4 ± 0.7	9.2 ± 0.8	<0.001
Weekend days (hh)	10.0 ± 1.4	10.3 ± 1.3	9.7 ± 1.5	<0.001
School Achievement	8.5 ± 1.0	8.5 ± 1.0	8.4 ± 1.0	0.467

Data are presented as mean ± SD of 690 (total sample), 357 (female) and 333 (male) independent measurements or as frequency (% of the total sample). A Pearson chi-square test was used to test the association of physical activity level with gender, while a t-test was used to compare all the other variables by gender.

No differences were found for weight and height between genders. The mean BMI corresponded to a normal weight status defined through the IOTF gender- and age-related cut-offs for both genders, despite its being higher in males (p = 0.019). In general, children had a medium adherence to the MD even by gender, with females being more adherent to the principles of the MD (p = 0.034). On the other hand, gender frequencies appear to differ by PAL ($\chi^2 = 17.1$, $df = 3$, $p < 0.001$), which was representative of a medium/high active lifestyle for both genders. According to the school-age children recommendations, children slept the recommended hours per night (9–11 h), and the sleep duration was found to be higher in females (p = 0.010 for the average total sleep and $p < 0.001$ for both weekdays and weekend days). School achievement was similar between genders, showing a good school performance of participants.

Irrespective of gender, 500 children (72.5%) had a low or normal weight, while 190 children were overweight-obese (Table 2). The two BMI groups frequencies appear to differ by gender ($\chi^2 = 8.7$, $df = 1$, $p = 0.003$), sleep duration ($\chi^2 = 9.7$, $df = 2$, $p = 0.008$), and school achievement categories ($\chi^2 = 12.0$, $df = 2$, $p = 0.002$), while they were similar for adherence to the MD, physical activity level, and sleep pattern. In addition, children in the under-normal weight group slept on average more hours per night (p = 0.005), and similar results were observed considering only weekdays or weekend days (p = 0.017 and p = 0.033, respectively).

Table 2. Dietary habits, lifestyle, school achievement, and sleeping behaviors by BMI.

Variable	Total Sample (n = 690)	Under-Normal Weight (n = 500)	Overweight—Obese (n = 190)	p Value
Gender				0.003
Female	357 (51.7)	276 (40.0)	81 (11.7)	
Male	333 (48.3)	224 (32.5)	109 (15.8)	
KIDMED Score				0.881
Low	64 (9.3)	46 (6.7)	18 (2.6)	
Medium	381 (55.2)	279 (40.4)	102 (14.8)	
High	245 (35.5)	175 (25.4)	70 (10.1)	
Physical Activity Level				0.729
Low	92 (13.3)	66 (9.6)	26 (3.8)	
Medium	129 (18.7)	96 (13.9)	33 (4.8)	
High	372 (53.9)	272 (39.4)	100 (14.5)	
Very high	97 (14.1)	66 (9.6)	31 (4.5)	
Sleep Duration				0.008
Low	149 (21.6)	94 (13.6)	55 (8.0)	
Recommended	525 (76.1)	392 (56.8)	133 (19.3)	
High	16 (2.3)	14 (2.0)	2 (0.3)	
Sleep Pattern				0.518
EE	211 (30.6)	149 (21.6)	62 (9.0)	
EL	123 (17.8)	93 (13.5)	30 (4.3)	
LE	125 (18.1)	86 (12.5)	39 (5.7)	
LL	231 (33.5)	172 (24.9)	59 (8.6)	
Sleep Time Quantity				
Mean sleep (hh)	9.5 ± 0.8	9.6 ± 0.8	9.4 ± 0.8	0.005
Week days (hh)	9.3 ± 0.8	9.4 ± 0.8	9.2 ± 0.8	0.017
Weekend days (hh)	10.0 ± 1.4	10.1 ± 1.4	9.8 ± 1.4	0.033
School Achievement				0.002
Mostly 10 and 9	360 (52.2)	279 (40.4)	81 (11.7)	
Mostly 8 and 7	314 (45.5)	213 (30.9)	101 (14.6)	
Mostly 6 or less	16 (2.3)	8 (1.2)	8 (1.2)	

Data are presented as frequency (% of the total sample) or as mean ± SD out of 690 (total sample), 500 (under weight and normal weight children), and 190 (overweight and obese children) independent measurements. A Pearson chi-square test was used to test the association of all categorical variables with BMI groups, while a *t*-Test was used to compare Sleep Time Quantity between BMI groups.

In relation to dietary habits, as shown in Table 3, only 9% of children showed a low adherence to the MD, while 55% showed a medium adherence, and 36% a high adherence. Associations were observed between adherence to MD and gender ($\chi^2 = 8.5$, $df = 2$, $p = 0.015$), MD and physical activity level ($\chi^2 = 23.3$, $df = 6$, $p = 0.001$), MD and school achievement categories ($\chi^2 = 10.9$, $df = 4$, $p = 0.028$). Children with a low adherence to the MD had also a lower mean sleep duration ($p = 0.010$) and a lower sleep time during weekdays ($p = 0.002$).

Consistently with their adherence to the MD, children showed positive eating habits, with only small variations registered by gender. The KIDMED questionnaire responses to each single question for the total sample and by gender are presented in Figure 1.

Fruit and fruit juices were consumed daily by 83% of children, 48% had a second portion every day, and 35% ate nuts regularly. In addition, 73% of children had fresh or cooked vegetables regularly once a day, and 44% ate more than one portion of vegetables each day. In relation to protein-based food, 47% of participants ate fish regularly and 53% had pulses more than once a week. Pasta or rice was consumed almost every day by 84% of children. Almost 90% of children had breakfast regularly, 62% consumed cereals or grains for breakfast, 74% milk or dairy products, and 60% commercially baked goods or pastries. In addition, 36% ate two yoghurts and/or some cheese daily, and 88% used olive oil as a condiment when eating at home. Considering unhealthy habits, only 7% of students went more than once per week to a fast food restaurant, and 26% had sweets and/or candy several times every day.

Table 3. Dietary habits, lifestyle, school achievement, and sleeping behaviors by adherence to the Mediterranean diet (MD).

Variable	Total Sample (n = 690)	Low Adherence (n = 64)	Medium Adherence (n = 381)	High Adherence (n = 245)	p Value
Gender					0.015
Female	357 (51.7)	25 (3.6)	190 (27.5)	142 (20.6)	
Male	333 (48.3)	39 (5.7)	191 (27.7)	103 (14.9)	
BMI category					0.087
Underweight	51 (7.4)	4 (0.6)	27 (3.9)	20 (2.9)	
Normal weight	449 (65.1)	42 (6.1)	252 (36.5)	155 (22.5)	
Overweight	157 (22.8)	15 (2.2)	92 (13.3)	50 (7.2)	
Obese	33 (4.8)	3 (0.4)	10 (1.4)	20 (2.9)	
Physical Activity Level					0.001
Low	92 (13.3)	12 (1.7)	54 (7.8)	26 (3.8)	
Medium	129 (18.7)	17 (2.5)	81 (11.7)	31 (4.5)	
High	372 (53.9)	29 (4.2)	205 (29.7)	138 (20.0)	
Very high	97 (14.1)	6 (0.9)	41 (5.9)	50 (7.2)	
Sleep Duration					0.315
Low	149 (21.6)	19 (2.8)	81 (11.7)	49 (7.1)	
Recommended	525 (76.1)	45 (6.5)	289 (41.9)	191 (27.7)	
High	16 (2.3)	0 (0.0)	11 (1.6)	5 (0.7)	
Sleep Pattern					0.101
EE	211 (30.6)	17 (2.5)	111 (16.1)	83 (12.0)	
EL	123 (17.8)	6 (0.9)	65 (9.4)	52 (7.5)	
LE	125 (18.1)	15 (2.2)	69 (10.0)	41 (5.9)	
LL	231 (33.5)	26 (3.8)	136 (19.7)	69 (10.0)	
Sleep Time Quantity					
Mean sleep (hh)	9.5 ± 0.8	9.2 ± 0.8^{a}	9.5 ± 0.8^{b}	9.6 ± 0.8^{b}	0.010
Week days (hh)	9.3 ± 0.8	9.0 ± 0.7^{a}	9.3 ± 0.8^{b}	9.4 ± 0.7^{b}	0.002
Weekend days (hh)	10.0 ± 1.4	9.7 ± 1.9	10.0 ± 1.4	10.1 ± 1.3	0.182
School Achievement					0.028
Mostly 10 and 9	360 (52.2)	22 (3.2)	205 (29.7)	133 (19.3)	
Mostly 8 and 7	314 (45.5)	39 (5.7)	170 (24.6)	105 (15.2)	
Mostly 6 or less	16 (2.3)	3 (0.4)	6 (0.9)	7 (1.0)	

Data are presented as frequency (% of the total sample) or as mean ± SD out of 690 (total sample), 64 (children with a low adherence to the Mediterranean Diet (MD)), 381 (children with a medium adherence to the Mediterranean Diet), and 245 (children with a high adherence to the Mediterranean Diet) independent measurements. A Pearson chi-square test was used to test the association of all categorical variables with adherence to Mediterranean Diet, while an ANOVA with a Bonferroni post hoc test was used to compare Sleep Time Quantity among adherence to MD groups ("a,b": different letters in the same raw indicate significant differences among adherence groups).

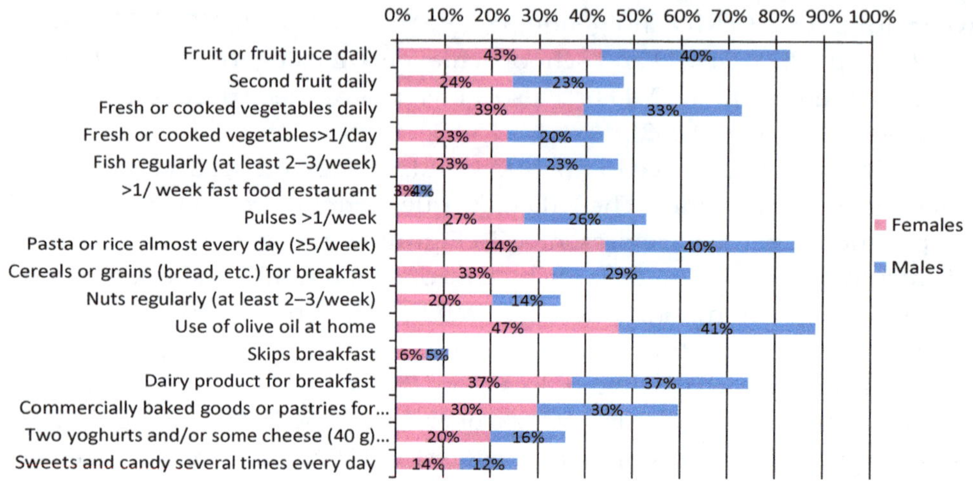

Figure 1. Responses to the KIDMED questionnaire of all children and by gender (percentage in respect to the total sample).

4. Discussion

This study describes the relationship among body mass index, diet quality, physical activity level, and sleep duration in a sample of healthy children (aged 9–11 years) attending an educational school program in Parma, Italy.

The amount of children classified as overweight or obese was 28%, a slightly lower percentage than the value (29%) observed in the region, where the city of Parma is located (Emilia-Romagna) [20]. In turn, the regional prevalence of overweight and obesity is lower when compared to the national situation (31%) [20]. The present study involved about 700 children and the prevalence of overweight and obesity is confirmed to be lower that observed in the data from another study, with a very similar sample size, conducted in Italy [27]. Our results showed a significantly higher overweight and obesity prevalence in boys than in girls, which is consistent with recent investigations [1].

In our study, children showed a medium adherence to the MD, with females significantly more faithful to the principles of the MD, showing a higher attention towards healthy behaviors. However, among 33 studies analyzing gender differences in MD adherence, only 7 studies were able to significantly spot it, and 6 out of 7 reported a higher adherence in girls [28]. In the studied population, the mean MD score (6.5) was higher than that observed in the most recent studies carried out in Italy [28]. Ferranti and colleagues [25] found a mean MD adherence of 4.3 in a population of more than 1500 adolescents. In another study, conducted on a Sicilian adolescent population, the mean MD score was 5.8 in rural areas and 4.8 in urban areas [29].

The detailed analysis obtained from each single question of the KIDMED questionnaire showed positive dietary behaviors for breakfast, fruit, vegetable, and olive oil consumption. However, some other aspects can still be improved through specific educational interventions, targeted for example to promoting fish, pulse, and nuts consumption, the intake of which is lower than the national recommendations, consistently with results from other Italian surveys [20,27]. No evidence was found of an association between BMI and MD score, in partial agreement with other studies. Actually, only 10 out of 26 papers published on the topic reported an inverse association of MD adherence with BMI values [28].

A significant association was observed between MD scores and PAL. This result is aligned with the findings of 14 out of 17 studies found in the literature and investigating the association of MD adherence with lifestyle aspects in children and adolescents [28]. Our study population showed a medium-high active lifestyle with only 13% classified as low PAL. This last result is slightly better than the national data [20], reporting 16% of "non-active" children. This may be partially due to the Giocampus experience, during which children received, each school year, a 2-h/week professionally guided program of physical activity that was found to improve their motor abilities [15], and may increase children's sensibility towards active lifestyles. In agreement with national data [20], a significantly more active lifestyle was observed for males.

No evidence was found of any association between BMI and PAL. In contrast, a highly significant negative association was found between BMI and sleep hours, although more than 76% of children declared sleeping the recommended amount of hours per night. Moreover, children with a lower sleep duration were also characterized by a low adherence to the MD, while children with a medium or high adherence to the MD slept for a similar number of hours, considering both mean and weekdays sleep quantity. These finding are aligned with results from the study by Ferranti and colleagues [25], where shorter sleep durations and poor sleep were associated with higher BMI and with unhealthy eating behaviors in adolescents. The results of this study are in agreement with the national survey "Okkio alla salute" [20], where the prevalence of overweight and obesity is significantly higher in children who sleep less hours per night. Moreover, results from the Quebec Longitudinal Study in preadolescents showed that, for each hour less of sleep per night at 10 years of age, a child was 1.5 times more likely of being overweight or 2.1 times of being obese at 13 years of age [30]. Adolescents with a longer wakefulness had a higher intake of high density snacks [31]. Moreover, results from a longitudinal study in the United States highlight bedtime as a potential target for weight management during adolescence and during the transition to adulthood [32]. In general, the importance of sleep patterns in the lifestyle of children is accepted worldwide, despite obvious cultural differences among countries [31].

In our study, we did not find any association between sleep patterns and overweight/obesity in agreement with Ferranti and colleagues [25]. However, He and colleagues [32] found that a high habitual variability in sleep patterns, but not the habitual sleep duration, was related to increased energy and food intake in adolescents, suggesting that the maintenance of a regular sleep pattern may decrease the risk of obesity.

Finally, both high adherence to the MD and normal body weight status seem to be correlated to high school achievement, suggesting a link between healthy lifestyle and academic performance. Recently, Tonetti and colleagues [33] found that a higher BMI was associated with a poorer school performance in Italian high school students when controlling for sleep quality, sleep duration, and socioeconomic status.

The main limitations of this study are linked to the biases inherent in the use of self-reported data, such as dietary habits and physical activity level. Besides, non-response bias shall also be considered a limitation due to the fact that the sample of respondents might not be representative of the entire potential population, and the lack of information on the non-response children (33%) could not allow bias corrections. Another limitation is that children lifestyle behaviors are affected by parental habits, which were not investigated in the present study.

5. Conclusions

In conclusion, this study investigated lifestyle behaviors of a sample of primary school Italian children who were enrolled in the fifth and last year of the Giocampus school program, in Parma, Italy. The prevalence of overweight and obesity was lower in this group when compared to both the regional and national situations. In addition, the adherence to the MD and the PAL were higher than the ones reported in nationwide surveys, suggesting that the Giocampus school programme may represent a relevant contribution to the attainment of healthy lifestyles in children. Additionally, the high/very high mean amount of sleep hours highlighted a healthy lifeslyle pattern and, interestingly, was negatively and significantly associated with body weight.

Based on these observations, the prevention of child obesity requires a multidisciplinary approach that considers not only physical activity and a healthy diet but also great care in defining sleeping habits. Promoting virtuous sleep behaviors may represent an important and relatively low-cost strategy for reducing the incidence of childhood obesity.

Further studies are recommended to better understand the role of sleep duration and sleep related behaviors in child energy balance.

Acknowledgments: We gratefully acknowledge all actors of the GIOCAMPUS Project, including children, teachers and families involved in it. Moreover, we gratefully thank Cinzia Franchini, and Rossella Santoro for their support in data acquisition.

Author Contributions: AR helped in designing research, performed the study, analyzed data, and wrote the manuscript. MVC helped in performed the study and contributed to write the manuscript. LP designed research, helped in data interpretation, and contributed to manuscript revision. GM helped in designing research and in data interpretation. LP analyzed data, helped in data interpretation, and contributed to manuscript revision. EV helped in data acquisition and data interpretation. FB helped in designing research and in data interpretation. FS designed research, contributed to data interpretation, contributed to writing the manuscript, and had primary responsibility for the final version of the manuscript.

References

1. Binkin, N.; Fontana, G.; Lamberti, A.; Cattaneo, C.; Baglio, G.; Perra, A.; Spinelli, A. A national survey of the prevalence of childhood overweight and obesity in Italy. *Obes. Rev.* **2010**, *11*, 2–10. [CrossRef] [PubMed]

2. Nardone, P.; Buoncristiano, M.; Lauria, L. OKkio alla SALUTE: Sintesi dei Risultati 2016. Italian Ministry of Health, 2017. Available online: http://www.salute.gov.it/imgs/C_17_notizie_2935_listaFile_itemName_24_file.pdf (accessed on 17 April 2017).
3. Di Renzo, L.; Tyndall, E.; Gualtieri, P.; Carboni, C.; Valente, R.; Ciani, A.S.; Tonini, M.G.; De Lorenzo, A. Association of body composition and eating behavior in the normal weight obese syndrome. *Eat. Weight Disord.* **2016**, *21*, 99–106. [CrossRef] [PubMed]
4. Golley, R.K.; Maher, C.A.; Matricciani, L.; Olds, T.S. Sleep duration or bedtime[quest] Exploring the association between sleep timing behavior, diet and BMI in children and adolescents. *Int. J. Obes.* **2013**, *37*, 546–551. [CrossRef] [PubMed]
5. Granich, J.; Rosenberg, M.; Knuiman, M.; Timperio, A. Understanding children's sedentary behavior: A qualitative study of the family home environment. *Health Educ. Res.* **2010**, *25*, 199–210. [CrossRef] [PubMed]
6. Serra-Majem, L.; Trichopoulou, A.; de la Cruz, J.N.; Cervera, P.; Álvarez, A.G.; La Vecchia, C.; Lemtouni, A.; Trichopoulos, D. Does the definition of the Mediterranean diet need to be updated? *Public Health Nutr.* **2004**, *7*, 927–929. [CrossRef] [PubMed]
7. Sofi, F.; Macchi, C.; Abbate, R.; Gensini, G.F.; Casini, A. Mediterranean diet and health status: An updated meta-analysis and a proposal for a literature-based adherence score. *Public Health Nutr.* **2014**, *17*, 2769–2782. [CrossRef] [PubMed]
8. St-Onge, M.-P.; Shechter, A. Sleep Restriction in Adolescents: Forging the Path Towards Obesity and Diabetes? *Sleep* **2013**, *36*, 813–814. [CrossRef] [PubMed]
9. St-Onge, M.P. The role of sleep duration in the regulation of energy balance: Effects on energy intakes and expenditure. *J. Clin. Sleep Med.* **2013**, *9*, 73–80. [CrossRef] [PubMed]
10. Westerlund, L.; Ray, C.; Roos, E. Associations between sleeping habits and food consumption patterns among 10–11-year-old children in Finland. *Br. J. Nutr.* **2009**, *102*, 1531–1537. [CrossRef] [PubMed]
11. Miller, A.L.; Lumeng, J.C.; LeBourgeois, M.K. Sleep patterns and obesity in childhood. *Curr. Opin. Endocrinol. Diabetes Obes.* **2015**, *22*, 41–47. [CrossRef] [PubMed]
12. WHO Regional Office for Europe. *WHO European Action Plan for Food and Nutrition Policy, 2007–2012*; WHO Regional Office for Europe: Copenhagen, Danmark, 2008.
13. Tremblay, A.; Lachance, É. Tackling obesity at the community level by integrating healthy diet, movement and non-movement behaviors. *Obes. Rev.* **2017**, *18*, 82–87. [CrossRef] [PubMed]
14. Rosi, A.; Brighenti, F.; Finistrella, V.; Ingrosso, L.; Monti, G.; Vanelli, M.; Vitale, M.; Volta, E.; Scazzina, F. Giocampus school: A "learning through playing" approach to deliver nutritional education to children. *Int. J. Food Sci. Nutr.* **2016**, *67*, 207–215. [CrossRef] [PubMed]
15. Chiodera, P.; Volta, E.; Gobbi, G.; Milioli, M.A.; Mirandola, P.; Bonetti, A.; Delsignore, R.; Bernasconi, S.; Anedda, A.; Vitale, M. Specifically designed physical exercise programs improve children's motor abilities. *Scand. J. Med. Sci. Sports* **2008**, *18*, 179–187. [CrossRef] [PubMed]
16. WHO. *Physical Status: The Use and Interpretation of Anthropometry*; WHO, Technical Report Series N 854; WHO: Geneva, Switzerland, 1995.
17. Censi, L.; Spinelli, A.; Roccaldo, R.; Bevilacqua, N.; Lamberti, A.; Angelini, V.; Nardone, P.; Baglio, G. Dressed or undressed? How to measure children's body weight in overweight surveillance? *Public Health Nutr.* **2013**, *17*, 2715–2720. [CrossRef] [PubMed]
18. Cole, T.J.; Lobstein, T. Extended international (IOTF) body mass index cut-offs for thinness, overweight and obesity. *Pediatr. Obes.* **2012**, *7*, 284–294. [CrossRef] [PubMed]
19. Serra-Majem, L.; Ribas, L.; Ngo, J.; Ortega, R.M.; Garcia, A.; Perez-Rodrigo, C.; Aranceta, J. Food, youth and the Mediterranean diet in Spain. Development of KIDMED, Mediterranean Diet Quality Index in children and adolescents. *Public Health Nutr.* **2004**, *7*, 931–935. [CrossRef] [PubMed]
20. Nardone, P.; Spinelli, A.; Buoncristiano, M.; Lauria, L.; Pizzi, E.; Andreozzi, S.; Galeone, D. *Il Sistema di Sorveglianza OKkio alla SALUTE: Risultati 2014. [Surveillance System OKkio alla SALUTE: 2014 Results.]*; Istituto Superiore di Sanità: Firenze, Italy, 2016; p. 63.
21. Kowalski, K.C.; Crocker, P.R.E.; Donen, R.M. The Physical Activity Questionnaire for Older Children (PAQ-C) and Adolescents (PAQ-A) Manual. Available online: http://www.dapa-toolkit.mrc.ac.uk/documents/en/PAQ/PAQ_manual.pdf (accessed on 17 April 2017).

22. SINU. *Livelli di Assunzione di Riferimento di Nutrienti ed Energia per la Popolazione Italiana—IV Revisione*; Società Italiana di Nutritione Umana: Firenze, Italy, 2014.
23. Institute of Medicine. *Dietary Reference Intakes for Energy, Carbohydrate, Fiber, Fat, Fatty Acids, Cholesterol, Protein, and Amino Acids (Macronutrients)*; The National Academies Press: Washington, DC, USA, 2005; pp. 1–1331.
24. Hirshkowitz, M.; Whiton, K.; Albert, S.M.; Alessi, C.; Bruni, O.; DonCarlos, L.; Hazen, N.; Herman, J.; Adams Hillard, P.J.; Katz, E.S.; et al. National Sleep Foundation's updated sleep duration recommendations: Final report. *Sleep Health* **2015**, *1*, 233–243. [CrossRef]
25. Ferranti, R.; Marventano, S.; Castellano, S.; Giogianni, G.; Nolfo, F.; Rametta, S.; Matalone, M.; Mistretta, A. Sleep quality and duration is related with diet and obesity in young adolescent living in Sicily, Southern Italy. *Sleep Sci.* **2016**, *9*, 117–122. [CrossRef] [PubMed]
26. Touchette, É.; Mongrain, V.; Petit, D.; Tremblay, R.E.; Montplaisir, J.Y. Development of sleep-wake schedules during childhood and relationship with sleep duration. *Arch. Pediatr. Adolesc. Med.* **2008**, *162*, 343–349. [CrossRef] [PubMed]
27. Roccaldo, R.; Censi, L.; D'Addezio, L.; Toti, E.; Martone, D.; D'Addesa, D.; Cernigliaro, A. Adherence to the Mediterranean diet in Italian school children (The ZOOM8 Study). *Int. J. Food Sci. Nutr.* **2014**, *65*, 621–628. [CrossRef] [PubMed]
28. Iaccarino Idelson, P.; Scalfi, L.; Valerio, G. Adherence to the Mediterranean Diet in children and adolescents: A systematic review. *Nutr. Metab. Cardiovasc. Dis.* **2017**, *27*, 283–299. [CrossRef] [PubMed]
29. Grosso, G.; Marventano, S.; Buscemi, S.; Scuderi, A.; Matalone, M.; Platania, A.; Giorgianni, G.; Rametta, S.; Nolfo, F.; Galvano, F.; et al. Factors associated with adherence to the Mediterranean diet among adolescents living in Sicily, southern Italy. *Nutrients* **2013**, *5*, 4908–4923. [CrossRef] [PubMed]
30. Seegers, V.; Petit, D.; Falissard, B.; Vitaro, F.; Tremblay, R.E.; Montplaisir, J.; Touchette, E. Short Sleep Duration and Body Mass Index: A Prospective Longitudinal Study in Preadolescence. *Am. J. Epidemiol.* **2011**, *173*, 621–629. [CrossRef] [PubMed]
31. Chaput, J.P.; Katzmarzyk, P.T.; LeBlanc, A.G.; Tremblay, M.S.; Barreira, T.V.; Broyles, S.T.; Fogelholm, M.; Hu, G.; Kuriyan, R.; Kurpad, A.; et al. Associations between sleep patterns and lifestyle behaviors in children: An international comparison. *Int. J. Obes. Suppl.* **2015**, *5* (Suppl. 2), S59–S65. [CrossRef] [PubMed]
32. He, F.; Bixler, E.O.; Berg, A.; Imamura Kawasawa, Y.; Vgontzas, A.N.; Fernandez-Mendoza, J.; Yanosky, J.; Liao, D. Habitual sleep variability, not sleep duration, is associated with caloric intake in adolescents. *Sleep Med.* **2015**, *16*, 856–861. [CrossRef] [PubMed]
33. Tonetti, L.; Fabbri, M.; Filardi, M.; Martoni, M.; Natale, V. The association between higher body mass index and poor school performance in high school students. *Pediatr. Obes.* **2016**, *11*, e27–e29. [CrossRef] [PubMed]

8

The Association of Breakfast Frequency and Cardiovascular Disease (CVD) Risk Factors among Adolescents in Malaysia

Norashikin Mustafa [1], Hazreen Abd Majid [2,3], Zoi Toumpakari [1], Harriet Amy Carroll [1], Muhammad Yazid Jalaludin [4], Nabilla Al Sadat [2] and Laura Johnson [1,*]

1 Centre for Exercise Nutrition and Health Sciences, School for Policy Studies, University of Bristol, Bristol BS8 1TZ, UK; norashikinmus@gmail.com (N.M.); z.toumpakari@bristol.ac.uk (Z.T.); hc12591@my.bristol.ac.uk (H.A.C.)

2 Centre for Population Health (CePH) and Department of Social & Preventive Medicine, Faculty of Medicine, University of Malaya, 50603 Kuala Lumpur, Malaysia; hazreen@ummc.edu.my (H.A.M.); drnabilla@gmail.com (N.A.S.)

3 Faculty of Public Health, Universitas Airlangga, Surabaya 60115, Indonesia

4 Department of Paediatrics, Faculty of Medicine, University of Malaya, 50603 Kuala Lumpur, Malaysia; yazidj@ummc.edu.my

* Correspondence: Laura.Johnson@bristol.ac.uk

Abstract: Breakfast frequency is associated with cardiovascular disease (CVD) risk in Western populations, possibly via the types of food eaten or the timing of food consumption, but associations in Malaysian adolescents are unknown. While the timing of breakfast is similar, the type of food consumed at breakfast in Malaysia differs from Western diets, which allows novel insight into the mechanisms underlying breakfast–CVD risk associations. We investigated foods eaten for breakfast and associations between breakfast frequency and CVD risk factors in the Malaysian Health and Adolescents Longitudinal Research Team study (MyHeARTs). Breakfast (frequency of any food/drink reported as breakfast in 7-day diet history interviews) and CVD risk factors (body mass index (BMI), waist circumference, fasting blood glucose, triacylglycerol, total cholesterol, high-density lipoprotein (HDL), low-density lipoprotein (LDL), and systolic and diastolic blood pressure) were cross-sectionally associated using linear regression adjusting for potential confounders (n = 795, age 13 years). Twelve percent of adolescents never ate breakfast and 50% ate breakfast daily, containing mean (SD) 400 (±127) kilocalories. Commonly consumed breakfast foods were cereal-based dishes (primarily rice), confectionery (primarily sugar), hot/powdered drinks (primarily Milo), and high-fat milk (primarily sweetened condensed milk). After adjustment, each extra day of breakfast consumption per week was associated with a lower BMI (−0.34 kg/m^2, 95% confidence interval (CI) −0.02, −0.66), and serum total (−0.07 mmol/L 95% CI −0.02, −0.13) and LDL (−0.07 mmol/L 95% CI −0.02, −0.12) cholesterol concentrations. Eating daily breakfast in Malaysia was associated with slightly lower BMI and total and LDL cholesterol concentrations among adolescents. Longitudinal studies and randomized trials could further establish causality.

Keywords: breakfast; obesity; cardiovascular; health; BMI; waist circumference; cholesterol; blood pressure; MyHeARTs

---

1. Introduction

Cardiovascular disease (CVD) is the number one cause of death globally [1]. In Malaysia, CVD is the biggest cause of mortality, accounting for 36% of total deaths [2]. Although the incidence of CVD (e.g., myocardial infarction and stroke) does not emerge until adulthood, CVD risk factors often present during adolescence [3]. For example, Malaysian children and adolescents have the highest prevalence of overweight and obesity across the South and Southeast Asian countries, at 22.5% (95% confidence interval (CI) 19.1–26.1) in boys and 19.1% (95% CI 16.1–22.6) in girls [4].

Over 50 cross-sectional studies, primarily in Europe and the United States, have reported consistent inverse associations between breakfast skipping and increased risk of overweight and obesity (odds ratio (OR) 1.55, 95% CI 1.46, 1.65) [5]. Outside of Europe and the United States, a meta-analysis of 19 cross-sectional studies in Asian populations also reported an increased risk of overweight and obesity (OR 1.76, 95% CI 1.48, 2.08) for breakfast skippers versus consumers [6], suggesting that the association is not limited to Western populations. Several causal mechanisms have been hypothesized to explain why eating breakfast may protect against CVD risk (Figure 1). In pathway 1, eating breakfast is hypothesized to reduce subsequent snacking, resulting in lower overall daily energy intake, thus maintaining energy balance and a lower body weight. Although in observational studies, breakfast is typically associated with higher total daily energy intakes [7]. In pathway 2, breakfast is associated with better food choices. For example, the kinds of foods typically eaten at breakfast in the United States and Europe tend to have cardio-protective properties e.g., wholegrain cereals that are high in fiber and micronutrients [8]. However, as foods typically eaten for breakfast vary widely across cultures, consistent associations of breakfast frequency across diverse countries could point to the timing of eating as more important than the type of food eaten. In pathway 3, it is hypothesized that eating in the morning is specifically better suited to circadian rhythms in metabolism, such that food ingested earlier in the day is metabolized more efficiently. The hypothesized circadian pathway is supported by acute randomized crossover experiments in adults, whereby the timing of food intake (but not the type of food consumed) is manipulated such that delaying breakfast is related to poorer appetite control, lower resting energy expenditure, impaired fasting lipid profiles, and reduced postprandial insulin sensitivity [9–12]. However more recent longer-term free-living trials that manipulated the timing of the first meal or randomized participants to receive simple advice to "eat breakfast" or not, have cast doubt on whether observational associations are causal but instead confounded i.e., eating breakfast may simply be an indicator of a generally healthy lifestyle [13–15]. Further research exploring breakfast frequency and the types of food eaten for breakfast in non-western populations is required to further understand existing observed associations.

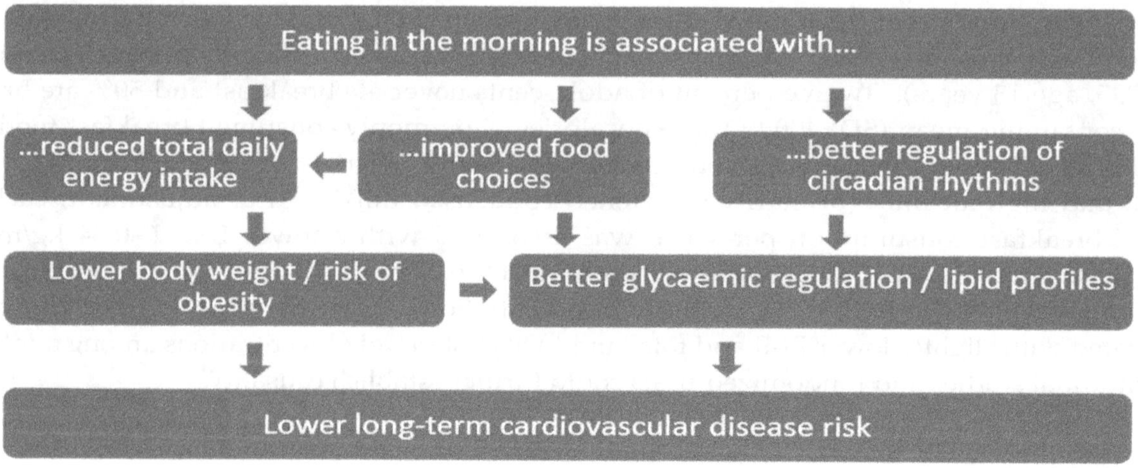

Figure 1. Hypothesized mechanisms for associations of breakfast with cardiovascular disease risk.

Most research on breakfast and health has been conducted in adults, with some work in children, but far less research has been dedicated to adolescents. However, adolescence represents a unique phase of life involving rapid growth, hormonal fluctuations, insulin resistance [16,17], and circadian dysregulation [18]. Considering the insulin resistance and circadian dysregulation can be influenced by breakfast consumption [19], it is important to understand the role of breakfast consumption on health in adolescents. In children aged 9–10 years in the 2011–2013 multi-country ISCOLE study, eating breakfast frequently (6–7 days/week), which varied from 58% in Brazil to 95% in Colombia, was associated with lower body mass index (BMI) z scores in some but not all countries [20]. This observation is supported by a systematic review including 10 longitudinal studies of children and adolescents of which eight provided evidence of inverse associations of more frequent breakfast consumption and adiposity [21]. In Malaysia, four cross-sectional studies have identified breakfast as the most frequently skipped meal among children and adolescents [22–25], with the prevalence of skipping breakfast varying from 17% [25] to 40% [24]. Only one cross-sectional study has examined breakfast consumption in relation to adiposity and obesity among Malaysian 12–19 year old adolescents [26]. Adolescents consuming breakfast five or more days/week had lower body weight, BMI, waist circumference, body fat mass, and percentage of body fat compared to those consuming breakfast less than five days/week. Overall, observational evidence on the association of a higher breakfast frequency with lower adiposity in adolescents is consistent worldwide.

Given that higher adiposity is associated with poorer CVD risk profiles [27], and breakfast frequency is associated with adiposity, one might expect to see similar associations with breakfast frequency and cardiovascular risk. However, evidence for associations of breakfast consumption with other CVD risk factors is less consistent. For example, fasted blood glucose concentrations were lowest among U.K. adolescents [28] and European boys [29] reporting daily breakfast consumption, but there was no evidence of a similar cross-sectional association among U.S. [30], Finnish [31], Taiwanese [32], or Japanese [33] adolescents. Lower systolic blood pressure has been observed among daily breakfast consumers in Taiwan [32] and in a European sample of boys, but no evidence of a similar cross-sectional association was observed among European girls and U.K., Japanese [33], U.S., Finnish, or Iranian [34] samples. Among Australian 9–15 year old children and adolescents followed-up as adults (aged 26–36 years), persistent breakfast skipping (defined as not eating between 0600 h and 0900 h as a child and adult) compared to consuming breakfast consistently was longitudinally associated with a higher waist circumference (mean difference 4.6, 95% CI 1.72, 7.53 cm), fasting serum insulin (mean difference 2.02, 95% CI 0.75, 3.29 mU/L), total cholesterol (mean difference 0.40, 95% CI 0.13, 0.68 mmol/L), and low density lipoprotein (LDL) cholesterol (mean difference 0.40, 95% CI 0.16, 0.64 mmol/L) concentrations [35]. Among Swedish 16 year-olds followed-up to age 43 years, eating breakfast only showed robust evidence of association with hyperglycemia (OR 1.75, 95% CI 1.01, 3.02), but not low high density lipoprotein (HDL) concentrations or hypertension [36]. Differences in sample sizes (ranging from 367 to 13,486 participants), diverse definitions of breakfast habits, and variation in adjustment for confounders may explain the inconsistency in findings to date.

Another possible explanation for inconsistent associations between breakfast consumption and CVD risk in adolescents is a lack of concurrent information on breakfast composition or diet quality. Existing evidence has typically relied on simple self-reported questions on usual breakfast frequency leaving it unclear how regular breakfast consumption relates to the types of food specifically eaten in the morning. Detailed dietary assessment methods like a food diary, 24-h diet recall, or diet history provide data on both the time of consumption and the food and nutrient content of breakfast, enabling both the frequency and composition of breakfast to be characterized and separate possible mechanisms to be explored. Finally, a proposed method for improved causal inference in observational research, by reducing the possibility that associations are confounded, is to explore the consistency of associations across high, middle- or low-income countries where the confounding structure may differ [37]. Therefore, adding to the existing evidence base on associations between breakfast and CVD risk, that is primarily in Western populations, by using Malaysian data may improve our understanding of the importance of breakfast.

No study to date has investigated the association of breakfast and CVD risk in Malaysian adolescents. In addition, few previous studies were able to explore what is eaten for breakfast in addition to breakfast frequency. The purpose of our study was to provide a detailed description of what adolescents ate for breakfast and investigate the association of breakfast frequency with CVD risk factors among adolescents using data from the Malaysian Health and Adolescent Longitudinal Research study

(MyHeARTs), including 7-day diet history enabling adjustment for potential confounders including concurrent diet quality.

2. Methods

2.1. Study Overview and Population

MyHeARTs is a prospective cohort study of 1351 schoolchildren (aged 13 years old at baseline) that attended 15 public secondary schools from central (Kuala Lumpur and Selangor) and northern (Perak) regions of Peninsular Malaysia. A detailed description of the MyHeARTs can be found elsewhere [38]. All procedures in MyHeARTs were approved by the Medical Ethics Committee, University Malaya Medical Centre according to the Declaration of Helsinki. Participation in the study was voluntary and written informed assent and consent was obtained from participants and parents/guardians of participants, respectively.

2.2. Dietary Assessment

Dietary intake was assessed using a seven-day diet history, which has been shown to give the most valid estimates of energy intake in children and adolescents (Burrows et al. 2010). Dietitians conducted open-ended interviews with the students to collect information on foods and drinks consumed during breakfast, mid-morning snack, lunch, afternoon tea, dinner and supper over the previous seven days. Pictures of local food and household measurement items were used to assist participants in estimating portion sizes consumed. Food and drink energy and nutrient intakes were calculated using the Nutritionist Pro™ Diet Analysis (Axxya Systems, Redmond, WA, USA) and Nutrient Composition of Malaysian Foods [39,40].

To compute breakfast consumption, energy intake from all foods or drink reported during the meal-slot identified as breakfast was combined on each day. Frequency of breakfast intake (days/week) was calculated as the number of days where any food or drinks were reported at breakfast. This was categorized for descriptive analyses by grouping into daily, 4–6 days/week, 1–3 days/week, and 0 days/week. The types of food and drink reported were investigated by grouping food items into 44 groups and then analyzing the frequency that each food group was reported across all food items in each breakfast occasions. Under-reporting of energy intake was assessed by comparing reported energy intake to estimated basal metabolic rate and participants defined as under-reporters (n = 497) were excluded [41]. Excluded participants were 43% male, 57% urban, 78% Malay, 12% Chinese, 7% Indian, and 2% other ethnicity, with age mean 12.9 (±0.3) years, BMI mean (±SD) 22.2 (±5.6) kg/m^2, and a mean daily energy intake of 1126 (±278) kcal.

A dietary pattern score for each adolescent was derived using reduced rank regression [42]. The score is a weighted linear combination of the 44 food groups (Supplementary Table S1) which predict the maximum variation in intermediate variables hypothesized to be on the pathway between food group intake and cardiovascular health, i.e., energy density (kJ/gram), fiber density (g/MJ), and percentage of energy intake from fat (%). A high pattern score represents an energy dense, low-fiber diet, which is characterized by high consumption of processed meat, bread products, chocolate, egg dishes and energy-dense Malaysian kuih (Malaysian snacks and desserts), and a low consumption of fruit, vegetables and vegetables dishes, and soups (unpublished results).

2.3. Anthropometric and Clinical Measurements

Height was measured without socks and shoes using a calibrated vertical stadiometer (Seca Portable 217, Seca, Birmingham, UK). Weight was measured with light clothing using a digital electronic weighing scale (Seca 813, Seca, Birmingham, UK). Body mass index was calculated as weight in kilograms divided by the square of height in meters (kg/m^2). Waist circumference was measured to the nearest millimeter using a non-elastic Seca measuring tape (Seca 201, Seca, Birmingham, UK). Systolic and diastolic blood pressure were calculated as the average of three readings using a stethoscope and a mercury sphygmomanometer. Fasting (≥10 h) venous blood samples were obtained from each participant and analyzed for serum total cholesterol, LDL cholesterol, HDL cholesterol, triacylglycerol (TAG), and blood glucose concentrations. More information on the way anthropometric and clinical measures were obtained can be found elsewhere [38].

2.4. Confounders

Physical activity was self-reported using the physical activity questionnaire (in Malay) for older children (PAC-Q). Sex, ethnicity (Malay, Chinese, Indian, other), smoking status (yes/no), and alcohol intake (yes/no) were self-reported in student questionnaires.

2.5. Statistical Analysis

Variables are described using mean (SD) if continuous and normal, or frequency (%) if categorical. Normality was checked via visual inspection of histograms. Analysis of variance (ANOVA) was performed to test the mean difference between breakfast frequency groups and continuous CVD risk factors. Tests for linear trend were performed using a likelihood ratio test comparing a model containing breakfast frequency (days/week) as a continuous variable with a model containing breakfast frequency as a categorical variable (daily, 4–6 days/week, 1–3 days/week, and 0 days/week). The chi-squared test was used to test for associations between breakfast frequency groups and categorical confounders. Multiple linear regression analysis was used to examine the independent relationship between breakfast frequency (days/week) and CVD risk factors. Risk factors analyzed as dependent variables were BMI, waist circumference, fasting serum glucose, TAG, total cholesterol, HDL and LDL concentrations, and systolic and diastolic blood pressure. Model 1 included only breakfast frequency as an independent variable. Model 2 included breakfast frequency, sex, ethnicity, physical activity level, smoking status, and alcohol intake. Model 3 included model 2 variables as well as BMI. Model 4 included model 3 variables together with total energy (kcal/day), total carbohydrate (% daily energy), total protein (% energy), total fat (% energy), total cholesterol (mg/1000 kcal), total saturated fatty acid (% energy), total sodium (mg/1000 kcal), total calcium (mg/1000 kcal), total iron (mg/1000 kcal), total fiber (g/1000 kcal), and total sugar (% energy). Model 5 included model 4 variables together with dietary pattern score. Statistical analyses were performed using SPSS (version 21, IBM), Stata (version 15, StataCorp LLC, College Station, Texas, USA), and SAS (version 9.4, Marlow, Buckinghamshire, UK).

3. Results

Figure 2 shows that 795 participants had complete data based on the variables of interest and were included in the current analysis. The characteristics of participants overall and stratified by breakfast frequency are presented in Table 1. Fifty one percent of the sample were daily breakfast eaters, 25% consumed breakfast 4–6 days/week, 15% consumed breakfast 1–3 days/week, and 10% of the sample never consumed breakfast. Adolescents of Indian ethnicity were more likely to be daily breakfast eaters (71%) compared to the overall sample, while no Chinese adolescents were identified as breakfast skippers. Boys were more likely than girls to consume breakfast daily (58% vs. 47%). Few differences in breakfast frequency were observed for any other individual characteristics.

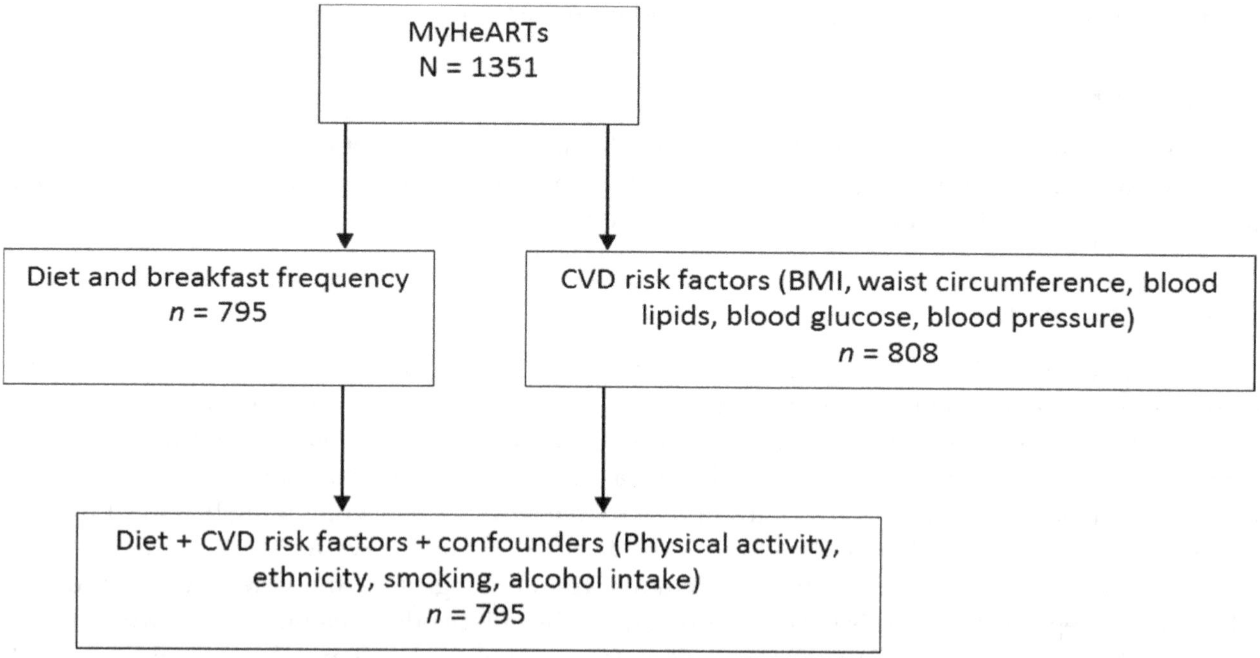

Figure 2. Number of participants with data available based on the variables of interest. CVD: cardiovascular disease; MyHeARTs: Malaysian Health and Adolescents Longitudinal Research Team study.

In terms of diet, adolescents who consumed breakfast but infrequently (1–3 days/week) consumed the least total daily energy, calcium, and sugar compared to both breakfast skippers and daily consumers (Table 1). Daily breakfast consumers had a positive dietary pattern score i.e., a more energy dense and lower fiber density diet, compared to infrequent breakfast eaters and breakfast skippers who, on average, had a negative dietary pattern score. Breakfasts reported in MyHeARTs contained a mean (SD) 400 ± 127 kcal. The most frequent food groups of all food items reported at breakfast were cereal-based mixed meals (19%), chocolate and confectionery (14%), hot and powdered drinks (13%), high fat milk (12%), and bread (6%) (Figure 3). Cereal-based mixed meals, were mainly rice in coconut milk (34% of cereal based mixed meals food items), fried rice (30%), and fried noodles (12%) (Supplementary Material Table S1). Chocolate and confectionery refer to granulated sugar (99% of chocolate and confectionery items reported at breakfast), while hot and powdered drinks, are mostly Milo (a chocolate and malt powder drink) (40%) and malted milk powder (38%). High fat milk and cream was primarily sweetened condensed milk (90% of items in that group) (Supplementary Material Table S1).

Table 1. Characteristics of MyHeARTs participants by breakfast frequency groups.

		Breakfast Frequency				
	Total	0 days/week	1–3 days/week	4–6 days/week	Daily	*p*-Value
All children, n (%)	795 (100)	76 (10)	115 (15)	196 (25)	408 (51)	-
Age (years), mean (SD)	12.9 (0.3)	12.9 (0.3)	12.9 (0.4)	12.8 (0.3)	12.9 (0.3)	-
Sex						
Boys, *n* (%)	298 (37)	32 (10)	36 (12)	58 (19)	172 (58)	0.01 [a]
Girls, *n* (%)	497 (63)	44 (9)	79 (16)	138 (28)	236 (47)	
Urbanicity						
Urban, *n* (%)	401 (50)	17 (4)	53 (13)	114 (28)	217 (54)	<0.001 [a]
Rural, *n* (%)	394 (50)	59 (15)	62 (16)	82 (21)	191 (48)	
Ethnicity						
Malay, *n* (%)	650 (82)	68 (10)	100 (15)	162 (25)	320 (49)	0.03 [a]
Chinese, *n* (%)	44 (6)	0 (0)	8 (18)	12 (27)	24 (55)	
Indian, *n* (%)	69 (14)	5 (7)	3 (4)	12 (17)	49 (71)	
Others, *n* (%)	32 (6)	3 (9)	4 (13)	10 (31)	15 (47)	
Smoking status						
Yes, *n* (%)	73 (9)	11 (15)	12 (16)	13 (18)	37 (51)	0.23 [a]
No, *n* (%)	722 (91)	65 (9)	103 (14)	183 (25)	371 (51)	
Alcohol intake						
Yes, *n* (%)	23 (3)	3 (13)	5 (22)	4 (17)	11 (48)	0.55 [a]
No, *n* (%)	772 (97)	73 (9)	110 (14)	192 (25)	397 (51)	
Physical activity (in last 7 days)						

Table 1. *Cont.*

	Total	Breakfast Frequency				*p*-Value
		0 days/week	1–3 days/week	4–6 days/week	Daily	
Never n (%)	237 (30)	27 (11)	35 (15)	55 (23)	120 (51)	0.35 [a]
1–2 times last week *n* (%)	361 (45)	32 (8)	58 (16)	89 (25)	182 (50)	
3–4 times last week *n* (%)	113 (14)	8 (7)	13 (12)	31 (27)	61 (54)	
5–6 times last week *n* (%)	34 (4)	2 (6)	8 (24)	8 (24)	16 (47)	
7+ times last week *n* (%)	50 (6)	7 (14)	1 (2)	13 (26)	29 (58)	
Total daily intake						
Energy (kcal/day)	1673 (332)	1744 (433)	1573 (276)	1594 (267)	1726 (339)	<0.001 [b]
Protein (% of total energy)	15 (2)	15 (2)	15 (2)	15 (2)	15 (2)	0.63 [b]
Fat (% of total energy)	29.930 (5)	30 (5)	30 (4)	30 (5)	30 (4)	0.87 [b]
Carbohydrate (% of total energy)	55 (5)	55 (5)	56 (5)	55 (5)	55 (6)	0.62 [b]
Cholesterol (mg/1000 kcal)	133 (52)	137 (58)	139 (50)	131(47)	132 (54)	0.53 [b]
SFA (% of total energy)	6 (2)	6 (2)	5 (2)	6 (3)	6 (2)	0.14 [b]
Sodium (mg/1000 kcal)	1387 (345)	1328 (380)	1363 (352)	1400 (329)	1399 (344)	0.32 [b]
Calcium (mg/1000 kcal)	226 (91)	229 (116)	195 (827)	222 (81)	236 (92)	<0.001 [b]
Iron (mg/1000 kcal)	9 (3)	9 (3)	8 (6)	8 (2)	9 (2)	0.42 [b]
Crude fiber (g/1000 kcal)	2 (1)	2 (1)	2 (1)	2 (11)	2 (1)	0.51 [b]
Sugar (% of total energy)	8 (4)	8 (4)	7 (3)	9 (4)	8 (4)	0.04 [b]
Dietary pattern score (SD units)	0.01 (1.10)	−0.06 (1.18)	−0.09 (1.02)	−0.12 (1.081)	0.12 (1.10)	0.05 [b]

[a] Pearson's chi-squared; [b] ANOVA. Abbreviations—ANOVA: analysis of variance; SD: standard deviation; SFA: saturated fatty acid.

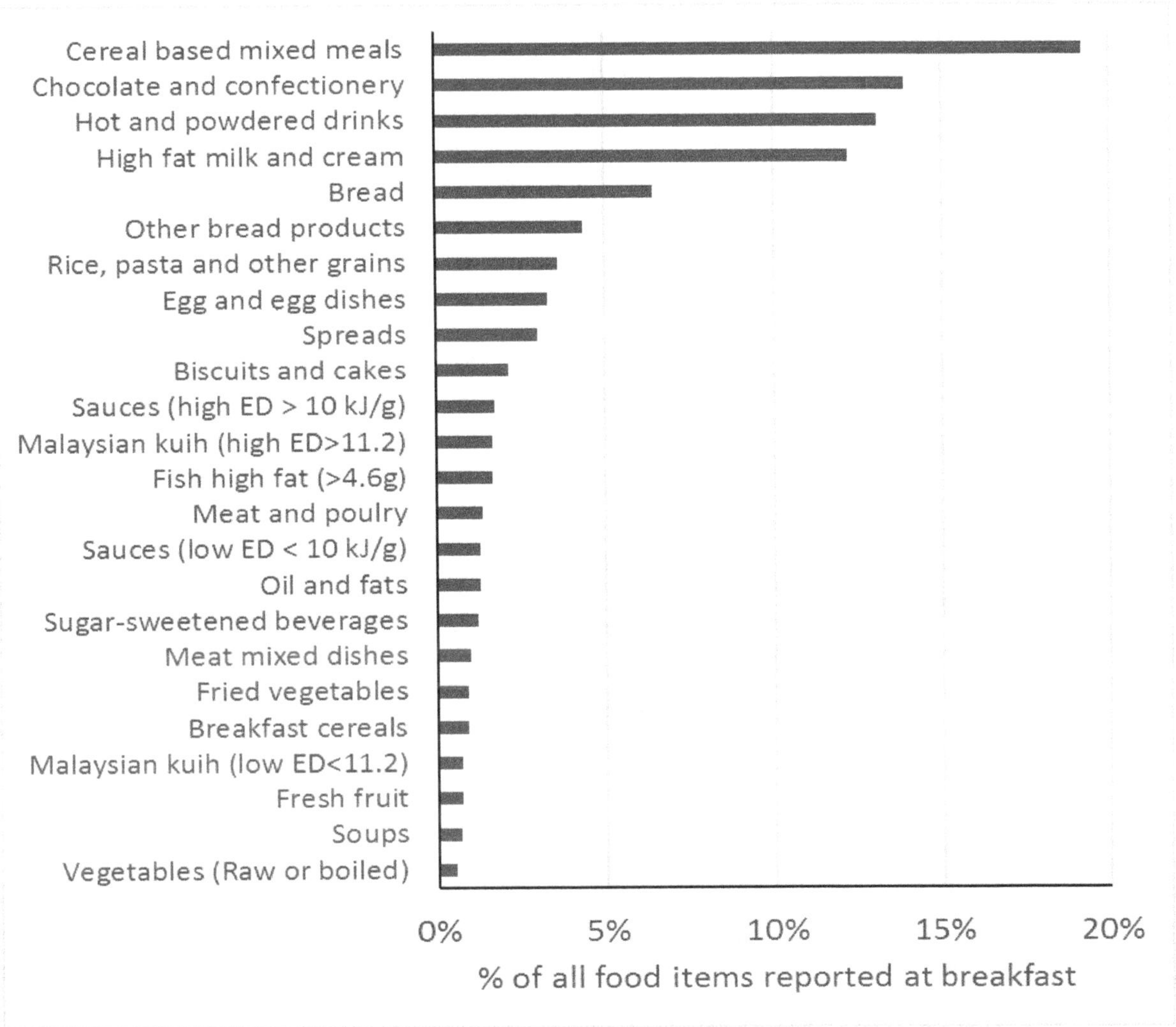

Figure 3. Food groups eaten for breakfast. Bars represent percentage of each food group from all food items reported in breakfast occasions (n = 15,507 food items reported at breakfast). Only food groups contributing 1% or more to all food items are displayed. Energy density (ED).

3.1. *Mean of Cardiovascular Disease Risk Factors*

A description of CVD risk factors by breakfast frequency is presented in Table 2. Compared to daily breakfast consumers, those who never ate breakfast had slightly higher serum total cholesterol concentrations (4.6 vs. 4.8 mmol/L, $p = 0.01$), driven by higher LDL cholesterol (2.7 vs. 2.9 mmol/L, $p = 0.01$) (Figure 4). These associations were linear across the breakfast categories. Unlike the other CVD risk variables, there was weak evidence ($p_{trend} = 0.06$) that the relationship between breakfast consumption and BMI may be non-linear. Those consuming breakfast daily had the lowest BMI (19.2 kg/m^2), but participants who consumed breakfast infrequently (1–3 days/week), rather than never, had the highest BMI (20.9 kg/m^2; Table 2 and Figure 4). There was no evidence of other CVD risk factors, i.e., fasting serum glucose, TAG, or HDL concentration and blood pressure, varying by breakfast frequency, though there was some weak evidence suggesting that waist circumference was 2 cm smaller in daily vs. never breakfast consumers ($p = 0.06$).

Table 2. Description of cardiovascular disease (CVD) risk factors by breakfast frequency (n = 795).

	Breakfast Frequency					
	0 days/week (n = 76)	**1–3 days/week (n = 115)**	**4–6 days/week (n = 196)**	**Daily (n = 408)**	**p-Value (ANOVA)**	p_{trend}
	Mean (SD)	**Mean (SD)**	**Mean (SD)**	**Mean (SD)**		
BMI (kg/m^2)	19.9 (5.7)	20.9 (5.3)	20.0 (4.4)	19.2 (4.7)	0.003	0.06
WC (cm)	70.1 (12.9)	71.0 (13.4)	69.0 (10.6)	67.9 (11.6)	0.06	0.91
FBG (mmol/L)	4.9 (0.4)	4.9 (0.4)	4.9 (0.4)	4.9 (0.8)	0.79	0.61
TC (mmol/L)	4.8 (1.0)	4.6 (0.9)	4.7 (0.8)	4.6 (0.8)	0.01	0.32
HDL(mmol/L)	1.5 (0.3)	1.5 (0.3)	1.4 (0.3)	1.5 (0.3)	0.56	0.38
LDL (mmol/L)	2.9 (0.9)	2.8 (0.8)	2.8 (0.7)	2.7 (0.7)	0.01	0.41
SBP (mmHg)	109 (13)	111 (11)	109 (11)	109 (11)	0.32	0.31
DBP (mmHg)	67 (13)	68 (10)	67 (10)	68 (10)	0.45	0.34
TAG (mmol/L)	0.98 (0.60)	0.92 (0.45)	0.99 (0.47)	0.91 (0.46)	0.24	0.23

Abbreviations—ANOVA: analysis of variance; BMI: body mass index; DBP: diastolic blood pressure; FBG: fasting plasma glucose; HDL: high-density lipoprotein; LDL: low-density lipoprotein; TC: total cholesterol; SBP: systolic blood pressure; SD: standard deviation; TAG: triacylglycerol; WC: waist circumference.

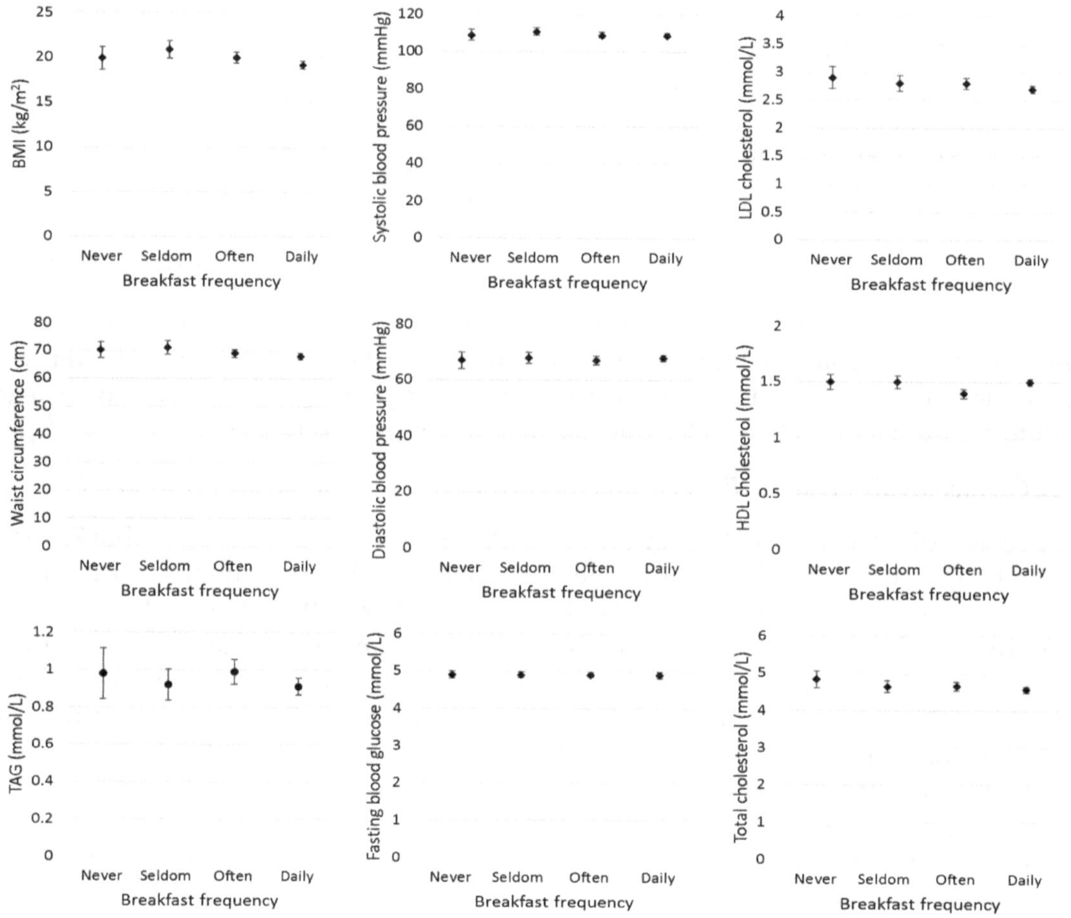

Figure 4. Baseline associations between breakfast frequency and cardiovascular disease (CVD) risk factors in MyHeARTs. Never = 0 days a week, n = 76; Seldom = 1–3 days a week, n = 115; Often = 4–6 days a week, n = 196; Daily = 7 days a week, n = 408. Abbreviations—BMI: body mass index; HDL: high-density lipoprotein; LDL: low-density lipoprotein; TAG: triacylglycerol.

3.2. *Association of Breakfast Consumption and cardiovascular disease (CVD) Risk Factors*

Table 3 shows associations between breakfast frequency and CVD risk factors, before and after adjusting for potential confounders. In the fully adjusted models, each extra day of breakfast was associated with a lower BMI by 0.2 kg/m^2 (95% CI −0.4, −0.1) and lower total cholesterol concentration of −0.03 mmol/L (95% CI −0.06, −0.01). The lower total cholesterol concentration was driven by LDL cholesterol, which was lower by the same order of magnitude for each extra day of breakfast (β −0.03, 95% CI −0.06, −0.01). Waist circumference was 0.5 cm (95% CI −0.84, −0.16 cm) lower per extra day of eating breakfast per week in model 2, but the association was reduced to 0.06 cm/breakfast/week after adjustment for BMI (model 3, Table 3). No evidence of association was observed for fasting serum glucose or TAG concentration, serum HDL cholesterol concentration, and blood pressure.

Table 3. Multiple linear regression analysis of association of breakfast frequency and risk factors of cardiovascular disease independent of potential confounding among participants (n = 795).

	β (95% CI)	*p*-Value
	Body mass index (kg/m^2)	
Model 1 [a]	−0.21 (−0.35, −0.07)	0.004
Model 2 [b]	−0.20 (−0.34, −0.06)	0.01
Model 4 [d]	−0.20 (−0.34, −0.05)	0.01
Model 5 [f]	−0.18 (−0.33, −0.04)	0.01
	Waist circumference (cm)	
Model 1 [a]	−0.44 (−0.78, −0.10)	0.01
Model 2 [b]	−0.50 (−0.84, −0.16)	0.004
Model 3[c]	−0.06 (−0.21, 0.09)	0.40
Model 4 [e]	−0.07 (−0.22, 0.08)	0.36
Model 5 [g]	−0.06 (−0.21, 0.09)	0.43
	Fasting glucose concentration (mmol/L)	
Model 1 [a]	0.00 (−0.02, 0.02)	0.80
Model 2 [b]	0.00 (−0.02, 0.02)	0.88
Model 3 [c]	0.00 (−0.02. 0.02)	0.79
Model 4 [e]	0.00 (−0.02, 0.02)	086
Model 5 [g]	0.00 (−0.02, 0.02)	0.82
	Total cholesterol concentration (mmol/L)	
Model 1 [a]	−0.04 (−0.06, −0.01)	0.004
Model 2 [b]	−0.04 (−0.06, −0.01)	0.003
Model 3 [c]	−0.04 (−0.06, −0.01)	0.01
Model 4 [e]	−0.03 (−0.06, −0.01)	0.01
Model 5 [g]	−0.03 (−0.06, −0.01)	0.01
	High-density lipoprotein cholesterol concentration (mmol/L)	
Model 1 [a]	0.00 (−0.01, 0.01)	0.68
Model 2 [b]	0.00 (−0.01, 0.01)	0.66
Model 3 [c]	0.00 (−0.01, 0.01)	0.57
Model 4 [e]	0.00 (−0.01, 0.01)	0.80
Model 5 [g]	0.00 (−0.01, 0.01)	0.82

Table 3. *Cont.*

	β (95% CI)	*p*-Value
Low-density lipoprotein cholesterol concentration (mmol/L)		
Model 1 [a]	−0.03 (−0.06, −0.01)	0.002
Model 2 [b]	−0.04 (−0.06, −0.01)	0.001
Model 3 [c]	−0.03 (−0.05, −0.01)	0.03
Model 4 [e]	−0.03 (−0.05, −0.01)	0.01
Model 5 [g]	−0.03 (−0.05, −0.01)	0.01
Systolic blood pressure (mmHg)		
Model 1 [a]	−0.18 (−0.51, 0.15)	0.28
Model 2 [b]	−0.14 (−0.46, 0.18)	0.389
Model 3 [c]	0.04 (−0.25, 0.34)	0.78
Model 4 [e]	0.07 (−0.23, 0.37)	0.65
Model 5 [g]	0.07 (−0.23, 0.37)	0.65
Diastolic blood pressure (mmHg)		
Model 1 [a]	0.11 (−0.19, 0.41)	0.48
Model 2 [b]	0.12 (−0.18, 0.42)	0.44
Model 3 [c]	0.26 (−0.03, 0.55)	0.08
Model 4 [e]	0.27 (−0.03, 0.56)	0.08
Model 5 [g]	0.27 (−0.02, 0.57)	0.07
Triacylglycerol concentration (mmol/L)		
Model 1 [a]	−0.01 (−0.02, 0.01)	0.26
Model 2 [b]	−0.01 (−0.02, 0.01)	0.34
Model 3 [c]	0.00 (−0.01, 0.01)	0.92
Model 4 [e]	0.00 (−0.02, 0.01)	0.82
Model 5 [g]	0.00 (−0.01, 0.01)	0.90

Abbreviations—CI: confidence interval. [a] Model 1 includes only breakfast frequency. [b] Model 2 includes breakfast frequency, physical activity, smoking status, alcohol intake, ethnicity, and sex. [c] Model 3 includes variables in model 2 plus BMI. [d] Model 4 includes variables from model 2 plus total daily energy (kcal), total daily carbohydrate (%), total daily protein (%), total daily fat (%), total daily cholesterol (mg/1000 kcal), total daily saturated fatty acid (%), total daily sodium (mg/1000 kcal), total daily calcium (mg/1000 kcal), total daily iron (mg/1000 kcal), total daily fiber (g/1000 kcal), and total daily sugar (%). [e] Model 4 includes variables from model 3 plus total daily energy (kcal), total daily carbohydrate (%), total daily protein (%), total daily fat (%), total daily cholesterol (mg/1000 kcal), total daily saturated fatty acid (%), total daily sodium (mg/1000 kcal), total daily calcium (mg/1000 kcal), total daily iron (mg/1000 kcal), total daily fiber (g/1000 kcal), and total daily sugar (%). [f] Model 5 includes variables from model 4 [d] plus dietary pattern score. [g] Model 5 includes variables from model 4 [e] plus dietary pattern score.

4. Discussion

In this cross-sectional analysis of a large sample of Malaysian adolescents with detailed dietary data and a broad range of CVD risk factors, we found evidence that breakfast frequency was inversely associated with BMI and fasting total and LDL cholesterol concentrations, but not waist circumference, fasting glucose, HDL or TAG concentrations, or blood pressure.

Among Malaysian adolescents in our study, 10% were breakfast skippers and 51% were daily breakfast consumers, which is similar to a previously reported prevalence in a different Malaysian sample of 12–19 year-olds [26]. A higher prevalence of breakfast skipping has been observed among U.S. and Finnish adolescents (i.e., 13–16% and 16–24% respectively [31,43]) as well as higher prevalence of daily breakfast consumption in other populations (i.e., 94% among U.K. primary school children and 89% among Taiwanese primary school children [28,32]). Differences in daily breakfast consumption could partly be explained by a lack of a consistent definition of breakfast in the literature [44]. For example, some studies defined breakfast based on the time of the day food was consumed, e.g., between 0600 h and 0900 h [35], while others based their definitions on the frequency of breakfast (self-identified by the participant) during the week [29,32,34] or only during weekdays [31]. In addition, adolescents with the same breakfast frequency may be in different groups across studies, e.g., breakfast skippers in the current study are those who never consumed breakfast, while in other studies those who never consumed breakfast are combined with irregular consumers [29].

4.1. *Breakfast Associations with Cardiovascular Disease Risk Factors*

Our findings agree with previous observational studies across the world showing consistent inverse associations between frequency of breakfast consumption and BMI [5,6]. Only one study previously investigated Malaysian adolescents (n = 236) [26], finding breakfast consumption to be associated with lower BMI, concordant with our analysis. Interestingly, we did not find strong evidence for a linear relationship potentially suggesting that never eating breakfast is not problematic per se, but rather irregular consumption of breakfast on some days but not others makes energy balance more difficult to regulate. Nurul-Fadhilah et al. [26] further found an inverse relationship between breakfast consumption and waist circumference, which our analysis supports, but the association was not robust to adjustment for BMI. Similar waist circumferences were found between the two studies for infrequent breakfast consumers (~70 cm) but the waist circumference observed in frequent breakfast consumers differed, where Nurul-Fadhilah et al. [26] found lower waist circumferences (~64 cm) compared with MyHeARTs (~68 cm). The differences in these findings may be explained by the comparatively homogenous sample (mostly Malay from Kelantan) with a smaller sample size compared to the larger and more diverse MyHeARTs sample.

Our study found frequent breakfast consumption was associated with lower total cholesterol driven by lower LDL cholesterol concentrations compared to infrequent breakfast consumption. These findings are in agreement with some [29,35], but not all [28–30,33] previous studies. However the effect sizes in our analyses were small and likely not clinically meaningful (~0.03 mmol/L difference in plasma total and LDL cholesterol concentrations for each extra day of breakfast), as ≥1.0 mmol/L reduction in LDL concentration is needed to reduce the risk of all-cause mortality by 10% in adults [45].

Previous research has reported inconsistent associations between breakfast consumption and HDL cholesterol concentrations [30–33]. Our analyses however provided no evidence of association in accordance with several studies [30,31,33,35]. Whilst others found statistically significant associations [32,46], the differences in HDL cholesterol concentrations observed elsewhere were small and unlikely to be clinically meaningful at reducing CVD risk (difference of <2 mg/dL). Importantly, all categories of breakfast consumption in this study were associated with plasma HDL cholesterol concentrations within the range associated with lowest CVD and mortality risk in adults [47]. Such findings may suggest that there is limited power in detecting associations between CVD risk markers such as HDL concentrations in an overall healthy sample. Despite the inconsistencies in statistical significance between studies, taken together there appears to be no meaningful association between HDL cholesterol concentrations and breakfast consumption in adolescents, in line with our results.

We did not observe evidence of association between breakfast consumption and blood pressure, which may partially be explained by the similar sodium intakes between breakfast consumption categories. As with HDL cholesterol concentrations, previous research has provided mixed results regarding the relationship between breakfast consumption and blood pressure in adolescents. Ahadi et al. [34] found breakfast consumption to be associated with lower blood pressure, supporting previous research showing a reduced risk of hypertension [31]. The latter study however only showed lower hypertension risk in girls who were semi-regular breakfast consumers. Our findings do however support other research demonstrating no association between breakfast consumption and diastolic [28,30,36,46] and systolic [30,36,46] blood pressure.

Our analysis did not find an association between breakfast consumption frequency and plasma TAG concentrations, supporting most other studies [28–30,48]. Smith et al. [35] found breakfast skipping to be longitudinally associated with increased serum TAG concentrations compared to regular breakfast consumption, potentially suggesting changes to TAG concentrations occur over a longer period. Such a time effect may be physiologically plausible; blood TAG concentrations are typically due to greater adiposity, but such an effect is not necessarily immediate. Since breakfast skipping has consistently been associated with greater adiposity [5], it may be that the associations with TAG are chronic adaptations to higher fat mass.

Lower fasting glucose concentrations have previously been associated with regular breakfast consumption in adolescents in some [28,29,36] but not all [30,32] studies, with others finding mixed results [31,35]. Our analyses provide no evidence for an association. However, we were unable to investigate markers of insulin resistance (e.g., Homeostatic model assessment HOMA) due to lack of insulin data; such a measure provides useful data due to the insulin resistance exhibited during adolescence [16,17]. This may explain the more consistent finding (compared to fasting plasma glucose concentrations alone) of regular breakfast consumption being associated with lower insulin resistance in adolescents [28–30,35].

There is a lack of causal data in adolescents pertaining to glycemic regulation and breakfast consumption. In adults, short-term experimental manipulations to meal regularity (including breakfast omission) have detrimental effects on acute postprandial glycemic and insulinemic responses [9,49], although longer-term breakfast consumption versus omission does not appear to negatively influence glycemic regulation [13]. Equally, in schoolchildren, fasted plasma glucose concentrations were unaffected by participation (compared to non-participation) in a nine-month school breakfast program [50], supporting our analysis. Such findings suggest chronic adaptations to blood glucose possibly occur mitigating the acute-effects of breakfast omission.

4.2. *Comparisons of Breakfast Definitions*

The differences in the way breakfast is defined and how frequencies are combined in each study make it hard to directly compare associations with health and may be responsible for the disparate findings [51]. For example Nurul-Fadhilah et al. [26] used two broad categories of breakfast, i.e., <5 days/week versus ≥5 days/week, which could explain the evidence for association observed for waist circumference, in comparison to the weaker evidence observed in our study, which included a greater number of breakfast categories. Furthermore, our study adjusted for aspects of adiposity and diet quality, which was not the case in previous studies showing associations for fasting glucose concentrations and blood pressure [28,32]. Different ranges of CVD risk factors could also explain the diverse findings; for example, mean diastolic blood pressure was higher among U.K. primary children [28] compared to our sample. Additional explanations could be the inclusion of younger and smaller sample sizes [28,30] and the inclusion of healthier adolescents compared to the average population [33].

4.3. *Breakfast Composition and Meal Timing*

Overall, our findings show some, albeit limited, evidence for a protective association between breakfast consumption and some CVD risk factors, such as BMI, and total and LDL cholesterol concentrations. One reason for which breakfast might be protective is the consumption of particular foods during breakfast. The fiber contained in cereal and the high protein content of eggs have been shown to increase satiety and improve appetite control [44,52,53]. This may explain the protective effect of breakfast in some populations. For example, European children and adolescents typically consume micronutrient-dense breakfast cereal (with milk) and bread [54], while in our sample the most commonly consumed breakfast foods were cooked rice dishes, sugar, malt drinks, and sweetened condensed milk. Considering the differences in the types of foods consumed at breakfast between populations, it is more likely that, if causal, breakfast relates to health because of the timing of food intake in relation to circadian metabolic rhythms rather than the type of food consumed.

The timing of eating has been associated with improved gluco-regulatory responses in adults (e.g., Farshchi et al. [9]). Improved postprandial metabolic responses may be of particular importance in adolescents because of the increased insulin resistance in this population compared to childhood and adulthood [16,17], as well as the circadian dysregulation, which often skews adolescents towards evening chronotypes [18] typically associated with poorer general health [55]. In adults, such circadian misalignment is causally implicated in poorer cardiometabolic health (e.g., Scheer et al. [56]), with observational research suggesting similar health outcomes in adolescents [57]. Compared to the evening, morning ingestion of nutrients results in lower postprandial glycemia and insulinemia, conducive to lower CVD risk [58], making breakfast a particularly important meal. Breakfast consumption may therefore act to improve cardiometabolic health via both circadian entrainment [59], and via exploiting the favorable postprandial response found when ingesting nutrients in the morning compared to the evening [60], though causal research specifically in adolescents is lacking and should be a priority for future studies.

4.4. Strengths and Limitations

One of the main strengths of our study is that the MyHeARTs is the largest study in Malaysia, involving adolescents from three main ethnicities, three regions, and the inclusion of rural and urban participants, providing superior representativeness than previous studies (e.g., Nurul-Fadhilah et al. [26]). The ethnic diversity in our analyses is a particular strength, demonstrating higher breakfast eating prevalence among Indian participants, and no cases of skipping breakfast every day in Chinese participants. Dietary intake was measured using a seven-day diet history, which is a valid method for estimating the energy and nutrient intake among adolescents (Burrows et al. 2010). A broad range of demographic data, with student lifestyle and information on parents enabled us to model the independent association of breakfast frequency with CVD risk factors, including multiple biomarkers.

Whilst the strengths of this study mean we have provided novel data on breakfast and cardiometabolic health in Malaysian adolescents, several limitations also need to be acknowledged. Breakfast is notoriously difficult to define, particularly in epidemiological studies due to limitations in data availability (e.g., wake time not being recorded). In our study, breakfast was self-defined by the participant. Recent research has aimed to define breakfast and has proposed a wake-time-dependent definition of within two or three hours of waking [44]. In data collection for MyHeARTs, dietitians asked participants when their breakfast time was, and if this was after 1030 h, the meal was not recorded as 'breakfast' but as a morning snack instead. Owing to early school start times in Malaysia (~0730 h), our definition of breakfast on week days is likely to have classified some breakfasts outside of 2–3 h of waking, thus capturing a slightly extended morning fast.

Future studies should further explore different types of breakfast which may help provide novel insights into the role of breakfast on cardiometabolic health. For example, in our sample, adolescents typically consumed foods such as rice and noodles for breakfast which, despite being high carbohydrates, differ in nutritional composition to typical breakfast foods in Europe, such as cereal, which is a vehicle for milk consumption in European children [54]. Differences in breakfast composition may help explain some of the aforementioned disparities compared to previous research. Future studies could explore this using meal coding, as has been done previously, to understand meal-based dietary patterns in adults [61,62]. Additionally, understanding breakfast composition may help elucidate whether the consistent associations with BMI are driven by breakfast food composition or timing of nutrient intake. In the case of the latter, this would explain why we observed a protective association with breakfast despite daily breakfast consumers having a more energy-dense, lower fiber overall dietary pattern score, which is associated with greater adiposity in the United Kingdom [63].

This may additionally suggest further cultural differences, as typically breakfast consumption in Western populations is associated with less obesogenic diets [64].

Physical activity and diet were both self-reported. Although validated methods were used to obtain these data minimizing risk of bias, there is known error within these measures, such as energy intake underreporting bias. As such, we aimed to control for dietary misreporting by excluding under-reporters. Finally, the cross-sectional and observational nature of the study prevents causal inference for the associations observed owing to the possibility of reverse causation and residual confounding. Thus, both longitudinal and randomized controlled studies are required in order to establish the causality of the relationship between breakfast consumption and lower CVD risk factors in this population. Longitudinal studies are particularly valuable in adolescents as some research has suggested breakfast skipping is cross-sectionally, but not longitudinally associated with higher BMI in adolescents with overweight, and vice versa in those in the normal BMI range [65]. Our study has provided valuable information for hypothesis generation to aid in developing such studies.

5. Conclusion

In conclusion, the present study suggests that adolescents in Malaysia who eat breakfast more frequently have a lower BMI, and lower plasma total and LDL cholesterol concentrations independent of a range of confounders. Our study results specifically highlight that the benefits of breakfast (if causal) are not limited to the types of foods typically eaten in Western populations such as breakfast cereals, milk, or bread, but may be independent of the type of food consumed and instead related to the timing of food intake. Furthermore, our data suggested that irregular habits may be more detrimental to CVD risk than uniform breakfast eating vs. skipping. Previous longitudinal studies or long-term randomized trials have not explored the potential impact of consistent versus irregular breakfast habits or been able to differentiate changes in the timing of eating from the type of food eaten. Future research should aim to examine whether the content, timing, or regularity of breakfast intake is associated with lower CVD risk both longitudinally and causally within trials in adolescents.

Author Contributions: N.M. and L.J. formulated the research question and designed the analysis; H.A.M., N.A.S., and M.Y.J. conceived the idea of the overall MyHeART study, obtained funding, and were involved with data collection; H.A.M. coordinated all main data entry; N.M. analyzed the data and wrote the first draft of the article. Z.T. and H.A.C. analyzed data. L.J. supervised the analyses. L.J., Z.T., and H.A.C. revised the article including comments from H.A.M. and M.Y.J. All authors approved the final manuscript.

Acknowledgments: We are grateful for the support and guidance provided by MyHeART study group members (Nik Rubiah Nik Abdul Rashid and Zarihah Mohd Zain (Ministry of Health, Malaysia), Maizurah Omar (USM), Mohamad Haniki Nik Mohamed (UIA), Khadijah Shamsuddin (UKM), Rosnah Sutan (UKM), and Sim Pei Ying, Ms Liyana Ramli, Tin Tin Su, Nahar Azmi, and Maznah Dahlui (University of Malaya).

References

1. Mendis, S.; Puska, P.; Norrving, B. *Global Atlas on Cardiovascular Disease Prevention and Control*; World Health Organization: Geneva, Switzerland.
2. Noncommunicable Diseases Country Profiles 2014. Available online: https://www.who.int/nmh/publications/ncd-profiles-2014/en/ (accessed on 30 June 2017).
3. Raitakari, O.T.; Juonala, M.; Kahonen, M.; Taittonen, L.; Laitinen, T.; Maki-Torkko, N.; Jarvisalo, M.J.; Uhari, M.; Jokinen, E.; Ronnemaa, T.; et al. Cardiovascular risk factors in childhood and carotid artery intima-media thickness in adulthood: the Cardiovascular Risk in Young Finns Study. *JAMA* **2003**, *290*, 2277–2283. [CrossRef]

4. Ng, M.; Fleming, T.; Robinson, M.; Thomson, B.; Graetz, N.; Margono, C.; Mullany, E.C.; Biryukov, S.; Abbafati, C.; Abera, S.F.; et al. Global, regional, and national prevalence of overweight and obesity in children and adults during 1980–2013: A systematic analysis for the Global Burden of Disease Study 2013. *Lancet* **2013**, *384*, 766–781. [CrossRef]
5. Brown, A.W.; Bohan Brown, M.M.; Allison, D.B. Belief beyond the evidence: using the proposed effect of breakfast on obesity to show 2 practices that distort scientific evidence. *Am. J. Clin. Nutr.* **2013**. [CrossRef] [PubMed]
6. Horikawa, C.; Kodama, S.; Yachi, Y.; Heianza, Y.; Hirasawa, R.; Ibe, Y.; Saito, K.; Shimano, H.; Yamada, N.; Sone, H. Skipping breakfast and prevalence of overweight and obesity in Asian and Pacific regions: A meta-analysis. *Prev. Med.* **2011**, *53*, 260–267. [CrossRef]
7. Purslow, L.R.; Sandhu, M.S.; Forouhi, N.; Young, E.H.; Luben, R.N.; Welch, A.A.; Khaw, K.T.; Bingham, S.A.; Wareham, N.J. Energy Intake at Breakfast and Weight Change: Prospective Study of 6,764 Middle-aged Men and Women. *Am. J. Epidemiol.* **2008**, *167*, 188–192. [CrossRef]
8. Mente, A.; de Koning, L.; Shannon, H.S.; Anand, S.S. A systematic review of the evidence supporting a causal link between dietary factors and coronary heart disease. *Arch. Intern. Med.* **2009**, *169*, 659–669. [CrossRef] [PubMed]
9. Farshchi, H.R.; Taylor, M.A.; Macdonald, I.A. Deleterious effects of omitting breakfast on insulin sensitivity and fasting lipid profiles in healthy lean women. *Am. J. Clin. Nutr.* **2005**, *81*, 388–396. [CrossRef] [PubMed]
10. Clayton, D.J.; Stensel, D.J.; James, L.J. Effect of breakfast omission on subjective appetite, metabolism, acylated ghrelin and GLP-17-36 during rest and exercise. *Nutrition* **2016**, *32*, 179–185. [CrossRef] [PubMed]
11. Bo, S.; Fadda, M.; Castiglione, A.; Ciccone, G.; De Francesco, A.; Fedele, D.; Guggino, A.; Parasiliti Caprino, M.; Ferrara, S.; Vezio Boggio, M.; et al. Is the timing of caloric intake associated with variation in diet-induced thermogenesis and in the metabolic pattern? A randomized cross-over study. *Int. J. Obes. (Lond)* **2015**, *39*, 1689–1695. [CrossRef] [PubMed]
12. Bandin, C.; Scheer, F.A.; Luque, A.J.; Avila-Gandia, V.; Zamora, S.; Madrid, J.A.; Gomez-Abellan, P.; Garaulet, M. Meal timing affects glucose tolerance, substrate oxidation and circadian-related variables: A randomized, crossover trial. *Int. J. Obes. (Lond)* **2015**, *39*, 828–833. [CrossRef]
13. Betts, J.A.; Richardson, J.D.; Chowdhury, E.A.; Holman, G.D.; Tsintzas, K.; Thompson, D. The causal role of breakfast in energy balance and health: a randomized controlled trial in lean adults. *Am. J. Clin. Nutr.* **2014**, *100*, 539–547. [CrossRef]
14. Chowdhury, E.A.; Richardson, J.D.; Holman, G.D.; Tsintzas, K.; Thompson, D.; Betts, J.A. The causal role of breakfast in energy balance and health: A randomized controlled trial in obese adults. *Am. J. Clin. Nutr.* **2016**, *103*, 747–756. [CrossRef]
15. Dhurandhar, E.J.; Dawson, J.; Alcorn, A.; Larsen, L.H.; Thomas, E.A.; Cardel, M.; Bourland, A.C.; Astrup, A.; St-Onge, M.P.; Hill, J.O.; et al. The effectiveness of breakfast recommendations on weight loss: a randomized controlled trial. *Am. J. Clin. Nutr.* **2014**, *100*, 507–513. [CrossRef]
16. Amiel, S.A.; Sherwin, R.S.; Simonson, D.C.; Lauritano, A.A.; Tamborlane, W.V. Impaired insulin action in puberty. A contributing factor to poor glycemic control in adolescents with diabetes. *N. Engl. J. Med.* **1986**, *315*, 215–219. [CrossRef]
17. Hannon, T.S.; Janosky, J.; Arslanian, S.A. Longitudinal study of physiologic insulin resistance and metabolic changes of puberty. *Pediatr. Res.* **2006**, *60*, 759–763. [CrossRef]
18. Crowley, S.J.; Acebo, C.; Carskadon, M.A. Sleep, circadian rhythms, and delayed phase in adolescence. *Sleep Med.* **2007**, *8*, 602–612. [CrossRef]
19. Jakubowicz, D.; Wainstein, J.; Landau, Z.; Raz, I.; Ahren, B.; Chapnik, N.; Ganz, T.; Menaged, M.; Barnea, M.; Bar-Dayan, Y. Influences of Breakfast on Clock Gene Expression and Postprandial Glycemia in Healthy Individuals and Individuals With Diabetes: A Randomized Clinical Trial. *Diabetes. Care* **2017**, *40*, 1573–1579. [CrossRef]
20. Zakrzewski, J.K.; Gillison, F.B.; Cumming, S.; Church, T.S.; Katzmarzyk, P.T.; Broyles, S.T.; Champagne, C.M.; Chaput, J.P.; Denstel, K.D.; Fogelholm, M.; et al. Associations between breakfast frequency and adiposity indicators in children from 12 countries. *Int. J. Obes. Suppl.* **2015**, *5*, S80–S88. [CrossRef] [PubMed]
21. Blondin, S.A.; Anzman-Frasca, S.; Djang, H.C.; Economos, C.D. Breakfast consumption and adiposity among children and adolescents: An updated review of the literature. *Pediatr. Obes.* **2016**. [CrossRef] [PubMed]

22. Chin, Y.S.; Mohd Nasir, M.T. Eating Behaviors among Female Adolescents in Kuantan District, Pahang, Malaysia. *Pak. J. Nutr.* **2009**, *8*, 425–432. [CrossRef]
23. Koo, H.-C.; Abdul Jalil, S.N.; Ruzita, A.T. Breakfast Eating Pattern and Ready-to-Eat Cereals Consumption among Schoolchildren in Kuala Lumpur. *Malays. J. Med. Sci.* **2015**, *22*, 32–39.
24. Law, L.S.; Mohd-Nasir, M.T.; Hazizi, A.S. Factors associated with breakfast skipping among school going adolescents in Sarawak, Malaysia. *Malays. J. Nutr.* **2013**, *19*, 401–407.
25. Ming, F.M.; Ying, G.C.; Kassim, S.Z.M. Eating patterns of school children and adolescent in Kuala Lumpur. *Malays. J. Nutr.* **2006**, *12*, 1–10.
26. Nurul-Fadhilah, A.; Teo, P.S.; Huybrechts, I.; Foo, L.H. Infrequent breakfast consumption is associated with higher body adiposity and abdominal obesity in Malaysian school-aged adolescents. *PLoS ONE* **2013**, *8*, e59297. [CrossRef]
27. Abdelaal, M.; le Roux, C.W.; Docherty, N.G. Morbidity and mortality associated with obesity. *Ann. Transl. Med.* **2017**, *5*, 161. [CrossRef] [PubMed]
28. Donin, A.S.; Nightingale, C.M.; Owen, C.G.; Rudnicka, A.R.; Perkin, M.R.; Jebb, S.A.; Stephen, A.M.; Sattar, N.; Cook, D.G.; Whincup, P.H. Regular Breakfast Consumption and Type 2 Diabetes Risk Markers in 9- to 10-Year-Old Children in the Child Heart and Health Study in England (CHASE): A Cross-Sectional Analysis. *PLoS Med.* **2014**, *11*, e1001703. [CrossRef] [PubMed]
29. Hallström, L.; Labayen, I.; Ruiz, J.R.; Patterson, E.; Vereecken, C.A.; Breidenassel, C.; Gottrand, F.; Huybrechts, I.; Manios, Y.; Mistura, L.; et al. Breakfast consumption and CVD risk factors in European adolescents: the HELENA (Healthy Lifestyle in Europe by Nutrition in Adolescence) Study. *Publi. Health Nutr.* **2013**, 1296–1305. [CrossRef]
30. Marlatt, K.L.; Farbakhsh, K.; Dengel, D.R.; Lytle, L.A. Breakfast and fast food consumption are associated with selected biomarkers in adolescents. *Prev. Med. Rep.* **2016**, *3*, 49–52. [CrossRef]
31. Jaaskelainen, A.; Schwab, U.; Kolehmainen, M.; Pirkola, J.; Jarvelin, M.R.; Laitinen, J. Associations of meal frequency and breakfast with obesity and metabolic syndrome traits in adolescents of Northern Finland Birth Cohort 1986. *Nutr. Metab. Cardiovasc. Dis.* **2013**, *23*, 1002–1009. [CrossRef]
32. Ho, C.-Y.; Huang, Y.-C.; Lo, Y.-T.C.; Wahlqvist, M.L.; Lee, M.-S. Breakfast is associated with the metabolic syndrome and school performance among Taiwanese children. *Res. Dev. Dis.* **2015**, *43*, 179–188. [CrossRef]
33. Yoshinaga, M.; Hatake, S.; Tachikawa, T.; Shinomiya, M.; Miyazaki, A.; Takahashi, H. Impact of Lifestyles of Adolescents and Their Parents on Cardiovascular Risk Factors in Adolescents. *J. Atheroscler. Thromb.* **2011**, *18*, 981–990. [CrossRef] [PubMed]
34. Ahadi, Z.; Qorbani, M.; Kelishadi, R.; Ardalan, G.; Motlagh, M.E.; Asayesh, H.; Zeynali, M.; Chinian, M.; Larijani, B.; Shafiee, G.; et al. Association between breakfast intake with anthropometric measurements, blood pressure and food consumption behaviors among Iranian children and adolescents: The CASPIAN-IV study. *Publ. Health* **2015**, *129*, 740–747. [CrossRef] [PubMed]
35. Smith, K.J.; Gall, S.L.; McNaughton, S.A.; Blizzard, L.; Dwyer, T.; Venn, A.J. Skipping breakfast: longitudinal associations with cardiometabolic risk factors in the Childhood Determinants of Adult Health Study. *Am. J. Clin. Nutr.* **2010**, *92*, 1316–1325. [CrossRef]
36. Wennberg, M.; Gustafsson, P.E.; Wennberg, P.; Hammarstrom, A. Poor breakfast habits in adolescence predict the metabolic syndrome in adulthood. *Publ. Health Nutr.* **2015**, *18*, 122–129. [CrossRef]
37. Brion, M.J.; Lawlor, D.A.; Matijasevich, A.; Horta, B.; Anselmi, L.; Araujo, C.L.; Menezes, A.M.; Victora, C.G.; Smith, G.D. What are the causal effects of breastfeeding on IQ, obesity and blood pressure? Evidence from comparing high-income with middle-income cohorts. *Int. J. Epidemiol.* **2011**, *40*, 670–680. [CrossRef]
38. Hazreen, M.A.; Su, T.T.; Jalaludin, M.Y.; Dahlui, M.; Chinna, K.; Ismail, M.; Murray, L.; Cantwell, M.; Al Sadat, N.; MyHe, A.R.T.S.G. An exploratory study on risk factors for chronic non-communicable diseases among adolescents in Malaysia: overview of the Malaysian Health and Adolescents Longitudinal Research Team study (The MyHeART study). *BMC Publ. Health.* **2014**, *14*, S6. [CrossRef]
39. Nutritient Composition of Malaysian Foods. Available online: http://www.nutriscene.org.my/books/Tee%20et%20al%201997%20-%20Nutr%20Comp%20of%20Malaysian%20Foods.pdf (accessed on 26 April 2019).
40. Mohd Yusoff, N.A.; Safii, N.A.; Ghazali, R.; Ahmed, R.; Shahar, S. *Atlas of Food Exchanges and Portion Sizes*, 2nd ed.; MDC Publisher Sdn Bhd: Kuala Lumpur, Malaysia, 2009.

41. Abdul Majid, H.; Ramli, L.; Ying, S.P.; Su, T.T.; Jalaludin, M.Y.; Abdul Mohsein, N.A. Dietary Intake among Adolescents in a Middle-Income Country: An Outcome from the Malaysian Health and Adolescents Longitudinal Research Team Study (the MyHeARTs Study). *PLoS ONE* **2016**, *11*, e0155447. [CrossRef]
42. Johnson, L.; Toumpakari, Z.; Papadaki, A. Social Gradients and Physical Activity Trends in an Obesogenic Dietary Pattern: Cross-Sectional Analysis of the UK National Diet and Nutrition Survey 2008–2014. **2018**, *10*, 388. [CrossRef]
43. Timlin, M.T.; Pereira, M.A.; Story, M.; Neumark-Sztainer, D. Breakfast Eating and Weight Change in a 5-Year Prospective Analysis of Adolescents: Project EAT (Eating Among Teens). *Pediatrics* **2008**, *121*, e638–e645. [CrossRef]
44. O'Neil, C.E.; Byrd-Bredbenner, C.; Hayes, D.; Jana, L.; Klinger, S.E.; Stephenson-Martin, S. The Role of Breakfast in Health: Definition and Criteria for a Quality Breakfast. *J. Acad. Nutr. Diet.* **2014**, *114*, S8–S26. [CrossRef]
45. Soran, H.; Dent, R.; Durrington, P. Evidence-based goals in LDL-C reduction. *Clin. Res. Cardiol.* **2017**, *106*, 237–248. [CrossRef]
46. Shafiee, G.; Kelishadi, R.; Qorbani, M.; Motlagh, M.E.; Taheri, M.; Ardalan, G.; Taslimi, M.; Poursafa, P.; Heshmat, R.; Larijani, B. Association of breakfast intake with cardiometabolic risk factors. *J. Pediatr. (Rio. J.)* **2013**, *89*, 575–582. [CrossRef]
47. Marz, W.; Kleber, M.E.; Scharnagl, H.; Speer, T.; Zewinger, S.; Ritsch, A.; Parhofer, K.G.; von Eckardstein, A.; Landmesser, U.; Laufs, U. HDL cholesterol: reappraisal of its clinical relevance. *Clin. Res. Cardiol.* **2017**, *106*, 663–675. [CrossRef] [PubMed]
48. Silva, F.A.; Padez, C.; Sartorelli, D.S.; Oliveira, R.M.S.; Netto, M.P.; Mendes, L.L.; Candido, A.P.C. Cross-sectional study showed that breakfast consumption was associated with demographic, clinical and biochemical factors in children and adolescents. *Acta. Paediatr.* **2018**. [CrossRef] [PubMed]
49. Farshchi, H.R.; Taylor, M.A.; Macdonald, I.A. Regular meal frequency creates more appropriate insulin sensitivity and lipid profiles compared with irregular meal frequency in healthy lean women. *Eur. J. Clin. Nutr.* **2004**, *58*, 1071–1077. [CrossRef] [PubMed]
50. Ramirez-Lopez, E.; Grijalva-Haro, M.I.; Valencia, M.E.; Antonio Ponce, J.; Artalejo, E. Effect of a School Breakfast Program on the prevalence of obesity and cardiovascular risk factors in children. *Salud Publica Mex* **2005**, *47*, 126–133.
51. Dialektakou, K.D.; Vranas, P.B. Breakfast skipping and body mass index among adolescents in Greece: Whether an association exists depends on how breakfast skipping is defined. *J. Am. Diet. Assoc.* **2008**, *108*, 1517–1525. [CrossRef]
52. Bayham, B.E.; Greenway, F.L.; Johnson, W.D.; Dhurandhar, N.V. A randomized trial to manipulate the quality instead of quantity of dietary proteins to influence the markers of satiety. *J. Diabetes Complic.* **2014**, *28*, 547–552. [CrossRef]
53. Rebello, C.J.; Johnson, W.D.; Martin, C.K.; Xie, W.; O'Shea, M.; Kurilich, A.; Bordenave, N.; Andler, S.; Klinken, B.J.W.v.; Chu, Y.-F.; et al. Acute Effect of Oatmeal on Subjective Measures of Appetite and Satiety Compared to a Ready-to-Eat Breakfast Cereal: A Randomized Crossover Trial. *J. Am. Coll. Nutr.* **2013**, *32*, 272–279. [CrossRef] [PubMed]
54. Alexy, U.; Wicher, M.; Kersting, M. Breakfast trends in children and adolescents: frequency and quality. *Publ. Health Nutr.* **2010**, *13*, 1795–1802. [CrossRef] [PubMed]
55. Randler, C. Association between morningness-eveningness and mental and physical health in adolescents. *Psychol. Health Med.* **2011**, *16*, 29–38. [CrossRef]
56. Scheer, F.A.; Hilton, M.F.; Mantzoros, C.S.; Shea, S.A. Adverse metabolic and cardiovascular consequences of circadian misalignment. *Proc. Natl. Acad. Sci. USA* **2009**, *106*, 4453–4458. [CrossRef]
57. Kong, A.P.; Wing, Y.K.; Choi, K.C.; Li, A.M.; Ko, G.T.; Ma, R.C.; Tong, P.C.; Ho, C.S.; Chan, M.H.; Ng, M.H.; et al. Associations of sleep duration with obesity and serum lipid profile in children and adolescents. *Sleep Med.* **2011**, *12*, 659–665. [CrossRef] [PubMed]
58. Van Cauter, E.; Polonsky, K.S.; Scheen, A.J. Roles of circadian rhythmicity and sleep in human glucose regulation. *Endocr. Rev.* **1997**, *18*, 716–738. [CrossRef] [PubMed]
59. Mendoza, J. Circadian clocks: Setting time by food. *J. Neuroendocrinol.* **2007**, *19*, 127–137. [CrossRef] [PubMed]

60. Qian, J.; Scheer, F. Circadian System and Glucose Metabolism: Implications for Physiology and Disease. *Trends. Endocrinol. Metab.* **2016**, *27*, 282–293. [CrossRef] [PubMed]
61. Woolhead, C.; Gibney, M.J.; Walsh, M.C.; Brennan, L.; Gibney, E.R. A generic coding approach for the examination of meal patterns. *Am. J. Clin. Nutr.* **2015**, *102*, 316–323. [CrossRef]
62. Murakami, K.; Livingstone, M.B.E.; Sasaki, S. Establishment of a Meal Coding System for the Characterization of Meal-Based Dietary Patterns in Japan. *J. Nutr.* **2017**, *147*, 2093–2101. [CrossRef] [PubMed]
63. Johnson, L.; Mander, A.P.; Jones, L.R.; Emmett, P.M.; Jebb, S.A. Energy-dense, low-fiber, high-fat dietary pattern is associated with increased fatness in childhood. *Am. J. Clin. Nutr.* **2008**, *87*, 846–854. [CrossRef] [PubMed]
64. Matthys, C.; De Henauw, S.; Bellemans, M.; De Maeyer, M.; De Backer, G. Breakfast habits affect overall nutrient profiles in adolescents. *Publ. Health Nutr.* **2007**, *10*, 413–421. [CrossRef] [PubMed]
65. Berkey, C.S.; Rockett, H.R.; Gillman, M.W.; Field, A.E.; Colditz, G.A. Longitudinal study of skipping breakfast and weight change in adolescents. *Int. J. Obes. Relat. Metab. Disord.* **2003**, *27*, 1258–1266. [CrossRef] [PubMed]

9

Interventions Aimed at Increasing Dairy and/or Calcium Consumption of Preschool-Aged Children

Victoria Srbely [1], Imtisal Janjua [2], Andrea C. Buchholz [3] and Genevieve Newton [1,*]

[1] Department of Human Health & Nutritional Science, University of Guelph, Guelph, ON N1G2W1, Canada; vsrbely@uoguelph.ca

[2] Department of Biomedical Sciences, University of Guelph, Guelph, ON N1G2W1, Canada; ijanjua@uoguelph.ca

[3] Department of Family Relations and Applied Nutrition, University of Guelph, Guelph, ON N1G2W1, Canada; abuchhol@uoguelph.ca

* Correspondence: newton@uoguelph.ca

Abstract: Dairy product consumption is important during childhood, as dairy products provide nutrients to support growth and development. However, a high proportion of children globally are not meeting recommended daily intakes, which may have long-term health implications. Accumulating evidence suggests that interventions aimed at instilling healthy lifestyle habits are most effective when initiated during the preschool years. Therefore, the purpose of the review was to identify the characteristics of effective dairy and/or calcium interventions targeting preschool-aged children. A systematic literature review identified 14 intervention studies published between 1998–2018 addressing dairy/calcium intakes in the preschool population (1.5 to 5 years). Intervention reporting was assessed using intervention intensity, behavior change techniques and Workgroup for Intervention Development and Evaluation Research (WIDER), with the quality of studies evaluated using risk of bias and Grades of Recommendation, Assessment, Development and Evaluation (GRADE). Five of the 14 studies included in the review reported significant improvements in children's dairy (4/5) or calcium (1/5) intake. Characteristics that may enable intervention effectiveness include the delivery of interventions in one setting (preschool facility), using specific behavior change techniques (environmental restructuring and teach to use prompts/cues), and targeting both parent and child. Overall, the interventions assessed demonstrated variable success and highlighted the need for developing effective interventions designed to increase dairy and/or calcium intakes in preschool-aged children.

Keywords: intervention; nutrition; preschool; child; parent; dairy; calcium

1. Introduction

Consumption of dairy products is an important determinant of childhood health and development [1]. Dairy products such as milk, yogurt, and cheese have a rich nutrient profile which includes both macronutrients and micro-nutrients (calcium, vitamin D) that support the optimization and maintenance of good health [2]. Despite the importance of dairy consumption, studies have demonstrated that a significant number of North American children are not meeting recommended intakes, as based on the 2018 Canadian Food Guide [3]. In Canada, 37% of children aged four to nine years do not consume the recommended number of servings of milk and alternatives [3]. Furthermore, between 1977–2001, the proportion of children aged two to 18 years in the United States (U.S.) consuming milk decreased from 94% to 84%, the number of servings consumed decreased from 3.5 to

2.8/day, and the portion size of each serving decreased from 460 to 410 mL [4]. Similar findings have been reported in Europe. For example, the Individuelle Nationale sur les Consommations Alimentaires study conducted in France between 1999–2007 reported a decrease in milk and cheese consumption of 10% and 12%, respectively, in children aged 3 to 10 years old [5]. The Dortmund Nutritional and Anthropometric Longitudinally Designed Study (1986–2001) comprised of German children between the ages of 1–13 years old further demonstrated the global decline in dairy consumption by also reporting a negative trend in milk consumption (−6.5 g/day/study year for children aged 1 to 3; −2.8 to −7.4 g/day/study year for children aged 4 to 13) [5]. A decline in dairy intake from early childhood may have important implications on bone health [6], as well as on the risk of developing a number of costly chronic health conditions such as obesity [7,8], type 2 diabetes [9,10], hypertension [9], and colorectal cancer [11].

Accumulating evidence strongly suggests that interventions aiming to instill healthy lifestyle habits and prevent chronic diseases are most effective when initiated during preschool (≤5 y), as compared to school-age (>5 y) years [12]. For example, Skinner et al. found that the consumption of fruits among school-aged children was predicted by exposure to and consumption of a variety of fruits during preschool years [13]. Marshall et al. (2005) similarly reported that the intake of carbonated beverages, juice drinks, and sugar-sweetened beverages was inversely associated with milk intake in a study of 645 children aged 1 to 5, suggesting the displacement of milk by other beverages [14]. This displacement has potentially significant health consequences, as reported by Dubois et al. (2007), who found that 15.4% of preschoolers in the Québec Longitudinal Study of Child Development who were regular consumers of sugar-sweetened beverages were overweight at 4.5 years of age, as compared to only 6.9% of non-consumers [15]. Furthermore, U.S. data suggest that for each 30-mL reduction in milk consumption by children aged five to 18 years, sugar-sweetened beverage consumption increases by 126 mL, resulting in a net increase of 31 kcal and a loss of 34 mg of calcium for each 30 mL of milk displaced [16]. Collectively, these findings reinforce the need to investigate factors influencing children's dairy intakes during preschool years. Previously published systematic literature reviews have investigated the effects of dietary interventions aiming to increase dairy consumption; however, they targeted children aged 5 to 12 [17] and adolescents aged ≥12 to ≤18 [18], so there is a gap in knowledge regarding dairy intakes in the preschool population.

Enhancing dairy and calcium intake in preschool children is potentially an important step in optimizing children's bone health [6] and mitigating other long-term health consequences associated with insufficient intake. Therefore, the objective of this systematic literature review was to identify the characteristics that constitute effective dairy and/or calcium interventions targeting preschool-aged children. The results of this review will inform the development of future dairy/calcium intervention studies and public health education efforts.

2. Materials and Methods

2.1. Search Method

A list of search terms and keywords were adopted from recent and relevant reviews [17,18], and modified with assistance from an open education resources librarian. The search terms were comprehensive and inclusive, highlighting dairy and/or calcium consumption in preschool-aged children. The search terms were categorized under four headings:

1. Interventions (e.g., intervention, clinical trial, experimental studies)
2. Nutrition (e.g., diet, food, beverage)

3. Population (e.g., preschool, toddler and parent, family)
4. Dairy/Calcium (e.g., yogurt, dairy, milk).

The databases searched included ProQuest, Web of Science, Cochrane Database, Cumulative Index to Nursing and Allied Health Literature, CAB Direct, and PsycINFO. Varying combinations of search terms and keywords were applied to each of the six databases searched (see Supplementary Materials). This allowed for Medical Subject Headings (MeSH) terms to be used along with keywords, where permitted. The final literature search was conducted on 14 June 2018. It included all papers published between 1998–2018, and was restricted to English publications. Grey literature and reference lists of review papers were searched for additional intervention studies focused on dairy consumption. All of the study protocols were registered on 17 July 2018 in PROSPERO (international database of prospectively registered systematic reviews) under the study identification code CRD42018099909.

2.2. *Inclusion Criteria*

Inclusion criteria limited the selection of studies to: (i) intervention studies with or without control groups, (ii) intervention studies modifying dietary intakes (specifically including dairy and/or calcium intake as a measurement), (iii) the primary or secondary aim of the study being an increase in dairy and/or calcium consumption in preschool-aged children (1.5 to 5 years), including any studies that targeted families (parents and/or children), schools, and/or early education centers, and (iv) intervention studies reporting changes in dairy and/or calcium intakes at either the individual and/or group level.

2.3. *Exclusion Criteria*

Exclusion criteria included: (i) studies targeting clinical populations (i.e., obese or lactose intolerant groups), (ii) case studies, (iii) studies focused on breast-feeding, allergies, or calcium supplementation, (iv) studies aimed at changing the type of dairy consumption (i.e., regular-fat dairy to low-fat dairy, but not total dairy), (v) publications older than 20 years (i.e., published prior to 1998), and (vi) non-English publications.

2.4. *Data Extraction and Synthesis*

The Preferred Reporting Items for Systematic Reviews and Meta-Analyses (PRISMA) diagram summarizing the search outcomes is presented in Figure 1. A total of 7178 records were screened (7176 records identified through database searching, two records [19,20] identified through grey literature searching), with 138 articles assessed in full-text based on the specified inclusion and exclusion criteria. A total of 124 articles were excluded based on a lack of access to full-text English publication ($n = 18$), incorrect age range ($n = 38$), not aiming to increase the consumption of dairy and/or calcium ($n = 23$), aiming to change the type of dairy consumption ($n = 16$), focusing on dairy and/or calcium supplementation ($n = 6$), being a case study ($n = 1$), or no intervention ($n = 22$). A total of 14 intervention studies were included in the final analysis.

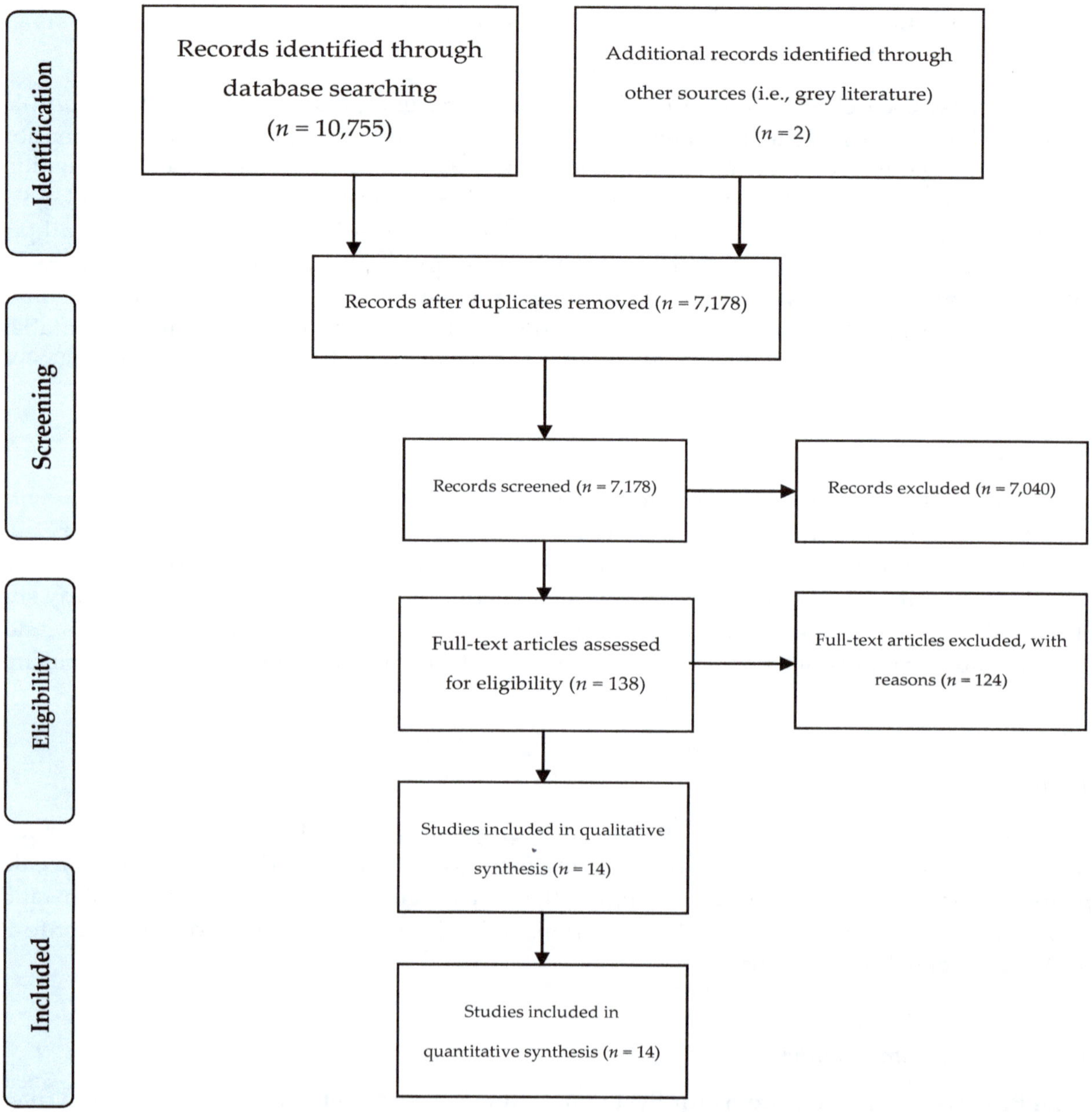

Figure 1. Preferred Reporting Items for Systematic Reviews and Meta-Analyses (PRISMA) four-phase flow diagram of the literature search results. From: Moher, D.; Liberati, A.; Tetzlaff, J.; Altman, D.G.; The PRISMA Group. Preferred reporting items for systematic reviews and meta-analyses: The PRISMA statement. *PLoS Med.* **2009**, *6*, e1000097, doi:10.1371/journal.pmed1000097 [21]. For more information, visit www.prisma-statement.org.

Two independent reviewers (VS, IJ) extracted data from the studies, including the author name and date, population characteristics, description of the intervention, relevant outcome measures, effect size, and effectiveness of the intervention (Table 1). Five assessment tools, including (1) Intervention Intensity Analysis, (2) Coventry, Aberdeen, and London—Refined Taxonomy of Behavior Change Techniques, (3) Workgroup for Intervention Development and Evaluation Research Recommendations, (4) Cochrane Collaboration Risk of Bias Tool, and (5) Grades of Recommendation, Assessment, Development and Evaluation were used to evaluate all of the intervention studies included in the analysis. The five assessment tools are described below.

Table 1. Dairy and calcium intervention studies targeting preschool-aged children: study data extraction table with effect size (*d*) and intervention effectiveness.

Study	Population	Description of Intervention (I = Intervention, C = Control)	Outcome Measure (s)	Intervention Outcome Measurement (s)	Effect Size (*d*)	Effective (Y/N) [1]
Akil (2013) [22]	Parents or caregivers of children aged 3 to 5 (*n* = 140)	I: Parents/caregivers and child followed ordinary HeadStart nutrition curriculum and participated in a nutrition education program (i.e., cooking classes, weekly nutrition newsletters) C: Parents/caregivers and children followed ordinary HeadStart nutrition curriculum	Daily number of servings of food groups (i.e., dairy, fruits, and vegetables)	N/A. Study does not report pre/post-intervention consumption.	ND [2]	N
Bender et al. (2013) [23]	Low income Hispanic mothers (18–35 years old) with children aged 3 to 5 (*n* = 33)	I: Two-phase intervention program; phase I included four biweekly interactive nutrition group lessons, and phase II included six monthly group community activities to reinforce target health behaviors (i.e., nutrition cooking classes)	Beverage (i.e., fruit juice, milk) serving size(s) and number of servings/day	Children's baseline milk consumption in ounces per day (mean (SD)): 14.3 (0.96) Post-intervention milk consumption in ounces per day (mean (SD)): 16.8 (2.1)	ND	N
Cason (2001) [19]	Children aged 3 to 5 (male = 2990, female = 3112)	I: Children participated in a multiple intelligences theory-based nutrition education curriculum (i.e., nutrition education lessons, food tasting)	Daily number of food group servings (i.e., meat, dairy, fruit)	Reported difference in daily servings of dairy in children as mean (SD). Pre-intervention was 0.99 (1.32) and post-intervention was 2.36 (1.54).	ND	Y
Harvey (2008) [24]	Low-income African-American and Hispanic parents (*n* = 25) Children aged 3 to 5 (female = 13, male = 12)	I: Parents participated in a weekly nutrition education intervention; they received weekly nutrition newsletters and tracked child daily dietary servings using a kid calendar	Weekly servings for dietary components (i.e., dairy, fruits, vegetables)	Reported changes in weekly servings of low-fat dairy as mean (SD). Baseline measure was 12.44 (7.10) and week 4 post-intervention was 18.04 (7.55).	ND	Y
Kopetsky (2017) [25]	Parent/caregiver (female = 7) Children aged 3 to 5 (male = 3, female = 3)	I: Parent and child attended five, 45-min nutrition education sessions on behavioral strategies (self-monitoring, parental modeling), attended education sessions on MyPlate food groups, and received weekly recipes in the mail C: Parent and child received weekly recipes in the mail	Dietary quality as measured by the Healthy Eating Index (HEI), 2010	HEI 2010 scores quality of dairy in the diet out of 10 points. Baseline and week 5 for dairy consumption (mean (SD)): Baseline: 8.2 (2.5) Week 5: 8.9 (2.0)	0.04	N

Table 1. *Cont.*

Study	Population	Description of Intervention (I = Intervention, C = Control)	Outcome Measure (s)	Intervention Outcome Measurement (s)	Effect Size (d)	Effective (Y/N) [1]
Korwanich et al. (2008) [26]	Parents (n = 219)	I: Nursery schools had implemented a newly developed healthy eating policy (i.e., advising on snack and beverage consumption at school, children engaged in nutrition education activities)	Frequency of dietary intakes per day (i.e., non-sugar milk, fresh fruit)	Frequency of non-sugar milk consumption within groups (mean (SD)). Baseline in intervention group was 0.94 (0.2) and post-intervention was 0.97 (0.2).	0.17	N
	Children aged 4 to 5 years (male = 111, female = 108)	C: No action provided in control schools				
Marquis et al. (2014) [27]	Parent/caregiver (n = 201)	I: Parents/caregivers attended weekly meetings for loan payments, entrepreneurship training, and nutrition education on child feeding practices	Frequency of dietary intakes per week (i.e., milk and milk products)	N/A. Study does not report pre/post-intervention consumption.	ND	Y
		C: Parents/caregivers received health education talks				
Munday et al. (2017) [28]	Parents/caregivers (n = 16) Children aged 3 to 5 (male = 13, female = 4)	I: Children participated in nutrition education sessions, food tasting sessions, sticker reward charts, kindergarten vegetable plots; parents/caregivers participated in cooking classes	Nutrient intake per day (i.e., calcium)	Reported calcium intakes as mean (SD). Baseline intake was 526 (198.4) and post-intervention was 608 (196.2).	ND	Y
O'Sullivan et al. (2016) [29]	Mothers of children aged 3 to 5 (n = 149)	I: Mothers received a community-based home visiting program (i.e., provided information and instruction on parenting practice, emotional support, and access to community services), participated in the Triple P Positive Parenting Program, received child developmental materials and book packs, and were encouraged to attend healthy eating workshops	Proportion of participants meeting daily recommendations (i.e., dairy)	Intakes reported as proportion of participants in the intervention group meeting daily dairy recommendations (mean (SD)). Proportions at each of 18, 24, and 36 months were 0.74 (±0.44), 0.64 (±0.48), and 0.66 (±0.48), respectively.	1.16 to 1.94	N
	Children aged 3 to 5 (n = 149)	C: Mothers received child developmental materials and book packs, and were encouraged to attend healthy eating workshops				

Table 1. *Cont.*

Study	Population	Description of Intervention (I = Intervention, C = Control)	Outcome Measure (s)	Intervention Outcome Measurement (s)	Effect Size (*d*)	Effective (Y/N) [1]
Roberts-Gray et al. (2016) [30]	Parent–child dyads (n = 608)	I: Parents received nutrition newsletters and participated in parent–child activity stations; children participated in parent–child activity stations and teacher–child classroom activities; nutrition workshops implemented at the organizational level	Number of dairy servings per day	Number of dairy servings per day (mean (SD)): pre-intervention 0.73 (0.7) and post-intervention 0.79 (0.07).	0.86	N
		C: No action provided in control schools				
Salehi et al. (2004) [31]	Parents or caregivers of children <5 years of age	I: Parents/caregivers were exposed to an educational program (i.e., educated on concepts of "food pyramid", taught daily requirements for milk and yogurt intakes)	Quantity of milk consumed (grams)	Reported quantity (g) of milk consumption at beginning of program compared to end. Beginning milk quantity (g) reported as mean (SD) was 50 (13.2), and end was 60 (9.5).	ND	N/A
	Children aged 3 to 5 (n = 811)	C: No action provided in control sub-tribes				
Schwartz et al. (2015) [32]	Children aged 3 to 5 (male = 40, female = 45)	I: Children were exposed to one of two feeding practices: (1) fruits, vegetables, and milk were served before the main meal (first course), and (2) fruits, vegetables, and milk were served before the main meal, and meats and grains were removed from the table after the first serving (combination)	Number of Child and Adult Care Food Program (CACFP) servings consumed per meal per day (i.e., milk)	N/A. Not reported as overall pre/post-test consumption.	−0.09 to 0.64	Y
Seward et al. (2018) [20]	Long day childcare services (n = 44)	I: Services were provided to staff, including training, receiving a resource pack to support the implementation of nutrition guidelines, having a dietitian complete an audit of the two-week menus, and being allocated an implementation support officer to provide advice and assistance	Number of dietary servings per day (i.e., dairy)	Reported as mean number of daily dairy servings consumed by children as mean (SD). Baseline was 0.55 (0.23) and post-intervention was 1.03 (0.57).	0.03	N
	Children aged 3 to 5 (n = 243)	C: Services posted a hard copy of the Caring for Children resource and received regular care from the local health district health promotion staff				

Table 1. *Cont.*

Study	Population	Description of Intervention (I = Intervention, C = Control)	Outcome Measure (s)	Intervention Outcome Measurement (s)	Effect Size (d)	Effective (Y/N) [1]
Vereecken et al. (2009) [33]	Parents (mother = 189, father = 11)	I: Children participated in guided and self-guided nutrition activities, were given feedback and reinforcement from teachers, and had access to cooking equipment and healthy foods; parents received nutrition newsletters, engaged in nutrition activities with children, and attended school activities with other parents	Average daily consumption of milk products (mL)	Reported changes in milk intakes in mL. Pre-intervention was 176 mL, and post-intervention was 153 mL. No SD reported.	−2.17	N
	Children aged 3 to 5 (male = 239, female = 237)	C: No action provided in control schools				

[1] Intervention effectiveness is defined as a statistically significant increase ($p < 0.05$) in a dairy or calcium outcome. [2] Abbreviation: ND, no data or not enough data available to calculate effect size.

2.5. Intervention Reporting

2.5.1. Intervention Intensity

Intervention intensity scales have been employed in scientific literature to enhance comparisons of interventions between studies [17]. An intervention intensity scale is a point-scale assessment tool that evaluates the characteristics and degree of an intervention [17]. The intensity score ranks the qualities of each individual intervention as high, medium, or low intensity, facilitating straightforward comparisons of different study designs and/or intervention settings [17].

The intervention intensity scale used was adapted from a recent review [18], assessing four characteristics of interventions on a 5-point ranking scale (1 = low, 2 = low-medium, 3 = medium, 4 = medium–high, and 5 = high), with the exception of "reach of the intervention strategies" [34]. The four characteristics are detailed below:

(1) *Duration of the intervention.* This category ranked the length of the intervention using the following scale: 1 = ≤6 weeks, 2 = 6 to 11 weeks, 3 = 12 weeks to 5 months, 4 = 6 to 12 months, and 5 = ≥12 months.

(2) *Frequency of contact with the intervention.* This characteristic assessed the frequency of contact between participants and the intervention. If the intervention employed multiple points of contact, an average contact score was computed. If the frequency of contact was not clearly stated by authors, the points of contact were divided by the overall duration of the intervention to determine an average frequency of contact. The ranking score that was used for frequency of contact with the intervention was 1 = annually, 2 = bimonthly to quarterly, 3 = monthly, 3.5 = twice a month, 4 = weekly, 4.5 = multiple times per week, and 5 = daily.

(3) *Level of personalization.* This characteristic describes the type and/or level of contact with the intervention. The ranking score used for the level of personalization included: 1 = environmental, 2 = group (parent or child), 2.5 = group (parent and child), 3 = environmental and group (parent or child), 3.5 = environmental and group (parent and child), 4 = group with an individual component (parent or child), 4.5 = group with an individual component (parent and child), and 5 = individual (parent and/or child) or individual, environmental, and group (parent and/or child). If the parent and child experienced different levels of personalization, they were scored independently, and the scores were averaged for a total personalization score out of 5. The more personalized the contact of the intervention, the higher the intensity score.

(4) *Reach of the intervention strategies.* This characteristic assessed the number of different settings (i.e., home, school) used by the researchers to reach their target audience, and used a scale where 1 = one setting, 3 = two settings, and 5 = three or more settings. The greater number of settings used with the intervention, the higher the intensity of the intervention.

The two reviewers (VS, IJ) scored the characteristics and provided an overall intervention intensity score for each intervention included in the analysis. The overall intensity score was the sum of the scores of the four characteristics, giving a total score out of 20. An overall intervention intensity score of greater than or equal to 13.5 was considered a high-intensity intervention, between 10.51–13.49 was rated as medium intensity, and a score of 10.5 or less indicated a low-intensity intervention.

2.5.2. Behavior Change Techniques

Michie et al. (2011) published the Coventry, Aberdeen, and London-Refined (CALO-RE) Taxonomy of Behavior Change Techniques to be used in assessment of interventions targeting healthy eating and physical activity [35]. The refined taxonomy published by Michie et al. (2011) was adopted from the taxonomy of theory-linked behavior change techniques developed by Abraham and Michie (2008) [36], which identified specific behavior change techniques in interventions that enabled effectiveness. The twofold rationale for the use of the CALO-RE Taxonomy is based on determining whether the differences in behavior change techniques observed across studies impacted the effectiveness of each intervention, and secondly, identifying which techniques affected the most significant behavioral change [36].

The CALO-RE Taxonomy provides a behavior change taxonomy of 40 items, which are defined in Supplementary Materials Table S1. Two independent reviewers (VS, IJ) evaluated the behavior change techniques applied in the intervention studies and resolved any discrepancies through discussion. Behavior change techniques three, six, 11, 12, 14, 17, 18, 31, 32, 33, 34, 37, and 40 were excluded from analysis, as these techniques were not employed in any of the interventions assessed.

2.5.3. WIDER Recommendations

The Workgroup for Intervention Development and Evaluation Research (WIDER) [37] developed a framework to assess and report the components of behavior change intervention studies, recommending a set of four criteria by which to evaluate techniques employed in behavior change interventions. The WIDER recommendations were developed to compare behavior change interventions across heterogeneous studies, with the goal of ensuring clarity in reporting of the components of behavior change techniques to ultimately improve the reproducibility of current intervention methods. The description of the four criteria of the WIDER recommendations are outlined in Supplementary Materials Table S2 and detailed below:

(1) The first recommendation addresses the description of the intervention(s) and the level of detail reported by authors. There are eight supplementary recommendations required for discussion throughout the intervention study, including the characteristics of those delivering the intervention, characteristics of the recipients, setting, mode of intervention delivery, intensity, duration, adherence to delivery protocols, and a detailed description of the intervention content for each study group.
(2) The second recommendation addresses the change process employed in the intervention and the design of the intervention. This recommendation requires a description of how the intervention was developed, the behavior change techniques used in the intervention, and the behavioral processes being targeted by the change techniques.
(3) The third recommendation addresses the extent to which the intervention protocols and/or manuals are accessible, as authors must provide easy access to the protocols/manuals for the interventions as supplementary materials (i.e., online).
(4) The fourth recommendation assesses the control group and the control conditions. Authors must describe the characteristics of the interveners delivering the control, characteristics of the control participants, setting, mode of delivery, intensity, duration, compliance to the delivery protocols, and a detailed description of the control content.

Two reviewers (VS, IJ) independently assessed all of the intervention studies using the four WIDER recommendations, and reported whether each intervention satisfied all of the subcomponents of the recommendations [38].

2.6. *Quality Criteria*

2.6.1. Risk of Bias

The Cochrane Risk of Bias Tool [39] was used to evaluate six types of bias in the individual studies, including selection bias, performance bias, attrition bias, reporting bias, detection bias, and other bias. Within the six types of bias, seven domains exist that aid in assessing the risk of each type of bias:

(1) *Selection bias*: assessed two domains: sequence generation and allocation concealment
(2) *Performance bias*: assessed the blinding procedures implemented in the study
(3) *Detection bias*: assessed the adequacy of the blinding of outcome assessors
(4) *Attrition bias*: assessed all the participant withdrawal from the study that lead to incomplete outcome data

(5) *Reporting bias*: identified the selective reporting of results
(6) *Other bias*: identified any other sources of bias that may be present in the literature, owing to a variety of circumstances or events.

The two reviewers (VS, IJ) evaluated the level of bias within each category for each individual study by assigning a material risk of bias score (high, low, or unclear) for each of the above criteria, including supporting rationale for this score. Material bias is defined as bias significant enough to affect the results and/or conclusions of the study. Examples of criteria used to assess material bias are included in Supplementary Materials Table S3.

The support for the bias judgment is derived from the study and is highlighted by verbatim quotes from the publication, where possible. In this section, review authors may include personal comments and any relevant information supporting the rationale for their judgments. The ambiguity of information within the study can be addressed by indicating 'probably done' or 'probably not done' in addition to an explanation for why they believe so. Lastly, if the primary authors did not provide sufficient information to enable review authors to make clearly defined judgments, this should be clearly indicated.

2.6.2. GRADE

The Grades of Recommendation, Assessment, Development, and Evaluation (GRADE) [40] is a systematic approach that is used to assess the quality of evidence across studies and evaluate the strength of clinical recommendations. Prior to their assessment of the quality of evidence, review authors identify the clinical outcomes on which they will be focusing. If applicable, three items must be clearly defined for each outcome, including the number of studies addressing the specific outcome of interest, the treatment comparison, and the number of participants in each comparison. Then, the quality of evidence addressing the outcomes is evaluated based on the type of evidence provided, quality points, consistency, directness, and effect size.

Two independent reviewers (VS, IJ) used the GRADE criteria to evaluate the quality of evidence across studies. The five GRADE criteria outlined by the British Medical Journal (BMJ) (2012) [40] are detailed in Supplementary Materials Table S4 and summarized below:

(1) *Type of evidence.* Scientific evidence derived from randomized control trials begins at a rating of four points; in contrast, evidence from observational studies is assigned a rating of two.
(2) *Quality points.* A total of three points can be deducted under this category based on inadequacies in follow-up procedures, sparse data, blinding, allocation concealment, and attrition.
(3) *Consistency.* Heterogeneous studies are evaluated under this category, as long as they all address the same outcomes and interventions. A quality point is deducted under this category for inconsistent results between studies while, in contrast, a quality point is added if a dose-response effect is observed or if adjustment of confounders increased the effect size.
(4) *Directness.* A maximum of two points can be deducted for issues affecting the generalizability of the results to the population of interest. Examples of issues affecting directness include co-interventions that are being tested alongside the intervention of interest, as well as the use of samples that are either too broad or too restricted.
(5) *Effect Size.* The GRADE criteria add a quality point for an odds ratio (OR) or relative risk (RR) $\geq$2 and adds two quality points for an OR or RR $\geq$5. One quality point is added for effect sizes >2 (or <0.5), while two quality points are added for effect sizes that are >5 (or <0.2) and are all statistically significant. No quality points are added for effect sizes <2 or statistically insignificant results.

When calculating the final GRADE score for each outcome, a score of at least four points indicates a high quality of evidence, three points suggests a moderate quality of evidence, two points reflects a low quality of evidence, and a score of one or less represents a very low quality of evidence. GRADE scores for independent outcomes are presented in table format, where explanations for the scores and judgments about the quality of evidence are provided. The overall interpretation of the GRADE score does not reflect the methodological quality of a single piece of literature, but rather is a measure of the quality rating of the overall evidence across studies addressing a specific outcome within the target population.

3. Results

3.1. *Intervention Studies*

3.1.1. Study Description

The present review identified 14 intervention studies published between 1998–2018 that aimed to increase dairy and/or calcium consumption. Of the 14 intervention studies identified, seven (50%) targeted total dairy intake, six (43%) targeted total milk intake, and one (7%) targeted calcium intake; all did so as part of a larger dietary intervention. All of the intervention studies targeted children between the ages of 1.5–5 years, their parents, and/or teachers, as it was acknowledged that interventions may engage the child's caregiver(s), but not be applied to the preschool-aged child(ren). The search methods were exhaustive and retrieved studies conducted globally, allowing for a comprehensive analysis of interventions for populations with differing baselines and habitual dairy and/or calcium intake.

3.1.2. Effectiveness

Intervention effectiveness was determined as a statistically significant ($p < 0.05$) increase in dairy and/or calcium intake. Of the 14 interventions included in the review, five were effective, eight were ineffective, and one did not provide any information on the effectiveness of the intervention (Table 1). Of the five effective interventions, one targeted both parent and child, two targeted only the parent, and two targeted the child alone; importantly, both interventions targeting the child demonstrated effectiveness. The overall intervention effectiveness results reported in this review were lower than those of previously published systematic literature reviews [17,18].

One intervention [30] did not report a statistically significant change in dairy consumption from baseline to six-week post-intervention follow-up, but reported a statistically significant increase in dairy consumption using a treatment-by-time interaction model at 28 weeks post-intervention booster follow-up. (A booster in this context is a reintroduction of the intervention some time after the initial intervention has concluded; it is used to determine whether the behavior changes that were taught/implemented in the initial intervention were maintained over time).

3.1.3. Sample Size, Control Groups, Effect Size

The sample size of intervention studies ranged from very small groups of parents ($n = 7$) and children ($n = 6$) as presented in the study of Kopetsky (2017) [25], to large groups of children ($n = 3112$) enrolled in the Food and Nutrition Services Food Stamp Nutrition Education Program as studied by Cason (2001) [19]. In addition, four (29%) interventions did not have a control group, while only seven (50%) interventions included in the review provided adequate information to calculate effect size. The other 50% had insufficient data (i.e., did not have a control group), or did not provide the data in the correct format to enable effect size calculation.

3.2. *Intervention Intensity*

The summary of the intervention intensity rating categories associated with effectiveness and overall intervention intensity results are presented in Tables 2 and 3, respectively. In this review, three (23%) interventions were of low intensity, five (~38%) interventions were of medium intensity, and five (~38%) interventions were of high intensity. More than half (60%) of the medium-intensity interventions and 66.7% of the low-intensity interventions reported statistically significant ($p < 0.05$) increases in dairy and/or calcium intakes, whereas none of the high-intensity interventions were effective at increasing dairy and/or calcium consumption.

Table 2. Intervention characteristics and intensity rating categories associated with intervention effectiveness ($n = 13$).

	Effective Interventions	Ineffective Interventions	Total [3]	% Effective [1]
Target of Intervention				
Mixed	5	8	13	38.5
Intervention Intensity				
Low	2	1	3	66.7
Medium	3	2	5	60.0
High	0	5	5	0.0
Duration				
<6 weeks	2	2	4	50.0
6 to 11 weeks	1	0	1	100.0
12 weeks to 5 months	-	-	-	-
6 to 12 months	1	5	6	16.7
>12 months	1	1	2	50.0
Frequency of Contact [2]				
Annually	-	-	-	-
Bimonthly to quarterly	-	-	-	-
Monthly	0	2	2	0.0
Biweekly	1	2	3	33.3
Weekly	2	5	7	28.6
Multiple times per week	2	0	2	100.0
Daily	-	-	-	-
Level of Personalization [2]				
Environmental	1	1	2	50.0
Group (Parent or Child)	3	3	6	50.0
Group (Parent and Child)	-	-	-	-
Environmental + Group (Parent or Child)	1	1	2	50.0
Environmental + Group (Parent and Child)	0	2	2	0.0
Group + Individual (Parent or Child)	1	1	2	50.0
Group + Individual (Parent and Child)	0	1	1	0.0
Individual or Individual + Environmental + Group	0	2	2	0.0
Reach				
1 setting	5	1	6	83.3
2 settings	0	5	5	0.0
3+ settings	0	2	2	0.0

[1] Intervention effectiveness is defined as a statistically significant increase ($p < 0.05$) in a dairy and/or calcium related outcome. [2] Total number of studies in Frequency of Contact and Level of Personalization will not sum to $n = 13$, because some studies used multiple frequencies of contact and multiple levels of personalization throughout the intervention. [3] Salehi et al. (2004) was excluded from the chart and analysis, as the authors did not provide the effectiveness of the intervention.

Table 3. Summary of overall intervention intensity results.

Study (n = 14)	Duration [4]	Frequency [4]	Personalization [4]	Reach [4]	Overall Intensity Score	Overall Intensity Rating [2]	Effective [3]	Group Score
Parent and Child								
Akil (2013) [22]	4	4	3	5	16	High	N	
Bender et al. (2013) [23]	4	3.25	2.5	5	14.75	High	N	
Kopetsky (2017) [25]	1	4	4.5	3	12.5	Medium	N	
Korwanich et al. (2008) [26]	4	4 [1]	3.5	3	14.5	High	N	13.5
Munday et al. (2017) [28]	2	4.5	3	1	10.5	Medium	Y	
Roberts-Gray et al. (2016) [30]	1	4	3.5	3	11.5	Medium	N	
Vereecken et al. (2009) [33]	4	4 [1]	3.5	3	14.5	High	N	
Parent								
Harvey (2008) [24]	1	4	2	1	8	Low	Y	
Marquis et al. (2014) [27]	5	4	2	1	12	Medium	Y	
Salehi et al. (2004) [31]	4	N/A	Unclear	1	N/A	N/A	N/A	12.2
O'Sullivan et al. (2016) [29]	5	3.5	5	3	16.5	High	N	
Child								
Cason (2001) [19]	4	3.5	3	1	11.5	Medium	Y	9.5
Schwartz et al. (2015) [32]	1	4.5	1	1	7.5	Low	Y	
Childcare Services								
Seward et al. (2018) [20]	4	3	1	1	9	Low	N	9

[1] Frequency of contact with intervention was estimated by review authors; points of contact were divided by the overall duration of the intervention to determine an average frequency of contact. [2] Overall intensity rating score breakdown: low intensity (≤10.5); medium intensity (10.51 to 13.49); high intensity (≥13.5). [3] Intervention effectiveness is defined as a statistically significant increase ($p < 0.05$) in a dairy and/or calcium-related outcome. [4] Intensity ranking scale: *Duration*: 1 = ≤6 weeks; 2 = 6 to 11 weeks; 3 = 12 weeks to 5 months; 4 = 6 to 12 months; 5 = ≥12 months; *Frequency*: 1 = annually; 2 = bimonthly to quarterly; 3 = monthly; 3.5 = twice a month; 4 = weekly; 4.5 = multiple times per week; 5 = daily; *Personalization*: 1 = environmental; 2 = group (parent or child); 2.5 = group (parent and child); 3 = environmental + group (parent or child); 3.5 = environmental + group (parent and child); 4 = group with an individual component (parent or child); 4.5 = group with an individual component (parent and child); 5 = individual (parent and/or child) or individual + environmental + group (parent and/or child); *Reach*: 1 = one setting; 3 = two settings; 5 = three or more settings.

When evaluating the individual intensity rating categories, no relationships appear to exist between duration, frequency of contact or level of personalization, and intervention effectiveness (Table 2). Only one intervention had a duration of 6 to 11 weeks and demonstrated effectiveness. Additionally, the two interventions [28,32] involving contact with participants multiple times per week were effective. None of the levels of personalization were consistently linked with effectiveness, as all were used in both effective and ineffective interventions. Consistent with a previously published systematic literature review [18], all of the studies in which the intervention was conducted and applied in only one setting/environment were effective. Of the six studies using a reach of one setting, five (83.3%) demonstrated significant increases in dairy and/or calcium consumption.

To further assess intervention intensity, the interventions were divided into four groups based on the target population(s): parent and child; parent; child; or childcare services (Table 3). Child-focused interventions had a group score of 9.5 (n = 2), indicating a low overall intervention intensity score; however, the interventions in both studies resulted in statistically significant increases in dairy consumption. Interventions that targeted both parent and child had the highest overall group intensity score of 13.5, although only one (14.3%) of the seven interventions resulted in significantly increased calcium consumption. Overall, there was heterogeneity in terms of effectiveness across different categories of intensity and with overall intensity.

3.3. Behavior Change Techniques

The interventions employed a variety of behavior change techniques (BCT). Table 4 outlines the frequency of BCT associated with intervention effectiveness. Salehi et al. (2004) [31] was not included in the BCT analysis, as information about intervention effectiveness was not provided.

Table 4. Behavior change techniques associated with intervention effectiveness.

Behavior Change Technique [1]	Effective (N = 5)	Ineffective (N = 8)	Total (N = 13) [2]	% Effective [3]
1. Provide information on consequences of behavior in general	3	5	8	37.5
2. Provide information on consequences of behavior to the individual	3	6	9	33.3
4. Provide normative information about others' behavior	1	0	1	100.0
5. Goal setting (behavior)	4	8	12	33.3
7. Action planning	5	8	13	38.5
8. Problem solving/barrier identification	2	3	5	40.0
9. Set graded tasks	0	1	1	0.0
10. Review of behavioral goals	1	4	5	20.0
13. Rewards contingent on successful behaviors	2	2	4	50.0
15. Generalization of target behavior	4	7	11	36.4
16. Self-monitoring of behavior	1	3	4	25.0
19. Provide feedback on performance	1	6	7	14.3
20. Provide information on when and where to perform the behavior	4	8	12	33.3
21. Provide instruction on how to perform the behavior	4	8	12	33.3
22. Model/demonstrate the behavior	3	7	10	30.0
23. Teach to use prompts/cues	4	3	7	57.1

Table 4. *Cont.*

Behavior Change Technique [1]	Effective (N = 5)	Ineffective (N = 8)	Total (N = 13) [2]	% Effective [3]
24. Environmental restructuring	5	3	8	62.5
25. Agree on behavioral contract	0	1	1	0.0
26. Prompt practice	4	8	12	33.3
27. Use of follow-up prompts	0	2	2	0.0
28. Facilitate social comparison	0	2	2	0.0
29. Plan social support/social change	2	8	10	20.0
30. Identification as a role model	2	7	9	22.2
35. Relapse prevention/coping planning	0	1	1	0.0
36. Stress management/emotional control training	0	1	1	0.0
38. Time management	0	1	1	0.0
39. General communication skills training	1	2	3	33.3

[1] Behavior change technique numbers three, six, 11, 12, 14, 17, 18, 31, 32, 33, 34, 37, and 40 were removed from the chart and analysis as no studies employed these techniques. [2] Salehi et al. (2004) was excluded from the chart and analysis, as the authors did not provide the effectiveness of the intervention. [3] Intervention effectiveness is defined as a statistically significant increase ($p < 0.05$) in a dairy or calcium outcome.

The most commonly used BCT, which was used in all 13 interventions, was action planning. Other commonly used BCTs were goal setting (behavior) ($n = 12$), providing information on when and where to perform the behavior ($n = 12$), providing instruction on how to perform the behavior ($n = 12$), and prompting practice ($n = 12$). There was one BCT that was used exclusively in the effective intervention by Marquis et al. (2014) [27], which was providing normative information about others' behavior (i.e., providing information about others' behaviors and whether they are common or uncommon in the population). Action planning and environmental restructuring were similarly used in all five effective studies, although both were also used in several ineffective studies. Action planning demonstrated 38.5% efficacy, and environmental restructuring demonstrated 62.5% efficacy. Goal setting (behavior) [19,24,27,28], generalization of the target behavior [19,24,27,28], providing information on when and where to perform the behavior [19,24,27,28], providing instruction on how to perform the behavior [19,24,27,28], teaching how to use prompts/cues [19,24,28,32], and prompt practice [19,24,27,28] were techniques used in four of the five effective interventions. Goal setting (behavior) demonstrated 33.3% efficacy, the generalization of target behavior demonstrated 36.4% efficacy, providing information on when and where to perform the behavior demonstrated 33.3% efficacy, providing instruction on how to perform the behavior had 33.3% efficacy, teaching to use prompts/cues demonstrated 57.1% efficacy, and prompting practice had 33.3% efficacy. The results demonstrate that intervention effectiveness is independent of BCT.

3.4. WIDER

Table 5 provides a summary of WIDER recommendations for each intervention study. Only seven of the 14 studies provided adequate descriptions of their intervention. Similarly, 57% of the studies adequately classified their change processes and design principles. Only three (21%) interventions provided access to intervention protocols, which made it difficult to further evaluate the risk of reporting bias. Four studies (29%) did not have a control group, which classified them under unclear risk of bias for random sequence generation and high risk of bias for allocation concealment. Of the 10 studies that had a control group, only three (30%) had an active control, with two of them providing adequate descriptions of the control.

Table 5. Summary of the Workgroup for Intervention Development and Evaluation Research (WIDER) recommendations.

Study (n = 14)	Description of Intervention	Classification of Change Process and Design Principles	Access to Intervention Manuals and/or Protocols	Description of Active Control Conditions
Akil (2013) [22]	N	N	N	N
Bender et al. (2013) [23]	Y	Y	N	No Control Group
Cason (2001) [19]	N	Y	N	No Control Group
Harvey (2008) [24]	N	N	N	No Control Group
Kopetsky (2017) [25]	Y	Y	N	Y
Korwanich et al. (2008) [26]	N	N	N	No Active Control
Marquis et al. (2014) [27]	Y	N	Y	No Active Control
Munday et al. (2017) [28]	Y	N	N	No Control Group
O'Sullivan et al. (2016) [29]	Y	Y	Y	No Active Control
Roberts-Gray et al. (2016) [30]	Y	Y	N	No Active Control
Salehi et al. (2004) [31]	N	Y	N	No Active Control
Schwartz et al. (2015) [32]	N	N	N	No Active Control
Seward et al. (2018) [20]	Y	Y	Y	Y
Vereecken et al. (2009) [33]	N	Y	N	No Active Control

3.5. *Risk of Bias*

All 14 intervention studies [19,20,22–33] included in the review were assessed for risk of bias. Figure 2 provides a summary of the authors' (VS, IJ) judgments regarding each risk of bias item for the included intervention studies. The study with the lowest overall risk of bias was O'Sullivan et al. (2016) [29], and the study with the highest overall risk of bias was Munday et al. (2017) [28]. Three studies, two of which were dissertations, had all categories classified as either high or unclear risk of bias [22–24]. Overall, most of the studies had a high or unclear risk of bias in a majority of the categories.

Figure 3 presents the percentages of each risk of bias item across the 14 intervention studies. There was a high percentage (71%) of studies with an unclear risk of bias for random sequence generation. Additionally, six studies inadequately described allocation concealment. All of the studies either had a high or unclear risk of bias in the blinding of participants and personnel. Similarly, only two studies had a low risk of bias in the blinding of outcome assessment. Compared to other categories, there was a high percentage (36%) of studies that had a low risk of bias in incomplete outcome data. For the selective reporting domain, 11 studies had an unclear risk of bias, as they failed to provide protocols, and thus reviewers were unable to make clear judgments about bias risk. Half of the studies (n = 7) had a high risk of other bias due to self-reporting, convenience sampling, crossover bias, and underreporting. A high risk of bias was reported in 50% of the studies across the categories 'other bias' and 'attrition bias', resulting in these two categories having the highest percentage of a high risk of bias. Similarly, the highest percentage (50%) of a low risk of bias was observed in the 'other bias' category. Overall, in four of the seven domains, the percentage of studies with an unclear risk of bias was 50% or greater.

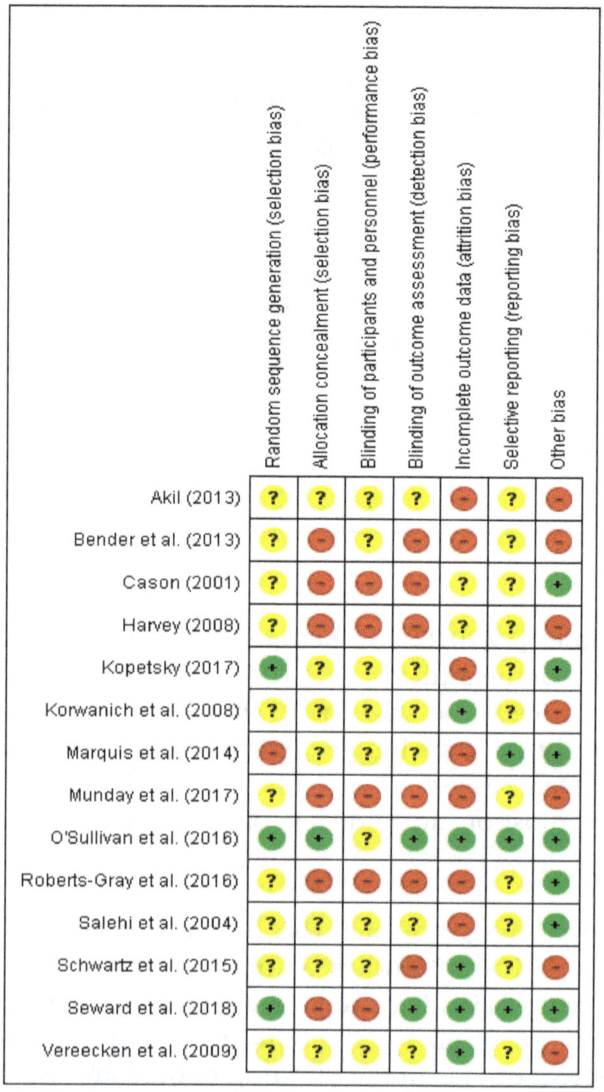

Figure 2. Risk of bias summary: review authors' judgments about each risk of bias item for each included intervention study. Red, yellow, and green circles represent high, unclear, and low risk of bias, respectively.

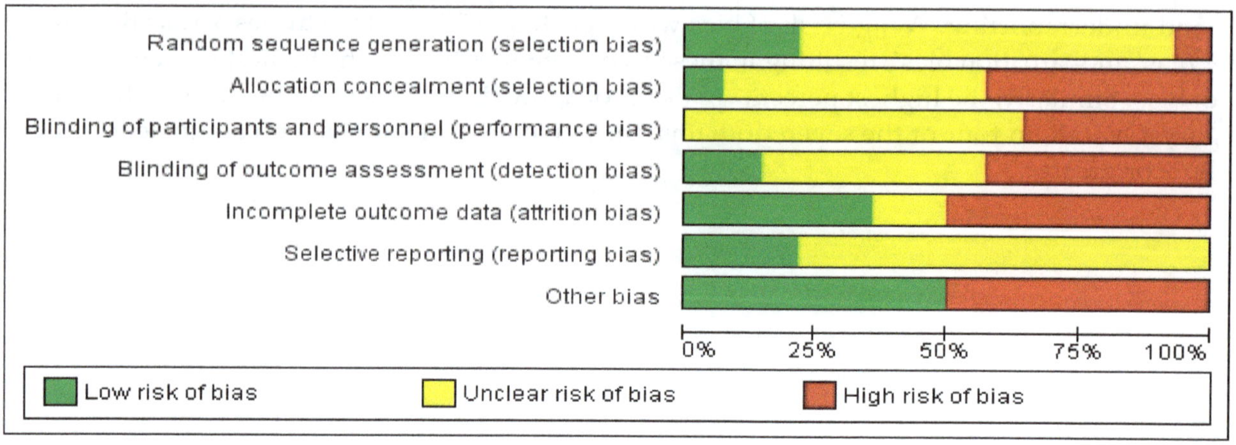

Figure 3. Risk of bias graph: review authors' judgments about each risk of bias item, which are presented as percentages across all of the included intervention studies (n = 14).

3.6. GRADE

Thirteen studies were included in the GRADE analysis. One study could not be included, as it was the only intervention assessing calcium intake as an outcome [28]. Table 6 provides a summary of GRADE results for the studies ($n = 7$) that had total dairy intake as an outcome. The overall quality of evidence across these studies was very low, as it received an overall score of zero. Table 7 provides a summary of GRADE results for the studies ($n = 6$) that had total milk intake as an outcome. Similar to total dairy intake, the overall quality of evidence across these studies was also very low, receiving an overall score of one.

Table 6. Summary of Grades of Recommendation, Assessment, Development and Evaluation (GRADE) results for total dairy intake outcome ($n = 7$). Intervention studies evaluated: Akil 2013 [22]; Cason 2001 [19]; Harvey 2008 [24]; Kopetsky 2017 [25]; O'Sullivan et al., 2016 [29]; Roberts-Gray et al., 2016 [30]; and Seward et al., 2018 [20].

GRADE Criteria	Rating	Support for Judgment	Overall Quality of Evidence
Type of Evidence	+4	All of the studies included were intervention studies.	High
Quality Points	−3	Multiple studies had <200 participants. The majority of studies had a high or unclear risk of bias for the blinding and allocation process, as well as attrition.	Low
Consistency	0	Most of the studies reported the ineffectiveness ($n = 5$) versus effectiveness ($n = 2$) of dairy intervention. Dairy outcomes assessed are relatively similar, as the majority of studies reported some variation of the number of servings of dairy consumed.	Moderate
Directness	−1	Generalizability of population was a limitation in several studies.	Moderate
Effect Size	0	$n = 3$ studies did not provide enough information to allow for the calculation of effect size. All of the other studies ($n = 4$) allowed for the calculation of effect size; not all of the effect sizes were >2 or <0.5 and significant.	Low
	Overall Score: 0		**Overall Quality of Evidence:** Very Low

Table 7. Summary of GRADE results for total milk intake outcome ($n = 6$). Intervention studies evaluated: Bender et al., 2013 [23]; Korwanich et al., 2008 [26]; Marquis et al., 2014 [27]; Salehi et al., 2004 [31]; Schwartz et al., 2015 [32]; and Vereecken et al., 2009 [33].

GRADE Criteria	Rating	Support for Judgment	Overall Quality of Evidence
Type of Evidence	+4	All of the studies included were intervention studies.	High
Quality Points	−1	All of the studies had a high or unclear risk of bias for blinding and allocation. Three studies had a low risk of attrition bias, with the other three studies having either a high or unclear risk of attrition bias. Generally, sparse data does not appear to be of concern, as the majority of studies had >200 participants.	Moderate
Consistency	−1	Most studies reported ineffectiveness ($n = 3$) versus effectiveness ($n = 2$) of dairy intervention, with one study not reporting effectiveness. Variability in reporting of milk outcomes; studies reported volumes of milk consumed, times consumed per day, or quantity of milk consumed in grams.	Low

Table 7. *Cont.*

GRADE Criteria	Rating	Support for Judgment	Overall Quality of Evidence
Directness	−1	Generalizability of population was a limitation in multiple studies.	Moderate
Effect Size	0	$n = 3$ studies did not provide enough information to allow for the calculation of effect size. All of the other studies ($n = 3$) allowed for the calculation of effect size; not all of the effect sizes were >2 or <0.5 and significant.	Low
	Overall Score: 1		**Overall Quality of Evidence:** Very Low

The type of evidence across both outcomes received a score of +4, as all of the studies that were included in the review were intervention studies. Total dairy intake received the lowest score (−3) for quality points, as a majority of the studies had <200 participants and had a relatively high risk of bias. Conversely, total milk intake had the lowest score (−1) for consistency, as there was variability in the reporting of milk outcomes. Both outcomes received the same scores for directness (−1) and effect size (0). Overall, these results demonstrate heterogeneity between intervention studies.

4. Discussion

The objective of this review was to identify the characteristics of effective interventions aimed at increasing dairy and/or calcium consumption in preschool-aged children. Intervention reporting was evaluated using intervention intensity analysis, behavior change technique taxonomy, and WIDER, with risk of bias and GRADE used to assess the quality of the intervention studies. Only five (35.7%) interventions included in the review reported significant increases in dairy and/or calcium consumption post-intervention, which was lower than the ~70% reported in previously published reviews in other populations [17,18]. Characteristics associated with effectiveness included those interventions delivered in one setting (i.e., preschools, early education centers and/or daycares) versus those delivered in multiple settings, those that included the selected behavior change techniques of environmental restructuring and teach to use prompts/cues, and those that targeted both the parent and child.

The most notable finding was the lack of effectiveness reported by intervention studies aiming to increase dairy and/or calcium intakes in preschool-aged children. The ineffectiveness of most interventions may be attributed to the lack of focus on dairy or calcium intake as the targeted message. All of the interventions in the final analysis included dairy and/or calcium intakes as part of a larger dietary intervention designed to encourage healthy eating and positive dietary habits in preschool-aged children. Hendrie et al. (2012) [17] concluded that interventions specifically targeting dairy or calcium intake independent of other dietary changes were more likely to be effective than those considering dairy/calcium intake in the context of a broader message, such as general healthy eating. These findings suggest that mixed dietary interventions may dilute the impact or preclude adequate communication and/or the adaption of more targeted health and dietary messages. A possible explanation could be that less time and/or effort are allocated to dairy-specific messaging when presented as part of a mixed dietary intervention. Resource availability may also be limited when engaging in broader dietary interventions, directly impacting dairy or calcium messaging and the extent of education and communication about dairy and calcium consumption. The effectiveness of increasing dairy and calcium consumption as part of a larger dietary intervention may be influenced by the behavior change techniques implemented. For example, behavior change techniques that are effective at increasing fruit and vegetable consumption may not be similarly effective at increasing dairy and calcium intake, and therefore may impact the communication of dairy and calcium health messages.

The ineffectiveness of dairy interventions may also be attributed to the heterogeneity of the interventions. The heterogeneity observed between populations may have introduced variability in the communication of dietary messages on the basis of cultural and/or societal norms. For example, Salehi et al. (2004) [31] conducted their interventions on Qashqa'i tribe families in Iran, while Marquis et al. (2014) [27] studied a cohort of rural Ghanaian children. Salehi et al. (2004) [31] aimed to change/improve the customs and cultural practices of the Qashqa'i tribe families through educational program topics such as sanitary waste disposal, water supply, and general dietary consumption guidelines. In contrast, Marquis et al. (2014) [27] focused on improving entrepreneurial training and nutrition education to increase household access to animal food products in rural Ghana. These examples highlight the differences in the availability of resources and/or food sources between cultures, and how this could impact the extent of the dietary health and messaging provided. Secondly, heterogeneity was also observed across participants, with variability in the targets of the interventions (i.e., parent and child, parent, child, or childcare services). The variability observed across intervention targets may significantly influence dietary messaging given that interventions targeting preschool children focus more on simply increasing dairy consumption, whereas those targeting adults are more likely to emphasize the importance or relevance of doing so. Thirdly, heterogeneity existed between the approaches used to communicate dietary messaging, including mass communication, targeted communication, or tailored communication [41]. Mass communication is more generic and most likely used in environmental or group interventions, as this type of communication enables general messages to be delivered to many individuals; in contrast, tailored communication is used when the health messages are specifically designed to individual need. The ineffectiveness and heterogeneity observed across interventions make it difficult to draw reliable conclusions, highlighting the need for future intervention designs to specifically and solely target dairy and/or calcium intake in preschoolers.

The characteristics of effective interventions were determined using intervention intensity analysis. No associations were observed between intervention intensity group scores and intervention effectiveness. Moreover, interventions targeting the parent and child demonstrated the highest intervention intensity scores, but only one of the seven studies demonstrated effectiveness. Both interventions targeting the child alone, by comparison, exhibited low intervention intensity scores, but were effective at increasing dairy intakes. These observations suggest that targeting the child alone may enhance the effectiveness of interventions; although, based on the young age of the preschool children, it is unreasonable to assume that these children would be able to change their intakes without the guidance from their parents and/or caregivers. Targeting both the parent and child may demonstrate higher efficacy in increasing dairy and/or calcium intakes in preschool children, as evidence suggests that parents play an important role in developing preschoolers' eating habits through a variety of mechanisms, including modeling of dietary behaviors [42,43], parental feeding behaviors [44,45], and the availability/accessibility of food products in the home environment [46,47]. Recent evidence from the Guelph Family Health Study, Canada, extended these findings: both mothers' and fathers' involvement of children in meal preparation was associated with lower child nutrition risk (mother beta = -3.45, $p = 0.02$; father beta = -1.74, $p = 0.01$) and healthy home environment scores (mother beta = -8.36, $p < 0.001$; father beta = -2.69, $p = 0.04$) [43]. These results demonstrate the strong parental influence on preschoolers' dietary intakes, supporting the need to target parents as well as children in interventions aiming to increase dairy and/or calcium intakes. Furthermore, when considered as independent categories, no associations were evident between intervention duration, frequency of contact or level of personalization, and overall intervention effectiveness. In contrast, intervention setting did appear to be associated with overall effectiveness, as it was observed that the majority of effective interventions used a reach of only one setting. This is consistent with Marquez et al. (2015) [18], who also reported an 81.8% intervention effectiveness using a reach of one setting, suggesting that a targeted and focused intervention delivered in a single setting may be preferable to interventions delivered across multiple settings. Based on the results of this study, interventions targeting dairy and/or calcium intake should focus on delivery in preschools, early education centers, and/or daycares. Nonetheless, despite the inclusion of 14 interventions in this analysis, the validity of our conclusions regarding the relationship between intervention intensity and effectiveness is limited by the small number of studies in any given category.

Analysis of behavior change techniques was used to investigate the relationship between the use of specific techniques and intervention effectiveness. Overall, the main finding from this analysis indicates some associations between the use of specific behavior techniques and intervention effectiveness. Specifically, environmental restructuring and teaching to use prompts/cues appear to be associated with overall intervention effectiveness. These two techniques are also related, because environmental restructuring prompts the participant to alter their environment to support the target behavior (i.e., put up posters/images) and teaching to use prompt/cues teaches the individual to identify environmental cues to prompt the target behavior. Given that these behavior change techniques are strongly associated with intervention effectiveness, altering the environment to support and encourage dairy/calcium consumption may be effective in the preschool population. As further support, Marquez et al. (2015) [18] reported 66.7% intervention effectiveness with the use of environmental restructuring, which is a result that is comparable to our review. Furthermore, no significant relationships were observed between the target population (i.e., parent and child, parent alone, child alone, or childcare services), the effectiveness of the intervention, and the use of behavior change techniques. These results are consistent with those of Marquez et al. (2015) [18], who concluded that parental involvement and support was not a significant predictor of intervention effectiveness. These findings are in contrast to those published by Hendrie et al. (2012) [17], who reported that effective studies implementing behavior change techniques specifically targeted the parents and/or family, while ineffective studies targeted only the child. Overall, intervention effectiveness appears to be independent of the majority of behavior change techniques, although environmental restructuring and teaching to use prompts/cues may encourage positive behavioral change in the preschool population.

Two assessment tools, risk of bias and GRADE, were used to evaluate the overall quality of the intervention studies included in the analysis. The majority of interventions demonstrated a high or unclear risk of bias in most or all of the risk of bias categories, with the quality appraisal of total dairy and total milk intake outcomes being very low based on the GRADE criteria. This demonstrates an overall lack of reliability and validity of intervention results and conclusions, suggesting a need to further develop standards and consistency in intervention design and the reporting of outcomes related to dairy/calcium intakes. Improving the reporting of outcomes will (i) enable the identification of the outcomes that are most meaningful and relevant in the preschool population, (ii) enable the development of a consensus in this field of research regarding definitions and measures of dairy/calcium outcomes (i.e., servings per day versus amount consumed), and (iii) identify those outcomes that are most likely to promote increases in the effectiveness of dairy/calcium interventions [48]. Finally, consistency in the reporting of outcomes and clarity in intervention design would enable a comparison of study designs, sample sizes, and target populations for the purpose of determining the factors promoting the effectiveness of dairy/calcium consumption in the preschool population. Improving clarity and transparency in outcome reporting and intervention design will in turn increase the reliability and the validity of conclusions about dairy/calcium intakes in preschoolers, and inform initiatives targeting positive health behaviors.

The results of the review should be interpreted considering the limitations. One limitation was a lack of disclosure in the methodology across interventions. This made it difficult to compare the different categories of intervention intensity and determine which behavior change techniques were implemented in interventions. Studies were restricted to those published in English, which may have limited the interventions selected for final analysis. As the primary focus of this review was on interventions aiming to increase dairy and/or calcium consumption, studies that were considered ineffective in this review may have demonstrated effectiveness in changing other dietary and/or physical activity targets in the intervention. Moreover, intervention effectiveness must also be considered in context of study design, as interventions specifically designed to increase dairy and/or calcium consumption may demonstrate increased effectiveness when compared to mixed interventions. Many studies did not report the actual quantities of participants' dairy/calcium intakes, making it difficult to report the degree of intervention efficacy. Lastly, gender bias may also be considered as a limitation, given that some studies included only one parent in the intervention, which was typically the mother. Despite these limitations, the use of several tools to both quantitatively and qualitatively review the included interventions provides a comprehensive critique of this body of literature and yields valuable insight into the characteristics of studies in this research domain.

5. Conclusions

Dietary interventions aiming to increase dairy and/or calcium consumption in preschool-aged children demonstrate variable success. The evidence presented in this review has identified characteristics that may enable the intervention effectiveness of increasing dairy and/or calcium intakes in preschoolers. This includes the delivery of interventions in one setting versus multiple settings, using specific behavior change techniques (such as environmental restructuring and teaching to use prompts/cues), and targeting both the parent and child. Future studies should modify interventions to exclusively target dairy and/or calcium intakes, reduce heterogeneity and/or bias, and improve transparency in the reporting of interventions. Further investigating the relationship and effect of target populations, specifically both parent and child, is another consideration, as it may be necessary and important to work with the parents and/or caregivers of these preschool children to ensure sustainable changes in dairy and/or calcium intakes. A potential avenue for future research includes exploring the use and effectiveness of booster periods for sustaining positive behavioral change over time in the preschool population. In the meantime, public health initiatives should aim to improve the dairy and calcium intake of preschool-aged children for the purpose of instilling healthy dietary habits at a young age, and mitigate the health consequences associated with insufficient intakes. Overall, the findings of this review demonstrate the need for developing effective interventions designed to increase dairy and/or calcium intakes in preschool-aged children.

Supplementary Materials:
Search Method and Inclusion/Exclusion Criteria; Table S1: Description of the 40 behavior change techniques used in the CALO-RE Taxonomy for assessment of interventions; Table S2: Description of the four criteria of the WIDER recommendations; Table S3: Description of the Risk of Bias assessment tool; Table S4: The GRADE scoring system used to evaluate the quality of scientific evidence.

Author Contributions: V.S.: literature searching, screening of articles, data extraction and analysis, manuscript writing, and editing; I.J.: literature searching, screening of articles, data extraction and analysis, writing of results, and manuscript editing; A.C.B.: study design, manuscript editing, supervised overall work; G.N.: study inception and design, manuscript editing, supervised overall work. All of the authors read and approved the final manuscript.

Acknowledgments: We thank Jess Haines and David W.L. Ma for providing feedback and comments that

References

1. Canadian Dairy Commission. Available online: http://www.cdc-ccl.gc.ca/CDC/index-eng.php?id=3805 (accessed on 2 November 2018).
2. National Health and Medical Research Council. *Australian Dietary Guidelines*; National Health and Medical Research Council: Canberra, Australia, 2013.
3. Garriguet, D. Nutrition: Findings from the Canadian Community Health Survey. Overview of Canadians' Eating Habits. Available online: www.statcan.gc.ca/pub/82-620-m/82-620-m2006002-eng.pdf (accessed on 2 November 2018).
4. Nielsen, S.J.; Popkin, B.M. Changes in beverage intake between 1977 and 2001. *Am. J. Prev. Med.* **2004**, *27*, 205–210. [CrossRef] [PubMed]

5. Dror, D.K.; Allen, L.H. Dairy product intake in children and adolescents in developed countries: Trends, nutritional contribution, and a review of association with health outcomes. *Nutr. Rev.* **2014**, *72*, 68–81. [CrossRef]
6. Rizzoli, R. Dairy products, yogurts, and bone health. *Am. J. Clin. Nutr.* **2014**, *99*, 1256S–1262S. [CrossRef]
7. Tremblay, A.; Gilbert, J.A. Human obesity: Is insufficient calcium/dairy intake part of the problem? *J. Am. Coll. Nutr.* **2011**, *30*, 449S–453S. [CrossRef] [PubMed]
8. Wang, H.; Troy, L.M.; Rogers, G.T.; Fox, C.S.; McKeown, N.M.; Meigs, J.B.; Jacques, P.F. Longitudinal association between dairy consumption and changes of body weight and waist circumference: The Framingham Heart Study. *Int. J. Obes.* **2014**, *38*, 299–305. [CrossRef] [PubMed]
9. Nicklas, T.A.; Qu, H.; Hughes, S.O.; He, M.; Wagner, S.E.; Foushee, H.R.; Shewchuk, R.M. Self-perceived lactose intolerance results in lower intakes of calcium and dairy foods and is associated with hypertension and diabetes in adults. *Am. J. Clin. Nutr.* **2011**, *94*, 191–198. [CrossRef]
10. O'Connor, L.M.; Lentjes, M.A.; Luben, R.N.; Khaw, K.T.; Wareham, N.J.; Forouhi, N.G. Dietary dairy product intake and incident type 2 diabetes: A prospective study using dietary data from a 7-day food diary. *Diabetologia* **2014**, *57*, 909–917. [CrossRef] [PubMed]
11. Larsson, S.C.; Bergkvist, L.; Rutegård, J.; Giovannucci, E.; Wolk, A. Calcium and dairy food intakes are inversely associated with colorectal cancer risk in the cohort of Swedish men. *Am. J. Clin. Nutr.* **2006**, *83*, 667–673. [CrossRef] [PubMed]
12. Davis, K.; Christoffel, K.K. Obesity in preschool and school-age children: Treatment early and often may be best. *Arch. Pediatr. Adolesc. Med.* **1994**, *148*, 1257–1261. [CrossRef]
13. Skinner, J.D.; Carruth, B.R.; Bounds, W.; Ziegler, P.; Reidy, K. Do food-related experiences in the first 2 years of life predict dietary variety in school-aged children? *J. Nutr. Educ. Behav.* **2002**, *34*, 310–315. [CrossRef]
14. Marshall, T.A.; Eichenberger Gilmore, J.M.; Broffitt, B.; Stumbo, P.J.; Levy, S.M. Diet quality in young children is influenced by beverage consumption. *J. Am. Coll. Nutr.* **2005**, *24*, 65–75. [CrossRef] [PubMed]
15. Dubois, L.; Farmer, A.; Girard, M.; Peterson, K. Regular sugar-sweetened beverage consumption between meals increases risk of overweight among preschool-aged children. *J. Am. Diet. Assoc.* **2007**, *107*, 924–934. [CrossRef]
16. Yen, S.T.; Lin, B.H. Beverage consumption among US children and adolescents: Full-information and quasi maximum-likelihood estimation of a censored system. *Eur. Rev. Agric. Econ.* **2002**, *29*, 85–103. [CrossRef]
17. Hendrie, G.A.; Brindal, E.; Baird, D.; Gardner, C. Improving children's dairy food and calcium intake: Can intervention work? A systematic review of the literature. *Public Health Nutr.* **2012**, *16*, 365–376. [CrossRef] [PubMed]
18. Marquez, O.; Racey, M.; Preyde, M.; Hendrie, G.A.; Newton, G. Interventions to increase dairy consumption in adolescents: A systematic review. *Infant Child Adolesc. Nutr.* **2015**, *7*, 242–254. [CrossRef]
19. Cason, K.L. Evaluation of a preschool nutrition education program based on the theory of multiple intelligences. *J. Nutr. Educ.* **2001**, *33*, 161–164. [CrossRef]
20. Seward, K.; Wolfenden, L.; Finch, M.; Wiggers, J.; Wyse, R.; Jones, J.; Yoong, S.L. Improving the implementation of nutrition guidelines in childcare centres improves child dietary intake: Findings of a randomised trial of an implementation intervention. *Public Health Nutr.* **2018**, *21*, 607–617. [CrossRef]
21. Moher, D.; Liberati, A.; Tetzlaff, J.; Altman, D.G.; Altman, D.; Antes, G.; Tugwell, P. Preferred reporting items for systematic reviews and meta-analyses: The PRISMA statement. *PLoS Med.* **2009**, *6*. [CrossRef] [PubMed]
22. Akil, N. Evaluation of Effectiveness of Classroom-Based Nutrition Intervention on Changes in Eating Behavior in African American Parents/Caregivers and Their Children. Master's Thesis, Wayne State University, Detroit, MI, USA, 2013. Available online: https://digitalcommons.wayne.edu/oa_theses/224 (accessed on 25 June 2018).
23. Bender, M.S.; Nader, P.R.; Kennedy, C.; Gahagan, S. A culturally appropriate intervention to improve health behaviours in Hispanic mother-child dyads. *Child. Obes.* **2013**, *9*, 157–163. [CrossRef]
24. Harvey, S.P. The Results of a Home-Based Physical Activity and Nutrition Program of Preschool Children and Parent Perceptions of Barriers. Ph.D. Thesis, University of Kansas, Lawrence, KS, USA, 2008.
25. Kopetsky, A. A Healthy Snacking Intervention in Preschool-Aged Children. Master's Thesis, University of Delaware, Newark, DE, USA, 2017.

26. Korwanich, K.; Sheiham, A.; Srisuphan, W.; Srisilapanan, P. Promoting healthy eating in nursery schoolchildren: A quasi-experimental intervention study. *Health Educ. J.* **2008**, *67*, 16–30. [CrossRef]
27. Marquis, G.S.; Colecraft, E.K. Community interventions for dietary improvement in Ghana. *Food Nutr. Bull.* **2014**, *35*, S193–S197. [CrossRef] [PubMed]
28. Munday, K.; Wilson, M. Implementing a health and wellbeing programme for children in early childhood: A preliminary study. *Nutrients* **2017**, *9*, 1031. [CrossRef]
29. O'Sullivan, A.; Fitzpatrick, N.; Doyle, O. Effects of early intervention on dietary intake and its mediating role on cognitive functioning: A randomised controlled trial. *Public Health Nutr.* **2016**, *20*, 154–164. [CrossRef] [PubMed]
30. Roberts-Gray, C.; Briley, M.E.; Ranjit, N.; Byrd-Williams, C.E.; Sweitzer, S.J.; Sharma, S.V.; Palafox, M.R.; Hoelscher, D.M. Efficacy of the Lunch is in the Bag intervention to increase parents' packing of healthy bag lunches for young children: A cluster-randomized trial in early care and education centers. *Int. J. Behav. Nutr. Phys. Act.* **2016**, *13*, 1–19. [CrossRef] [PubMed]
31. Salehi, M.; Kimiagar, S.M.; Shahbazi, M.; Mehrabi, Y.; Kolahi, A.A. Assessing the impact of nutrition education on growth indices of Iranian nomadic children: An application of a modified beliefs, attitudes, subjective-norms and enabling-factors model. *Br. J. Nutr.* **2004**, *91*, 779–787. [CrossRef]
32. Schwartz, M.B.; O'Connell, M.; Henderson, K.E.; Middleton, A.E.; Scarmo, S. Testing variations on family-style feeding to increase whole fruit and vegetable consumption among preschoolers in child care. *Child. Obes.* **2015**, *11*, 499–505. [CrossRef]
33. Vereecken, C.; Huybrechts, I.; van Houte, H.; Martens, V.; Wittebroodt, I.; Maes, L. Results from a dietary intervention study in preschools "Beastly Healthy at School". *Int. J. Public Health* **2009**, *54*, 142–149. [CrossRef]
34. Racey, M.; O'Brien, C.; Douglas, S.; Marquez, O.; Hendrie, G.; Newton, G. Systematic Review of School-Based Interventions to Modify Dietary Behavior: Does Intervention Intensity Impact Effectiveness? *J. Sch. Health* **2016**, *86*, 452–463. [CrossRef] [PubMed]
35. Michie, S.; Ashford, S.; Sniehotta, F.F.; Dombrowski, S.U.; Bishop, A.; French, D.P. A refined taxonomy of behaviour change techniques to help people change their physical activity and healthy eating behaviours: The CALO-RE taxonomy. *Psychol. Health* **2011**, *26*, 1479–1498. [CrossRef]
36. Abraham, C.; Michie, S. A Taxonomy of Behavior Change Techniques Used in Interventions. *Health Psychol.* **2008**, *27*, 379–387. [CrossRef] [PubMed]
37. Albrecht, L.; Archibald, M.; Arseneau, D.; Scott, S.D. Development of a checklist to assess the quality of reporting of knowledge translation interventions using the Workgroup for Intervention Development and Evaluation Research (WIDER) recommendations. *Implement. Sci.* **2013**, *8*, 1–5. [CrossRef] [PubMed]
38. Scott, S.; Albrecht, L.; O'Leary, K.; Ball, G.; Hartling, L.; Hofmeyer, A.; Dryden, D. Systematic review of knowledge translation strategies in the allied health professions. *Implement. Sci.* **2012**, *7*, 70. [CrossRef] [PubMed]
39. Cochrane Handbook for Systematic Reviews of Interventions. Available online: http://handbook-5-1.cochrane.org/ (accessed on 15 January 2018).
40. What Is GRADE? Available online: http://clincialevidence.bmj.com/x/set/static/ebm/learn/665072.html (accessed on 15 January 2018).
41. Hawkins, R.P.; Kreuter, M.; Resnicow, K.; Fishbein, M.; Dijkstra, A. Understanding tailoring in communicating about health. *Health Educ. Res.* **2008**, *23*, 454–466. [CrossRef] [PubMed]
42. Grimm, G.C.; Harnack, L.; Story, M. Factors associated with soft drink consumption in school-aged children. *J. Am. Diet. Assoc.* **2004**, *104*, 1244–1249. [CrossRef]
43. Watterworth, J.; Mackay, J.M.; Buchholz, A.C.; Darlington, G.; Randall Simpson, J.; Ma, D.W.L.; Haines, J.; Guelph Family Health Study. Food parenting practices and their associations with child nutrition risk status: Comparing mothers and fathers. *Appl. Physiol. Nutr. Metab.* **2017**, *42*, 667–671. [CrossRef]
44. Birch, L.L.; Fisher, J.O. Development of eating behaviours among children and adolescents. *Pediatrics* **1998**, *101*, 539–549.
45. Faith, M.S.; Scanlon, K.S.; Birch, L.L.; Francis, L.A.; Sherry, B. Parent-child feeding strategies and their relationships to child eating and weight status. *Obes. Res.* **2004**, *12*, 1711–1722. [CrossRef]
46. Hanson, N.I.; Neumark-Sztainer, D.; Eisenberg, M.E.; Story, M.; Wall, M. Associations between parental report of the home food environment and adolescent intakes of fruits, vegetables and dairy foods. *Public Health Nutr.* **2005**, *8*, 77–85. [CrossRef] [PubMed]

47. Kratt, P.; Reynolds, K.; Shewchuk, R. The role of availability as a moderator of family fruit and vegetable consumption. *Health Educ. Behav.* **2000**, *27*, 471–482. [CrossRef] [PubMed]
48. Tunis, S.R.; Clarke, M.; Gorst, S.L.; Gargon, E.; Blazeby, J.M.; Altman, D.G.; Williamson, P.R. Improving the relevance and consistency of outcomes in comparative effectiveness research. *J. Comp. Eff. Res.* **2016**, *5*, 193–205. [CrossRef] [PubMed]

Changes in Dietary Patterns from Childhood to Adolescence and Associated Body Adiposity Status

Danielle Biazzi Leal [1,2,*], Maria Alice Altenburg de Assis [1,2], Patrícia de Fragas Hinnig [1], Jeovani Schmitt [3], Adriana Soares Lobo [1], France Bellisle [4], Patrícia Faria Di Pietro [1], Francilene Kunradi Vieira [1], Pedro Henrique de Moura Araujo [3] and Dalton Francisco de Andrade [5]

1 Post Graduate Program in Nutrition, Health Sciences Center, Federal University of Santa Catarina, CCS/UFSC, Campus Trindade, Florianopolis 88040-900, Brazil; malicedeassis@gmail.com (M.A.A.d.A.); phinnig@yahoo.com.br (P.d.F.H.); adri_lobo@hotmail.com (A.S.L.); fariadipietro@gmail.com (P.F.D.P.); frankunradi@gmail.com (F.K.V.)

2 Post Graduate Program in Physical Education, Sports Center, Federal University of Santa Catarina, CDS/UFSC, Campus Trindade, Florianopolis 88040-900, Brazil

3 Post Graduate Program in Production Engineering, Technological Center, Federal University of Santa Catarina, University Campus Trindade, Florianopolis 88040-900, Brazil; jeovani.schmitt@yahoo.com.br (J.S.); phma05@gmail.com (P.H.d.M.A.)

4 Equipe de Recherche en Epidémiologie Nutritionnelle, Centre de Recherche en Epidémiologie et Statistiques, Université Paris 13, Inserm (U1153), Inra (U1125), Cnam, COMUE Sorbonne Paris Cité, Bobigny 93017, France; bellisle@uren.smbh.univ-paris13.fr

5 Informatics and Statistics Department, Technological Center, Federal University of Santa Catarina, University Campus Trindade, Florianopolis 88040-900, Brazil; daltoncasa@hotmail.com

* Correspondence: danibiazzi@yahoo.com.br

Abstract: The aims of this study were to identify cross-sectional dietary patterns (DPs) in a representative sample of 7–10-year-old schoolchildren, to examine how scores for these DPs tracked over a time period of five years (from age 7–10 years to 12–15 years), and to investigate longitudinal associations between changes in DPs scores and changes in BMI (Body Mass Index) *z*-scores. Children aged 7–10-years were examined in 2007 (n = 1158) and a subset of the sample participated in a follow-up in 2012 (n = 458). Factor analysis (FA) was applied to derive DPs at baseline. The change in DP from childhood to adolescence was analyzed by comparing factor scores using the complete cases, in which factor loadings were the ones evaluated at baseline. Associations of BMI change with DP change were assessed by multivariate linear regression. At baseline, four DP were identified that explained 47.9% of the food intake variance. On average, the factor scores of "DP II" (salty snacks, French fries, fast-food, sugary beverages) decreased in follow-up, while no changes were observed for "DP I" (rice, cooked beans, beef/poultry, leafy vegetables), "DP III" (fruits, cooked and leafy vegetables, fruit juices, pasta, milk, cheese), and "DP IV" (milk, coffee with milk, cheese, breads/biscuits). No significant linear association was shown between changes in BMI *z*-scores and changes in DP scores from childhood to adolescence. In conclusion, three out of four DP scores identified at baseline tracked slightly in adolescence.

Keywords: dietary patterns; tracking; children; adolescents; factor analysis

1. Introduction

Establishing healthy eating habits is important during childhood and adolescence, given that these behaviors may have cumulative effects on health and tend to be continued into adulthood [1,2]. The transition in diet from childhood to adolescence marks important changes due to individual factors such as physiological development related to growth and maturation, changes in parental influence, as well as the increasing independence and interaction of adolescents with their social environment [3,4]. Investigating eating behaviors in children longitudinally during the transition into adolescence is important in order to provide information on the nature of individual-level change over time and when, how, and why dietary changes occur [4].

The transition in a child's diet may be affected by socioeconomic and demographic changes within the family [4,5]. In addition, in many emerging and developing countries, as incomes rise and populations experience urbanization, there is a shift from traditional fiber and grain-rich diets to fat, sugar-rich, refined grains, animal fat, and protein diets [6], leading to obesity and diet-related chronic diseases [7].

In epidemiology, tracking is defined as the stability or maintenance of a given constant over time [8]. Dietary tracking values can therefore be considered to demonstrate the preservation of dietary habits, and the consumption of food or nutrients over a period of time [1]. Dietary patterns (DPs) are found to track during infancy [9], to older childhood [10], and from children to adults [1], and then remain stable in adulthood [11]. In children and adolescents there are mixed findings, with some studies reporting stability [1,4,12,13], and others showing changes in DPs [14–17]. The limited available prospective epidemiological evidence consistently indicates that DPs that are high in energy-dense, high-fat, and low-fiber foods predispose young people to overweight and obesity later in life [18–20].

DPs have been identified in some cross-sectional studies in Brazilian children and adolescents [21–26]. None of these studies has investigated the stability of DPs specifically from childhood to adolescence, and their relationship with changes in body mass index.

We have previously reported the association between dietary patterns (derived by latent class analysis) and overweight/obesity in a cross-sectional study of 7 to 10-year-old Brazilian schoolchildren [25]. In the present study, we assessed the stability of DPs in the same children five years later, using confirmatory factor analysis (FA). FA was also used at baseline, as this is currently the most popular method for identifying DPs.

The aims of the present study were (a) to identify cross-sectional DPs in a representative sample of schoolchildren aged 7–10 years old; (b) to examine how scores for these DPs tracked over a time period of five years (from age 7–10 years to 12–15 years) and (c) to investigate longitudinal associations between changes in DPs scores and changes in body mass index (BMI) *z*-scores.

2. Materials and Methods

2.1. Design and Study Population

A cross-sectional survey designed to investigate the prevalence of overweight/obesity and related behaviors of schoolchildren was conducted in Florianopolis (Brazil) from April to October 2007. The final sample consisted of 1232 children from 17 schools (782 children from 11 public schools and 450 children from six private schools). Detailed sampling procedures have been described elsewhere [27].

In 2012, an active search of all adolescents (12–15 years) surveyed in 2007 was performed using the Brazilian School Census (EducaCenso). However, the collection of data for this second study was restricted to students still enrolled in the same schools as the 2007 survey or transferred to other schools in the metropolitan area of the city. As the schoolchildren search did not occur in other regions of the state or the country, the eligible sample decreased. A total of 494 cohort members from 65 schools were identified and interviewed in 2012 (40.1% of the 2007 participants).

After excluding 74 children at baseline (boys $n = 44$, girls $n = 30$) and 36 adolescents at follow-up (boys $n = 21$, girls $n = 15$) with outlier's data for food intake (i.e., reporting fewer than three food items or with a total daily frequency intake of foods/beverages exceeding three standard deviation scores), 1158 children (581 boys and 577 girls) at baseline and 458 adolescents (213 boys and 245 girls) at follow-up were included in the dietary pattern analyses. Detailed sampling and reasons for follow-up losses are shown in the flowchart (Figure 1).

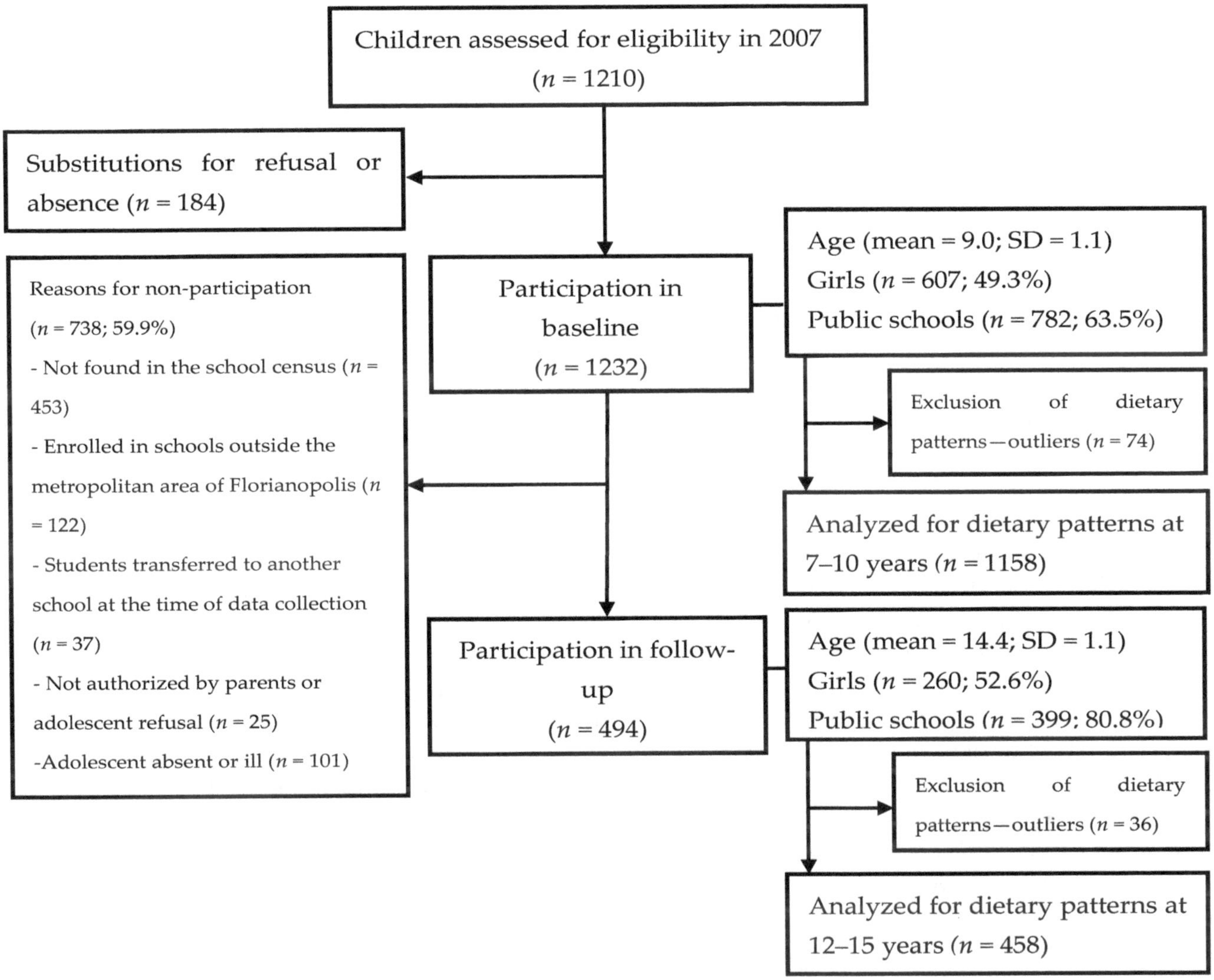

Figure 1. Flowchart of participants in the 2007 survey (7–10-year-olds) and in the 2012 survey (12–15-year-olds).

Both studies were conducted according to the guidelines set out in the Code of Ethics of the World Medical Association (Declaration of Helsinki) and all procedures involving human subjects were approved by the Human Studies Committee of the Federal University of Santa Catarina (07636813.3.0000.0121). Written informed consent was obtained from the parents and oral assent was obtained from the children.

2.2. Dietary Intake

At both time points, dietary data were obtained using the third version of the Previous Day Food Questionnaire (PDFQ-3) [28] based on a single day recall procedure, designed to investigate the consumption frequency of specific foods (not nutrients) as markers of (un)healthy diet and types of physical activities on the previous day. For example, a range of specific foods have been suggested as important dietary determinants of weight status in childhood and adolescence, including fruit and vegetables [29], fat [30], fast-food [31], and sugary drinks [32]. The PDFQ is a paper and pencil questionnaire, designed to be applied in the school setting as a supervised classroom exercise where children are guided by trained researchers following a standardized protocol [28]. The PDFQ-3 was previously validated in a sample of 6–11-year-old schoolchildren, with direct observation of the food eaten at school meals on the previous day as the gold standard, and demonstrated a reasonable average sensitivity (probability of correctly reporting a food intake) of 70.2% and an excellent average specificity (probability of correctly not reporting a food intake) of 96.2% [28]. The food section of the questionnaire covers six daily eating occasions (three main meals and three snacks) ordered chronologically (breakfast and mid-morning snack, lunch and afternoon snack, dinner and evening snack). Each meal and snack is illustrated with 21 pictures of foods/beverages or food groups (bread and biscuits, chocolate milk, coffee with milk, milk, yoghurt, cheese, rice, beans, pasta, beef and poultry, fish and seafood, leafy vegetables, cooked vegetables, vegetable soup, fruits, fruit juices, French fries, pizza and hamburgers, sweets, salty snacks, and soft drinks). The tool does not assess foods or food groups like water, cooking fats, fat, or sugary spreads on bread (e.g., butter or margarine, honey, jam, chocolate or nut-based products), fat content (e.g., low-fat milk or high-fat milk), types of soft drinks and fruit juices (e.g., regular or diet), or types of cooking methods (e.g., frying, baking, roasting).

The foods and food groups illustrated in PDFQ-3 were selected in order to represent the food patterns of children in this age group, foods presented in school menus, and foods recommended in the guidelines for the Brazilian population [33]. Supplementary Figure S1 shows one page of the questionnaire.

The PDFQ-3 was assessed once at each time point for every child, and the day at which the PDFQ-3 was assessed differed between children. This strategy was used in order to describe the daily variability of dietary intake on schooldays (Monday to Thursday) and non-school days (Sunday and holidays) allowing for the analysis of food consumption at the group level. In the 2007 survey, 71.3% (n = 826) of the participants reported food intake on weekdays/schooldays (16.8% on Monday; 22.1% on Tuesday; 17.2% on Wednesday; 15.2% on Thursday), and 28.7% (n = 332) on Sunday/holidays (non-schooldays). As the PDFQ-3 was applied in the school setting and there was no school on Saturdays and Sundays, it was not possible to obtain data representing food consumption for Fridays and Saturdays. Portion sizes were not assessed; therefore, the food intake could not be quantified by weight or energy and instead the (relative) frequency of intake was used as an indicator for the factors. However, number of servings per day (frequency) is routinely used to determine empirical dietary patterns [34–36]. The frequency of food intake was estimated as number of times per day, ranging from 0 to 6 for each food/beverage consumed, assuming that only one serving was consumed on each occasion.

2.3. *Physical Activity*

In the physical activity section of the PDFQ-3, schoolchildren were asked to report their physical activities (walking/running, playing with a dog, cycling, swimming, playing ball games, jumping rope, athletics, climbing stairs, roller skating/blading, dancing, and helping with household chores). The validation of the physical activity section of the questionnaire using comparisons between the scores generated by the instrument and the number of step counts obtained by pedometers showed mean values for sensitivity and specificity of 78% and 56%, respectively [37]. In the present study, metabolic equivalents (METs) were assigned to each activity reported using the Compendium of Energy Expenditures for Youth [38] and summed for all physical activities (PA) reported by each child. PA in terms of metabolic equivalents (PA MET) were categorized into tertiles (the first tertile was defined as lowest, second tertile as intermediary, and third tertile as highest METs). This scoring method was validated in Brazilian children in a previous study [39].

2.4. Anthropometric and Sociodemographic Measurements

The administrative department of each school provided information on the child's date of birth, sex, and type of school (an important marker of socioeconomic condition in Brazil). Trained research staff measured weight and height of participants following standard techniques [40] in both surveys. Theoretical and practical workshops on measurement techniques were held to standardize the anthropometric measurements in both surveys [41]. Anthropometric measurements were taken with the children wearing light clothes and without shoes. Weight was measured with a digital 180 kg scale (Marte®, model PP, 50 g precision). Height was measured with a portable stadiometer (Alturexata®, 1 mm precision). Body mass index (BMI) was computed as weight (in kg) divided by the square of height (in m). Parents completed a self-administered questionnaire reporting their weight, height, and monthly family income. Monthly family income was defined as a categorical variable taking into account the minimum wage at both time points (<3; ≥3 and <5; ≥5 and <10; ≥10). Maternal weight status was assessed by BMI based on self-reported weight (kg) and height (m). Type of school was constructed as a dichotomous variable (public or private). Children's age was computed as the difference between the date of birth and the date of measurements.

At both time points, children's BMI data was converted into z-scores (according to age and sex) based on the World Health Organization Growth References (WHO-2007) [42]. Weight status of children (baseline) and adolescents (follow-up) were then categorized as non-overweight (N-OW) (BMI-for-age < +1.0 SD) or overweight including obesity (OW) (BMI-for-age ≥ +1.0 SD). Underweight (0.8%) and normal weight children were grouped together into the N-OW category, while overweight (non-obese) and obese (6.7%) children were grouped into the OW category. Weight status change was based on individual changes from childhood to early adolescence. In the regression analysis, the change in BMI z-score (BMI z-score at follow-up − BMI z-score at baseline) was modeled as a continuous variable in order to consider the entire distribution of weight status among the whole study population.

2.5. Statistical Analysis

In order to identify DPs in a representative sample of 7–10-year-old schoolchildren, exploratory FA with principal component estimation was applied to the total sample at baseline (n = 1158). A polychoric correlation model for categorical ordered data was used. The number of factors to retain was first examined by the chi-squared test, which showed that the five-factor solution provided the best fit of the a priori model (baseline FA) ($\chi^2(12) = 31.51$, $p < 0.01$). However, the four-factor solution produced better interpretability, which was confirmed by the common practice to choose components with Eigenvalues >1.5 to limit the factors [43], and by the examination of the Scree plot (Figure S2). After the choice of the number of factors, the factor loadings of foods items were calculated. Those foods/beverages that showed low loadings for all factors were excluded from the analysis (yoghurt, sweets, fish and vegetable soup), as they did not explain any factor. After the exclusion of those foods, FA was performed again, and four major dietary patterns were considered as best representing the data. The varimax orthogonal rotation was carried out in order to simplify the interpretation of the data, maximizing the higher factor loadings and minimizing the lower ones. Variables with factor loadings ≥0.30 or ≤−0.30 were considered important for the interpretability of the factors. For the total sample in 2007, the factor scores for each DP were calculated at the individual level by summing the observed standardized frequencies of consumption per food/beverage, weighted according to the absolute factor loadings. The factor scores were standardized and the group mean factor scores were set to zero.

A confirmatory analysis for the complete cases (n = 458) in 2012 was used, in which all factor loadings were the ones evaluated at baseline. This allowed the comparisons in mean factor scores between the same children at follow-up. Using this approach, the changes in factor scores reflected actual differences in the intake frequency of foods/beverages identifying the factor (pattern) rather than a change in the individuals' relative rank position compared to the group mean intake frequency [44].

A high factor score for a given pattern indicated high frequency intake of the foods constituting that food pattern, and a low score indicated low frequency intake of those foods. Factors were labeled by numbers (I, II, III, IV) according to the variance explained and were interpreted according to the food groups that loaded highly on each pattern.

Tracking was defined as how stable the factor scores identified at baseline in the complete-cases sample remained at follow-up. Paired *t* test was used to determine whether the mean factor scores difference between the completers was zero. Spearman's correlation was calculated between the factor scores obtained at each time point. The power analysis of these effects was analyzed considering the effect size measured with Cohen's *d* parameters: <0.2 = small effect, 0.2 to 0.8 = medium, and >0.8 = large [45].

Multivariate linear regression was used to examine the changes in BMI *z*-scores (defined as the difference between BMI *z*-score at follow-up and at baseline) associated to changes in each dietary pattern scores (the difference between dietary patterns scores at follow-up and at baseline), simultaneously. The potential confounding variables in the multiple regression models were: child's age (continuous), sex, BMI *z*-scores (continuous), maternal BMI (continuous), type of school (private or public), monthly family income (categorical), day of the week (school days or Sunday/holidays), and tertiles of PA MET at baseline. The maternal BMI was included in the model, as there is a solid body of evidence on both genetic and environmental parental influence on children's dietary patterns [9,23]. All the covariates were chosen among a range of possible confounders because they were both associated with BMI and with food intake. Interaction terms were not used, as preliminary analyses did not find important examples of interaction, as well as to avoid over-adjustment and chance findings (data not shown).

To investigate if the DPs differed on school days compared with non-school days (Sunday and holidays), exploratory FA with principal component estimation was applied to baseline data for children who reported their food intake on school days using the same analytical approach described above for the complete baseline data. The factor scores obtained on school days were standardized and the group mean factor scores were set to zero and used as a reference. Then, the factor scores for non-school days were computed in a simple confirmatory FA model, in which the loadings on the four factors were those evaluated at school days. One-sample *t* test was used to test the differences between the mean factor scores for non-school days versus school days.

Considering that the sample size available for analyses was restricted to complete cases ($n = 458$), with 80% test power and alpha error of 5%, the study was able to detect an effect size of at least 0.131 for the two-tail paired *t*-test; at least 0.165 for the one-tail Spearman's rho; and at least 0.027 in the multivariate linear regression.

Statistical significance level was set at 5%. Statistical software R [46] was used for factor analysis and Stata 13.0 (Stata Corp., College Station, TX, USA) was used for descriptive and analytical statistics.

3. Results

The total baseline characteristics of participants at age 7 to 10 years ($n = 1158$), including children participating in the follow-up survey ($n = 458$) or lost to follow-up ($n = 700$), are shown in Table 1. There were no differences for age, sex, BMI, prevalence of overweight, mother's weight status, monthly family income, day of the week, and tertiles of PA MET. Nevertheless, a greater proportion of children enrolled in private schools were lost in the follow-up.

Table 1. Characteristics of the study participants by follow-up status.

	Not Followed-Up (n = 700)	Followed-Up (n = 458)	Total Baseline (n = 1158)
		Mean ± SD (95% CI)	
Age (years)	9.1 ± 1.2 (8.9–9.1)	9.0 ± 1.1 (8.9–9.2)	9.0 ± 1.1 (8.9–9.1)
BMI	17.8 ± 2.8 (17.5–18.0)	17.6 ± 2.9 (17.2–17.8)	17.7 ± 2.9 (17.5–17.7)
		% (95% CI)	
Sex			
Boys	49.4 (45.7–53.1)	46.5 (42.0–51.1)	48.3 (45.4–51.2)
Girls	50.6 (46.9–54.3)	53.5 (48.9–58.0)	51.7 (48.8–54.6)
Overweight [a]			
Yes	34.3 (30.9–37.9)	34.3 (30.1–38.8)	34.3 (31.6–37.1)
No	65.7 (62.1–69.1)	65.7 (61.2–69.9)	65.7 (62.9–68.4)
Type of school			
Public	70.4 (66.9–73.7)	86.2 (82.8–89.1)	76.7 (74.2–79.0)
Private	29.6 (26.3–33.1)	13.3 (10.9–17.2)	23.3 (21.0–25.8)
Mother's weight status [b]			
Thin	3.5 (2.3–5.2)	5.5 (3.7–8.1)	4.3 (3.2–5.7)
Normal weight	65.9 (62.2–69.4)	63.0 (58.4–67.5)	64.8 (61.9–67.6)
Overweight	22.6 (19.5–25.9)	20.8 (17.2–24.9)	21.9 (19.5–24.4)
Obese	8.0 (6.2–10.4)	10.6 (8.0–13.9)	9.1 (7.5–10.9)
Monthly family income (minimum wage) [c]			
<3	45.4 (41.4–49.5)	47.3 (42.4–52.3)	46.2 (43.1–49.3)
3–5	20.0 (16.9–23.4)	26.8 (22.7–31.4)	22.7 (20.2–25.5)
5–10	19.9 (16.9–23.4)	15.2 (12.0–19.1)	18.0 (15.8–20.6)
>10	14.7 (12.0–17.8)	10.7 (7.9–14.1)	13.1 (11.1–15.3)
Day of the week [d]			
Non-school days	32.9 (29.5–36.4)	22.3 (18.7–26.3)	28.7 (26.1–31.4)
School days	67.1 (63.6–70.5)	77.7 (73.7–81.3)	71.3 (68.7–73.9)
Tertiles of PA MET			
Lowest	35.0 (31.5–38.6)	32.5 (28.4–37.0)	34.0 (31.3–36.8)
Medium	32.4 (29.1–36.0)	33.0 (28.8–37.4)	32.6 (30.0–35.4)
Highest	32.6 (29.2–36.1)	34.5 (30.3–39.0)	33.3 (30.7–36.1)

PA MET: Physical activities in terms of metabolic equivalents; BMI: Body mass index; WHO: World Health Organization; [a] Overweight (including obesity BMI ≥ +1.0 z-scores—WHO-2007); [b] BMI based on self-reported data on weight and height and classified according to WHO recommendations (Thin—BMI <18.5 kg/m^2, Normal weight—BMI 18.5–24.9 kg/m^2, Overweight non-obese BMI 25–29.9 kg/m^2, Obese—BMI ≥30 kg/m^2); [c] 1 minimum wage = $US 204.30 ($BR 380): September 2007 exchange rate; [d] Day of the week. Missing mother's weight status data (4.0%); Missing income data (15.3%); Missing child's BMI (1.7%).

After computing the FA on the 17 foods/beverages at baseline, four DPs were identified with the highest Eigenvalues that accounted for 47.9% of the total variance of food intake and could be interpreted meaningfully in terms of nutritional characteristics. The detailed structures of the four DPs with their explained variance and loading coefficients are shown in Table 2. The "DP I" had positive high loadings on rice, cooked beans, leafy vegetables, and beef/poultry, while having negative loadings on pasta and fast-food, suggesting that the intake of these foods showed a deviation from this DP. The high loading foods on "DP II" included French fries, salty snacks, soft drinks, and fast-food. The "DP III" loaded highly on fruit juices, cooked vegetables, fruits, pasta, leafy vegetables, cheese and milk, with a negative loading on soft drinks. Finally, the "DP IV" loaded highly on coffee with milk, breads/biscuits, cheese and milk, with negative loadings on chocolate milk and fast-food (Table 2).

Table 2. Structures of four dietary patterns identified by factor analysis with principal component method in a representative sample of 7–10-year-old schoolchildren in 2007.

	Dietary Patterns 2007 (n = 1158)			
	DP I	DP II	DP III	DP IV
Variance explained (%)	17.5	10.7	10.0	9.7
Foods and food groups		**Factor loadings** [a]		
Beans (cooked)	**0.66**	−0.22	0.16	0.08
Beef/poultry	**0.30**	0.08	0.08	0.07
Bread/biscuits	0.04	−0.07	0.19	**0.54**
Cheese	**−0.34**	−0.28	**0.40**	**0.41**
Chocolate milk	−0.17	−0.09	0.21	**−0.58**
Coffee with milk	0.01	0.05	−0.08	**0.90**
Fast-food	**−0.41**	**0.31**	0.04	**−0.31**
French fries	−0.07	**0.85**	0.04	−0.10
Fruit juices	0.07	−0.07	**0.71**	−0.07
Fruits	0.16	0.03	**0.50**	0.00
Leafy vegetables	**0.57**	0.11	**0.40**	0.00
Milk	0.08	−0.08	**0.34**	**0.36**
Pasta	**−0.46**	0.22	**0.49**	0.15
Rice	**0.84**	−0.09	0.08	0.04
Salty snacks	0.08	**0.84**	−0.05	0.09
Soft drinks	−0.27	**0.49**	**−0.32**	−0.02
Vegetables (cooked)	0.21	−0.15	**0.54**	0.04

[a] Factor loading values in bold: ≥0.30 or ≤−0.30.

Table 3 shows mean factor scores of the four dietary patterns at the two time points in the complete cases (n = 458), spearman correlations coefficients between factor scores at the two time points, and the effect size for each analysis. Considering the difference between the mean factors scores at the two time points, our sample allows us to conclude that only the scores for DP II differed between the two time points, with a medium effect size. The sample size of the follow-up has sufficient power to show correlations between factor scores of DPs I, III, and IV at the two time points, with a medium effect size. These findings together imply that children presenting higher scores for DP I, DP III, and DP IV at baseline also showed higher scores for the respective DPs at follow-up, and the mean frequencies of consumption of foods constituting these patterns did not increase. On the other hand, no correlation was found for DP II scores between baseline and follow-up and the mean frequency of consumption of the foods constituting the pattern decreased (Table 3).

Table 3. Mean (standard deviation), spearman correlation coefficients, and effect size for corresponding factor scores at each time point in the complete cases (n = 458).

	DP I	DP II	DP III	DP IV
		Mean (SD)		
Baseline	−0.04 (1.2)	−0.02 (1.1)	0.07 (1.1)	0.03 (1.3)
Follow-up	0.06 (1.2)	−0.39 (1.0)	−0.07 (1.1)	−0.08 (1.1)
p	0.13	<0.01	0.03	0.15
Effect size	0.07	0.25	0.10	0.07
		Spearman Correlation		
Baseline vs. Follow-up	0.20	0.07	0.22	0.10
p	<0.01	0.12	<0.01	0.03
Effect size	0.41	0.14	0.45	0.20

After controlling for baseline BMI z-scores, maternal BMI, sex, age, type of school, family income, day of the week, and tertiles of PA MET, there was no significant linear association between changes in BMI z-scores and changes in DP scores from childhood to adolescence. The analysis of the change in DP scores showed a small effect size on the change of BMI z-scores (Table 4). Based on the weight status categories defined by WHO-2007, out of the 153 children classified as overweight or obese at baseline, 65.4% (n = 100) remained overweight/obese in adolescence (boys: 69.8%; girls: 59.7%). Out of the 297 children classified as non-overweight at baseline, 9.4% (n = 28) were found to be overweight/obese (boys: 4.8%; girls: 9.8%) at follow-up.

Table 4. Relation between changes in BMI z-scores and changes in factor scores from ages 7–10 years to 12–15 years in the complete cases.

Change in Dietary Pattern	Change in BMI z-Scores [a]		
	Coefficient	p	Effect Size
DP I	0.01	0.92	0.00
DP II	0.02	0.45	0.00
DP III	−0.04	0.19	0.00
DP IV	0.05	0.07	0.01

[a] Outcome change in BMI z-scores (n = 450) over the five years since baseline; Adjusted by age (continuous), sex, BMI z-score, maternal BMI, type of school, family income, day of the week (school days or non-school days), and tertiles of PA MET (all baseline).

The FA on the same 17 foods/beverages applied at baseline in the sample who reported food intake on school days also identified four DPs with higher Eigenvalues that explained 49.0% of the food intake variance (Table S1). One-sample t test showed that the two DP scores (DP I and DP II) for non-school days were statistically different from zero, i.e., food intake on non-school days differed from school days for these patterns (Table S2).

4. Discussion

The longitudinal analysis of the present study conducted with the complete cases of children and adolescents five years apart showed that, on average, the factor scores for "DP II" (French fries, salty snacks, soft drinks and fast-food) identified at baseline (in 7–10-year-old children) decreased in the follow-up sample (in 12–15-year-olds), whereas no changes were observed for "DP I" (rice, cooked beans, leafy vegetables, beef/poultry), "DP III" (fruit juices, cooked vegetables, fruits, pasta, leafy vegetables, cheese and milk), and "DP IV" (coffee with milk, breads/biscuits, cheese and milk).

Cross-sectional analysis of data obtained at baseline identified four DPs that satisfactorily captured eating behavior (47.9% of food intake variance explained) in this population-based sample of Brazilian schoolchildren. These DPs were also identified in our previous study that extracted DPs by Latent class analysis (LCA) based on the time-of-day of eating events [25] and resembled other patterns identified in Brazilian and international studies conducted in children and adolescents. "DP I" in the present study (including rice and beans) was also identified in studies based on the Brazilian Household Budget Surveys (2002–2003) [47] and (2008–2009) [23]. The latter, conducted in individuals over 10 years of age, confirmed the aggregation of DPs among members of the same family and extracted three major DPs by factor analysis: "Traditional snack" (coffee, rolls, oils and fats, cheese), "Traditional main meal" (rice, beans and other legumes, and meat) and "Fast-food snack" (sandwiches, processed meats, soft drinks, snacks, pizza) [23] in line with "DP I" and "DP II" (salty snacks, French fries, fast-food and sugary beverages) of the present study. The "DP II" in the present study shared various dietary items of high fat and high energy-density items with other studies of children and adolescents in Brazil [21,22], Colombia [48], Canada [49], and European countries [1,35,50,51]. Our "DP III" (fruit juices, cooked vegetables, fruits, pasta, leafy vegetables, cheese and milk) was similar to the "health aware/conscious" pattern associated with lower fat gain in girls between 9 and 11 years of age in the Avon Study in England [52,53].

On average, the factor scores for "DP II" (French fries, salty snacks, soft drinks, and fast-food) identified at baseline (in 7–10-year-old children) decreased in the follow-up sample (12–15-year-olds), whereas no changes were observed for "DP I" (rice, cooked beans, leafy vegetables, and beef/poultry), "DP III" (fruit juices, cooked vegetables, fruits, pasta, leafy vegetables, cheese and milk), and "DP IV" (coffee with milk, breads/biscuits, cheese and milk). Although food consumption was only assessed for one day in the present study and considerable within-subject variation in daily food consumption may occur, our results provide evidence of slight stability of three DP scores (DP I, III, IV) as well as change in "DP II" scores over the five-year follow-up period.

Direct comparisons of the present results with previous DP studies in children and adolescents should consider differences in study design, sample sizes, dietary assessment methods, and statistical methods to derive DPs and to estimate the tracking of DPs. Furthermore, the extent of changes of DP from childhood to adolescence may vary in different populations due to cultural, social, and economic factors. A review of the literature found that the tracking of DPs ranged from weak to moderate between childhood and adolescence [54].

The stability of the mean factor scores for "DP I" (rice, cooked beans, beef/poultry, leafy vegetables) and "DP IV" (milk, coffee with milk, cheese, and breads/biscuits) from childhood to adolescence may be explained by cultural factors. The components of these patterns are traditional foods eaten in Brazilian meals ("DP I" in lunch and/or dinner; "DP IV" in breakfast and/or snacks between meals). These patterns were also identified in cross-sectional studies conducted with children [22,24,25], adolescents [21,22,26], and adults [55] from different regions in Brazil.

We expected to observe an increase in scores for "DP II" (salty snacks, French fries, fast-food, and sugary beverages) at follow-up. However, this was not the case in our study, and the decrease in its factor scores at follow-up might result from a social desirability bias (underreporting). It is also possible that adolescents at follow-up consumed larger portions of the unhealthy foods constituting "DP II", but less frequently. We cannot investigate this hypothesis because the PDFQ-3 did not measure portion sizes. Therefore, energy intake could not be estimated and input variables for DP analysis could not be adjusted for energy intake. The issue of adjusting for energy intake is still controversial in studies of changes in DPs [34].

The present study did not find a significant linear association between changes in DP scores and changes in BMI *z*-scores. The longitudinal association of a high adherence to unhealthy DPs with increased risk of overweight and obesity was not verified in some earlier studies [12,56]. In the European DONALD study [57], a positive though small association between baseline consumption of high-energy convenience foods and the change in the percentage of body fat over a five-year follow-up was found among boys. A cohort of 5–12-year-old children from low- and middle-income families in Bogota showed that those in the highest quartile of adherence to a snacking pattern had a 0.09 kg/m^2 higher BMI gain and 0.012 mm higher gain in trunk adiposity per year compared to children in the lowest quartile [48].

The strengths of the present study were the longitudinal follow-up design based on a relatively large sample size at baseline, the use of the same validated questionnaire to assess food intake at the two time points, the use of potential confounding variables in the regression analysis, and the application of confirmatory FA to compute factor scores over time. An important feature of our analysis, which was rarely present in previous longitudinal studies on the tracking of DPs [19,44], is that we applied confirmatory FA to calculate factor scores at follow-up by using the factor loadings obtained at baseline. By using this approach to compute the factor scores, the problem of the data dependency and lower reproducibility of factors in different datasets is eliminated [44]. When exploratory FA is used to identify DPs and to investigate their stability over time, the correlation between foods is commonly used to create multiple continuous scores at each time point. A difficulty inherent in this approach is that the DPs obtained are not generally reproducible. The performance of separate exploratory FA at each time point to evaluate tracking may result in high correlations between pattern scores at baseline and at follow-up, despite large changes in the correlations between the specific food items that define a pattern [11].

We acknowledge some limitations in the present study. First, the retention rate in the follow-up study (40.1%) was low, limiting the generalizability of our results to the general population. It could be argued that changes in DP scores from childhood to adolescence were a result of attrition biases. However, children lost to follow-up did not differ significantly from the included participants in DP scores, demographic variables, and weight status at baseline. Therefore, we believe that the low correlations found between the baseline factor scores of DPs I, III, and IV and its scores at follow-up were not affected by such bias. We cannot exclude the possibility that the lack of association found between changes in DPs and changes in BMI *z*-score could be due to the underrepresentation of adolescents who studied in private schools (wealthier than adolescents from public schools in Brazil) in the follow-up study.

Second, as for all other dietary assessment studies, the self-reported food recall may potentially be subject to misreporting. The PDFQ-3 used in this study proved to be a valid instrument [28] and has been used to assess dietary patterns and behaviors [25,26,58]. The PDFQ-3 was designed to avoid the difficulties associated with children's assessments of portion size, and to simplify the memory task by prompting only the relevant food items eaten on the previous day. The cognitive task required for estimating portion size, frequency, and averaging may not be compatible with the perceptual and conceptual capacities of children who have not reached the stage of abstract reasoning at approximately 10–11 years of age [59,60]. Like some questionnaires validated in other countries [35,61], this approach keeps the questionnaire relatively brief and easy for the child to complete with minimal assistance. Also, the dietary information is derived from the children themselves (without help from parents or guardians). The use of the parent report of a child's diet has also been seen as a limitation [35,62]. In the age range of the present study (7–15 years), children spend a considerable amount of time unsupervised by their parents, who therefore could not validate the children's dietary recall.

The results are based on the frequency of food/beverage and food groups eaten on only one day in each time point in a group of children and conclusions may be applicable to the population rather than to individuals, since a single day of intake may not be representative of usual individual intake. The expected effect of use a food questionnaire that only covers one day of dietary intake is to attenuate the statistical association between changes in adherence to a dietary pattern and changes in BMI *z*-score [15,63].

The differences in DP between weekdays/schooldays and non-schooldays found in the present study should be highlighted, and in this sense our results are strengthened by a good coverage of the days of the week (school days), including one day of the weekend (Sunday) and holidays to cover the variation in diet at the group level. While the factor scores for "DP I" on weekdays/school days with high loadings for unhealthy foods (fast-foods, French fries, salty snacks, and soft drinks) increased on Sunday/non-school days ($p < 0.01$), the factor scores for "DP II" with high loadings for foods included in Brazilian traditional lunch and/or dinner (rice, beans, beef/poultry) decreased on Sunday/non-school days ($p < 0.01$), thus indicating that specific foods eaten on non-schooldays were less healthy. Changes in daily patterns such as not attending school on the weekend contribute significantly to changes in dietary patterns of food consumption, patterns of physical activity, and ultimately energy balance [64]. Previous research in children indicates that dietary quality is poorer on the weekends compared with weekdays, with significantly higher intakes of total sugars [62], sugar sweetened beverages, confectionery, and lower consumption of fruit and vegetables [62,65]. The potential influence of day-to-day variation of food consumption in the FA merits more attention in future research.

In future studies, information on children's diet from the PDFQ-3 should be integrated with a food frequency questionnaire filled in by parents to complement the measure of food items not covered by the child's questionnaire. In addition, the PDFQ-3 should be applied on various days of the week, including one day of the weekend at each time point, assuring that the child completes the PDFQ-3 on the same day of the week at each time point.

Additionally, although we adjusted for a variety of potential confounding variables, residual confounding cannot be ruled out. In particular, adjustments for social mobility, which expresses life-long changes in family income [5], and which might affect dietary habits and changes in weight status, were not possible due to the lack of information.

5. Conclusions

Four dietary patterns were identified at baseline in schoolchildren aged 7–10 years old: "DP I" (rice, cooked beans, beef/poultry, leafy vegetables), "DP II" (salty snacks, French fries, fast-food, sugary beverages), "DP III" (fruits, cooked and leafy vegetables, fruit juices, pasta, milk, cheese) and "DP IV" (milk, coffee with milk, cheese, breads/biscuits). Slight tracking was observed between factor scores for "DP I", "DP III", and "DP IV" from childhood to adolescence using the complete cases, while the factor scores for "DP II" decreased in follow-up. No significant linear association was shown between changes in BMI z-scores and changes in DP scores over a five-year period.

We cannot be certain that the level of tracking of dietary patterns found in the present study reflected a real finding or resulted from an artifact due to change in intake from a single day in childhood to a single day in adolescence. We intend to address this in the next follow-up of the study by taking repeated dietary assessments during childhood and adolescence.

Supplementary Materials:
Figure S1: The Previous Day Food Questionnaire (PDFQ-3), page 2., Figure S2: Scree plot for identification of dietary patterns (components) by factor analysis (FA) with principal component estimation, Table S1: Structures of four dietary patterns identified by factor analysis with the principal component method on baseline cross-sectional data on school days., Table S2: Factor scores on non-school days versus school days (reference) and significance of difference, as assessed by one-sample t test.

Acknowledgments: The survey was funded by the Brazilian National Council for Scientific and Technological Development—CNPq (grants 402322/2005-3 and 483955/2011-6), (M.A.A.d.A. grants no. 305148/2011-7 and 308352/2016-5). D.B.L. and A.S.L. received a fellowship from the Brazilian Federal Agency for the Improvement of Higher Education and the Foundation of Research from Santa Catarina State, respectively. The funding sources had no role in the study design; collection, analysis, and interpretation of data; writing of the report; or the decision to submit the article for publication.

Author Contributions: The authors' responsibilities were as follows: D.B.L. and P.F.H. participated in the concept, data analysis and interpretation, and preparation of the paper. M.A.A.d.A. participated in design, ethics submission, supervised the study implementation, interpretation and preparation of the paper. A.S.L., F.B., P.F.D.P. and F.K.V assisted with interpretation and reviewed the paper. D.F.A., J.S. and P.H.d.M.A. assisted with data analysis, interpretation and reviewed the paper. All authors had final approval of the submitted and published versions.

References

1. Mikkila, V.; Rasanen, L.; Raitakari, O.T.; Pietinen, P.; Viikari, J. Consistent dietary patterns identified from childhood to adulthood: The cardiovascular risk in Young Finns Study. *Br. J. Nutr.* **2005**, *93*, 923–931. [CrossRef] [PubMed]
2. Craigie, A.M.; Lake, A.A.; Kelly, S.A.; Adamson, A.J.; Mathers, J.C. Tracking of obesity-related behaviors from childhood to adulthood: A systematic review. *Maturitas* **2011**, *70*, 266–284. [CrossRef] [PubMed]
3. Due, P.; Krølner, R.; Rasmussen, M.; Andersen, A.; TrabDamsgaard, M.; Graham, H.; Holstein, B.E. Pathways and mechanisms in adolescence contribute to adult health inequalities. *Scand. J. Public Health* **2011**, *39*, 62–78. [CrossRef] [PubMed]
4. Totland, T.H.; Gebremariam, M.K.; Lien, N.; Bjelland, M.; Grydeland, M.; Bergh, I.H.; Klepp, K.I.; Andersen, L.F. Does tracking of dietary behaviors differ by parental education in children during the transition into adolescence? *Public Health Nutr.* **2013**, *16*, 673–682. [CrossRef] [PubMed]

5. Arruda, S.P.; da Silva, A.A.; Kac, G.; Goldani, M.Z.; Bettiol, H.; Barbieri, M.A. Socioeconomic and demographic factors are associated with dietary patterns in a cohort of young Brazilian adults. *BMC Public Health* **2014**, *14*, 654. [CrossRef] [PubMed]
6. Popkin, B.M.; Gordon-Larsen, P. The nutrition transition: An overview of world patterns of change. *Nutr. Rev.* **2004**, *62*, S140–S143. [CrossRef] [PubMed]
7. Hawkes, C.; Chopra, M.; Friel, S. Globalization, Trade, and the Nutrition Transition. In *Globalization and Health: Pathways, Evidence and Policy*; Labonté, R., Schrecker, C., Eds.; Routledge: New York, NY, USA, 2009; pp. 235–262.
8. Twisk, J.W.R. *Applied Longitudinal Data Analysis for Epidemiology: A Practical Guide*; Cambridge University Press: Cambridge, UK, 2007.
9. Robinson, S.; Marriott, L.; Poole, J.; Crozier, S.; Borland, S.; Lawrence, W.; Law, C.; Godfrey, K.; Cooper, C.; Inskip, H. Dietary patterns in infancy: The importance of maternal and family influences on feeding practice. *Br. J. Nutr.* **2007**, *98*, 1029–1037. [CrossRef] [PubMed]
10. Northstone, K.; Emmett, P.M. Are dietary patterns stable throughout early and mid-childhood? A birth cohort study. *Br. J. Nutr.* **2008**, *100*, 1069–1076. [CrossRef] [PubMed]
11. Northstone, K.; Emmett, P.M. A comparison of methods to assess changes in dietary patterns from pregnancy to 4 years post-partum obtained using principal components analysis. *Br. J. Nutr.* **2008**, *99*, 1099–1106. [CrossRef] [PubMed]
12. Oellingrath, I.M.; Svendsen, M.V.; Brantsaeter, A.L. Tracking of eating patterns and overweight: A follow-up study of Norwegian schoolchildren from middle childhood to early adolescence. *Nutr. J.* **2011**, *10*, 106. [CrossRef] [PubMed]
13. Bull, C.J.; Northstone, K. Childhood dietary patterns and cardiovascular risk factors in adolescence: Results from the Avon Longitudinal Study of Parents and Children (ALSPAC) cohort. *Public Health Nutr.* **2016**, *19*, 3369–3377. [CrossRef] [PubMed]
14. Lytle, L.A.; Seifert, S.; Greenstein, J.; McGovern, P. How do children's eating patterns and food choices change over time? Results from a cohort study. *Am. J. Health Promot.* **2000**, *14*, 222–228. [CrossRef] [PubMed]
15. Patterson, E.; Warnberg, J.; Kearney, J.; Sjostrom, M. The tracking of dietary intakes of children and adolescents in Sweden over six years: The European Youth Heart Study. *Int. J. Behav. Nutr. Phys. Act.* **2009**, *6*, 91. [CrossRef] [PubMed]
16. Demory-Luce, D.; Morales, M.; Nicklas, T.; Baranowski, T.; Zakeri, I.; Berenson, G. Changes in food group consumption patterns from childhood to young adulthood: The Bogalusa Heart Study. *J. Am. Diet. Assoc.* **2004**, *104*, 1684–1691. [CrossRef] [PubMed]
17. Harris, C.; Flexeder, C.; Thiering, E.; Buyken, A.; Berdel, D.; Koletzko, S.; Bauer, C.P.; Brüske, I.; Koletzko, B.; Standl, M.; et al. Changes in dietary intake during puberty and their determinants: Results from the GINIplus birth cohort study. *BMC Public Health* **2015**, *15*, 841. [CrossRef] [PubMed]
18. Ambrosini, G.L. Childhood dietary patterns and later obesity: A review of the evidence. *Proc. Nutr. Soc.* **2014**, *73*, 137–146. [CrossRef] [PubMed]
19. Ambrosini, G.L.; Emmett, P.M.; Northstone, K.; Jebb, S.A. Tracking a dietary pattern associated with increased adiposity in childhood and adolescence. *Obesity* **2014**, *22*, 458–465. [CrossRef] [PubMed]
20. Wilks, D.C.; Mander, A.P.; Jebb, S.A.; Thompson, S.G.; Sharp, S.J.; Turner, R.M.; Lindroos, A.K. Dietary energy density and adiposity: Employing bias adjustments in a meta-analysis of prospective studies. *BMC Public Health* **2011**, *11*, 48. [CrossRef] [PubMed]
21. Rodrigues, P.R.; Pereira, R.A.; Cunha, D.B.; Sichieri, R.; Ferreira, M.G.; Vilela, A.A.; Gonçalves-Silva, R.M. Factors associated with dietary patterns in adolescents: A school-based study in Cuiabá, Mato Grosso. *Rev. Bras. Epidemiol.* **2012**, *15*, 662–674. [CrossRef] [PubMed]
22. Santos, N.H.; Fiaccone, R.L.; Barreto, M.L.; Silva, L.A.; Silva Rde, C. Association between eating patterns and body mass index in a sample of children and adolescents in Northeastern Brazil. *Cad. Saude Publica* **2014**, *30*, 2235–2245. [CrossRef]
23. Massarani, F.A.; Cunha, D.B.; Muraro, A.P.; Souza Bda, S.; Sichieri, R.; Yokoo, E.M. Familial aggregation and dietary patterns in the Brazilian population. *Cad. Saude Publica* **2015**, *31*, 2535–2545. [CrossRef] [PubMed]
24. Carvalho, C.A.; Fonsêca, P.C.; Nobre, L.N.; Priore, S.E.; FranceschiniSdo, C. Methods of a posteriori identification of food patterns in Brazilian children: A systematic review. *Cien. Saude Colet.* **2016**, *21*, 143–154. [CrossRef] [PubMed]

25. Kupek, E.; Lobo, A.S.; Leal, D.B.; Bellisle, F.; de Assis, M.A. Dietary patterns associated with overweight and obesity among Brazilian schoolchildren: An approach based on the time-of-day of eating events. *Br. J. Nutr.* **2016**, *116*, 1954–1965. [CrossRef] [PubMed]
26. Pinho, M.G.M.; Adami, F.; Benedet, J.; Vasconcelos, F.A.G. Association between screen time and dietary patterns and overweight/obesity among adolescents. *Rev. Nutr.* **2017**, *30*, 377–389. [CrossRef]
27. Leal, D.B.; de Assis, M.A.; González-Chica, D.A.; da Costa, F.F.; de Andrade, D.F.; Lobo, A.S. Changes in total and central adiposity and body fat distribution among 7–10-year-old schoolchildren in Brazil. *Public Health Nutr.* **2015**, *18*, 2105–2114. [CrossRef] [PubMed]
28. Assis, M.A.; Benedet, J.; Kerpel, R.; Vasconcelos, F.A.G.; Di Pietro, P.F.; Kupek, E. Validation of the third version of the Previous Day Food Questionnaire (PDFQ-3) for 6-to-11-years-old schoolchildren. *Cad. Saude Publica* **2009**, *25*, 1816–1826.
29. Ledoux, T.A.; Hingle, M.D.; Baranowski, T. Relationship of fruit and vegetable intake with adiposity: A systematic review. *Obes. Rev.* **2011**, *12*, e143–e150. [CrossRef] [PubMed]
30. Pate, R.R.; O'Neill, J.R.; Liese, A.D.; Janz, K.F.; Granberg, E.M.; Colabianchi, N.; Harsha, D.W.; Condrasky, M.M.; O'Neil, P.M.; Lau, E.Y.; et al. Factors associated with development of excessive fatness in children and adolescents: A review of prospective studies. *Obes. Rev.* **2013**, *14*, 645–658. [CrossRef] [PubMed]
31. Rosenheck, R. Fast-food consumption and increased caloric intake: A systematic review of a trajectory towards weight gain and obesity risk. *Obes. Rev.* **2008**, *9*, 535–547. [CrossRef] [PubMed]
32. Hu, F.B. Resolved: There is sufficient scientific evidence that decreasing sugar-sweetened beverage consumption will reduce the prevalence of obesity and obesity related diseases. *Obes. Rev.* **2013**, *14*, 606–619. [CrossRef] [PubMed]
33. Ministério da Saúde. Guia Alimentar Para a População Brasileira. 2006. Available online: http://bvsms.saude.gov.br/bvs/publicacoes/guia_alimentar_populacao_brasileira_2008.pdf (accessed on 16 July 2015).
34. Newby, P.K.; Tucker, K.L. Empirically derived eating patterns using factor or cluster analysis: A review. *Nutr. Rev.* **2004**, *62*, 177–203. [CrossRef] [PubMed]
35. Pala, V.; Lissner, L.; Hebestreit, A.; Lanfer, A.; Sieri, S.; Siani, A.; Huybrechts, I.; Kambek, L.; Molnar, D.; Tornaritis, M.; et al. Dietary patterns and longitudinal change in body mass in European children: A follow-up study on the IDEFICS multicenter cohort. *Eur. J. Clin. Nutr.* **2013**, *67*, 1042–1049. [CrossRef] [PubMed]
36. Thorpe, M.G.; Milte, C.M.; Crawford, D.; McNaughton, S.A. A comparison of the dietary patterns derived by principal component analysis and cluster analysis in older Australians. *Int. J. Behav. Nutr. Phys. Act.* **2016**, *13*, 30. [CrossRef] [PubMed]
37. Cabral, L.G.A.; Costa, F.F.; Liparotti, J.R. Preliminary validation of the physical activity section of the previous day physical activity and food consumption questionnaire (PDPAFQ). *Rev. Bras. Ativ. Fis. Saude* **2011**, *16*, 100–106.
38. Ridley, K.; Ainsworth, B.E.; Olds, T.S. Development of a Compendium of Energy Expenditures for Youth. *Int. J. Behav. Nutr. Phys. Act.* **2008**, *5*, 1–8. [CrossRef] [PubMed]
39. De Jesus, J.M.; Assis, M.A.A.; Kupek, E. Assessment of physical activity in schoolchildren using a web-based questionnaire. *Rev. Bras. Med. Esporte* **2016**, *22*, 261–266.
40. Lohman, T.G.; Roche, A.F.; Martorell, R. *Anthropometric Standardization Reference Manual*; Human Kinetics: Champaign, IL, USA, 1988.
41. Frainer, D.E.; Adami, F.; Vasconcelos, F.A.; Assis, M.A.; Calvo, M.C.; Kerpel, R. Standardization and reliability of anthropometric measurements for population surveys. *Arch. Latinoam. Nutr.* **2007**, *57*, 335–342. [PubMed]
42. de Onis, M.; Onyango, A.W.; Borghi, E.; Siyam, A.; Nishida, C.; Siekmann, J. Development of a WHO growth reference for school-aged children and adolescents. *Bull. World Health Organ.* **2007**, *85*, 660–667. [CrossRef] [PubMed]
43. Khani, B.R.; Ye, W.; Terry, P.; Wolk, A. Reproducibility and validity of major dietary patterns among Swedish women assessed with a food-frequency questionnaire. *J. Nutr.* **2004**, *134*, 1541–1545. [PubMed]
44. Togo, P.; Osler, M.; Sørensen, T.I.; Heitmann, B.L. A longitudinal study of food intake patterns and obesity in adult Danish men and women. *Int. J. Obes. Relat. Metab. Disord.* **2004**, *28*, 583–593. [CrossRef] [PubMed]
45. Cohen, J. Statistical power analysis. *Curr. Dir. Psychol. Sci.* **1992**, *1*, 98–101. [CrossRef]

46. R Core Team. *R: A Language and Environment for Statistical Computing*; R Foundation for Statistical Computing: Vienna, Austria, 2016.
47. Nascimento, S.; Barbosa, F.S.; Sichieri, R.; Pereira, R.A. Dietary availability patterns of the Brazilian macro-regions. *Nutr. J.* **2011**, *10*, 79. [CrossRef] [PubMed]
48. Shroff, M.R.; Perng, W.; Baylin, A.; Mora-Plazas, M.; Marin, C.; Villamor, E. Adherence to a snacking dietary pattern and soda intake are related to the development of adiposity: A prospective study in school-age children. *Public Health Nutr.* **2014**, *17*, 1507–1513. [CrossRef] [PubMed]
49. Shang, L.; O'Loughlin, J.; Tremblay, A.; Gray-Donald, K. The association between food patterns and adiposity among Canadian children at risk of overweight. *Appl. Physiol. Nutr. Metab.* **2014**, *39*, 195–201. [CrossRef] [PubMed]
50. Craig, L.C.; McNeill, G.; Macdiarmid, J.I.; Masson, L.F.; Holmes, B.A. Dietary patterns of school-age children in Scotland: Association with socio-economic indicators, physical activity and obesity. *Br. J. Nutr.* **2010**, *103*, 319–334. [CrossRef] [PubMed]
51. Moreira, P.; Santos, S.; Padrao, P.; Cordeiro, T.; Bessa, M.; Valente, H.; Barros, R.; Teixeira, V.; Mitchell, V.; Lopes, C.; et al. Food patterns according to sociodemographics, physical activity, sleeping and obesity in Portuguese children. *Int. J. Environ. Res. Public Health* **2010**, *7*, 1121–1138. [CrossRef] [PubMed]
52. Smith, A.D.; Emmett, P.M.; Newby, P.K.; Northstone, K. Dietary patterns and changes in body composition in children between 9 and 11 years. *Food Nutr. Res.* **2014**, *58*. [CrossRef] [PubMed]
53. Emmett, P.M.; Jones, L.R.; Northstone, K. Dietary patterns in the Avon Longitudinal Study of Parents and Children. *Nutr. Rev.* **2015**, *73*, 207–230. [CrossRef] [PubMed]
54. Madruga, S.W.; Araújo, C.L.; Bertoldi, A.D.; Neutzling, M.B. Tracking of dietary patterns from childhood to adolescence. *Rev. Saude Publica* **2012**, *46*, 376–386. [CrossRef] [PubMed]
55. de Oliveira Santos, R.; Fisberg, R.M.; Marchioni, D.M.; Troncoso Baltar, V. Dietary patterns for meals of Brazilian adults. *Br. J. Nutr.* **2015**, *114*, 822–828. [CrossRef] [PubMed]
56. Alexy, U.; Sichert-Hellert, W.; Kersting, M.; Schultze-Pawlitschko, V. Pattern of long-term fat intake and BMI during childhood and adolescence—Results of the DONALD Study. *Int. J. Obes. Relat. Metab. Disord.* **2004**, *28*, 1203–1209. [CrossRef] [PubMed]
57. Alexy, U.; Libuda, L.; Mersmann, S.; Kersting, M. Convenience foods in children's diet and association with dietary quality and body weight status. *Eur. J. Clin. Nutr.* **2011**, *65*, 160–166. [CrossRef] [PubMed]
58. Assis, M.A.; Calvo, M.C.; Kupek, E.; Assis Guedes de Vasconcelos, F.; Campos, V.C.; Machado, M.; Costa, F.F.; de Andrade, D.F. Qualitative analysis of the diet of a probabilistic sample of schoolchildren from Florianópolis, Santa Catarina State, Brazil, using the Previous Day Food Questionnaire. *Cad. Saude Publica* **2010**, *26*, 1355–1365. [CrossRef] [PubMed]
59. Baranowski, T.; Domel, S. A cognitive model of children's reporting of food intake. *Am. J. Clin. Nutr.* **1994**, *59* (Suppl. 1), 212S–217S. [PubMed]
60. Livingstone, M.B.; Robson, P.J.; Wallace, J.M. Issues in dietary intake assessment of children and adolescents. *Br. J. Nutr.* **2004**, *92* (Suppl. 2), S213–S222. [CrossRef] [PubMed]
61. Magarey, A.; Golley, R.; Spurrier, N.; Goodwin, E.; Ong, F. Reliability and validity of the Children's Dietary Questionnaire: A new tool to measure children's dietary patterns. *Int. J. Pediatr. Obes.* **2009**, *4*, 257–265. [CrossRef] [PubMed]
62. Rothausen, B.W.; Matthiessen, J.; Andersen, L.F.; Brockhoff, P.B.; Tetens, I. Dietary patterns on weekdays and weekend days in 4–14-year-old Danish children. *Br. J. Nutr.* **2013**, *109*, 1704–1713. [CrossRef] [PubMed]
63. Junior, E.V.; Fisberg, R.M.; Cesar, C.L.G.; Marchioni, D.M.L. Sources of variation of energy and nutrient intake among adolescents in São Paulo, Brazil. *Cad. Saude Publica* **2010**, *26*, 2129–2137. [CrossRef]
64. McCarthy, S. Weekly patterns, diet quality and energy balance. *Physiol. Behav.* **2014**, *134*, 55–59. [CrossRef] [PubMed]
65. Svensson, A.; Larsson, C.; Eiben, G.; Lanfer, A.; Pala, V.; Hebestreit, A.; Huybrechts, I.; Fernández-Alvira, J.M.; Russo, P.; Koni, A.C.; et al. European children's sugar intake on weekdays versus weekends: The IDEFICS study. *Eur. J. Clin. Nutr.* **2014**, *68*, 822–828. [CrossRef] [PubMed]

11

Clustering of Multiple Energy Balance-Related Behaviors in School Children and its Association with Overweight and Obesity—WHO European Childhood Obesity Surveillance Initiative (COSI 2015–2017)

Silvia Bel-Serrat [1,*], Ana Ojeda-Rodríguez [1,2], Mirjam M. Heinen [1], Marta Buoncristiano [3], Shynar Abdrakhmanova [4], Vesselka Duleva [5], Victoria Farrugia Sant'Angelo [6], Anna Fijałkowska [7], Tatjana Hejgaard [8], Constanta Huidumac [9], Jolanda Hyska [10], Enisa Kujundzic [11], Sanja Musić Milanović [12,13], Guljemal Ovezmyradova [14], Napoleón Pérez-Farinós [15], Ausra Petrauskiene [16], Ana Isabel Rito [17], Lela Shengelia [18], Radka Taxová Braunerová [19], Harry Rutter [20], Celine M. Murrin [1], Cecily C. Kelleher [1] and João Breda [3]

1 National Nutrition Surveillance Centre, School of Public Health, Physiotherapy and Sports Science, University College Dublin, D4 Dublin, Ireland; aojeda.5@alumni.unav.es (A.O.-R.); mirjam.heinen@ucd.ie (M.M.H.); celine.murrin@ucd.ie (C.M.M.); cecily.kelleher@ucd.ie (C.C.K.)
2 Department of Nutrition, Food Science and Physiology, University of Navarra, 31008 Pamplona, Spain
3 Division of Noncommunicable Diseases and Promoting Health through the Life-course, WHO European Office for Prevention and Control of Noncommunicable Diseases, 125009 Moscow, Russia; marta.buoncristiano@gmail.com (M.B.); rodriguesdasilvabred@who.int (J.B.)
4 National Center of Public Health, Ministry of Health of the Republic of Kazakhstan, 010000 Astana, Kazakhstan; shynar_a@mail.ru
5 National Center of Public Health and Analyses, 1431 Sofia, Bulgaria; v.duleva@ncpha.government.bg
6 Primary Health Care, 1940 Floriana, Malta; victoria.farrugia-santangelo@gov.mt
7 Department of Cardiology, Institute of Mother and Child, 01-211 Warsaw, Poland; anna.fijalkowska@imid.med.pl
8 Danish Health Authority,2300 København, Denmark; thv@sst.dk
9 National Institute of Public Health, 050463 Bucharest, Romania; constanta.huidumac@insp.gov.ro
10 Institute of Public Health, 1001 Tirana, Albania; lhyska2002@yahoo.it
11 Institute of Public Health of Montenegro, 8100 Podgorica, Montenegro; enisa.kujundzic@ijzcg.me
12 Croatian Institute of Public Health, 10000 Zagreb, Croatia; sanja.music@hzjz.hr
13 School of Medicine, School of Public Health Andrija Štampar, University of Zagreb, 10000 Zagreb, Croatia
14 WHO Country Office in Turkmenistan, 744000 Ashgabat, Turkmenistan; ovezmyradovag@who.int
15 Spanish Agency for Food Safety and Nutrition (AESAN), 28071 Madrid, Spain; estrategianaos@mscbs.es
16 Department of Preventive Medicine, Lithuanian University of Health Sciences, 44307 Kaunas, Lithuania; Ausra.Petrauskiene@lsmuni.lt
17 National Institute of Health Doutor Ricardo Jorge, I.P., 1649-016 Lisbon, Portugal; ana.rito@insa.min-saude.pt
18 National Center for Disease Control and Public Health of Georgia, 0186 Tbilisi, Georgia; lelasheng@gmail.com
19 Obesity Management Centre, Institute of Endocrinology, 113 94 Prague, Czech Republic; rbraunerova@endo.cz
20 Department of Social and Policy Sciences, University of Bath, Claverton Down, Bath BA2 7AY, UK; h.r.rutter@bath.ac.uk
* Correspondence: silvia.belserrat@ucd.ie

Abstract: It is unclear how dietary, physical activity and sedentary behaviors co-occur in school-aged children. We investigated the clustering of energy balance-related behaviors and whether the identified clusters were associated with weight status. Participants were 6- to 9-year-old children (n = 63,215, 49.9% girls) from 19 countries participating in the fourth round (2015/2017) of the World Health Organization (WHO) European Childhood Obesity Surveillance Initiative. Energy balance-related behaviors were parentally reported. Weight and height were objectively measured. We performed cluster analysis separately per group of countries (North Europe, East Europe, South Europe/Mediterranean countries and West-Central Asia). Seven clusters were identified in each group. Healthier clusters were common across groups. The pattern of distribution of healthy and unhealthy behaviors within each cluster was group specific. Associations between the clustering of energy balance-related behaviors and weight status varied per group. In South Europe/Mediterranean countries and East Europe, all or most of the cluster solutions were associated with higher risk of overweight/obesity when compared with the cluster 'Physically active and healthy diet'. Few or no associations were observed in North Europe and West-Central Asia, respectively. These findings support the hypothesis that unfavorable weight status is associated with a particular combination of energy balance-related behavior patterns, but only in some groups of countries.

Keywords: cluster analysis; energy balance-related behaviors; physical activity; sedentary behavior; screen time; dietary intake; overweight; obesity; children

---

1. Introduction

Childhood obesity is one of the most serious public health problems of the 21st century [1]. Evidence from a major epidemiological study which evaluated worldwide trends of weight status from 1975 to 2016 revealed that obesity in children has multiplied eightfold in the last 40 years, with a plateauing of body mass index (BMI) in high-income countries [2]. Obesity is a major risk factor of multifactorial etiology. Modifiable factors such as dietary patterns, physical activity and sedentary behaviors play a key role in energy imbalance leading to overweight and obesity in children [3].

Low fruit and vegetable (F&V) intake [4,5], consumption of high energy-dense/nutrient-poor foods [6,7], low physical activity (PA) levels and high sedentary time [8,9] have individually been associated with childhood overweight and obesity in a large number of studies; however, their effects on children's lifestyles are multivariable and interrelated [10]. Previous studies have investigated the clustering of energy balance-related behaviors (EBRB) and its association with childhood obesity to gain some understanding about the potential interplay among different behavior patterns [11–18]. Healthy and unhealthy behaviors seem to co-exist in the same groups of children in complex ways that are not well understood [10]. For instance, it has been shown that isolated unhealthy behaviors may not be related to higher obesity risk when they are compensated with healthy behaviors [15]. However, evidence on the associations between behavior cluster patterns and overweight and obesity remains inconclusive [10]. While some studies have reported higher obesity risk in unhealthy clusters [11,13,14,18], other studies have found no association at all [15,16].

Evaluating the synergetic effect instead of the individual effects of EBRB will help researchers, health professionals and policy makers to understand which behaviors need to be approached simultaneously. This may be helpful to identify and to promote a healthy lifestyle as well as to assist in the development of successful obesity prevention programs. Therefore, this study aimed to identify clusters of EBRB based on dietary patterns, PA and sedentary behaviors, and to investigate their association with obesity, including overweight, in a large sample of children in the World Health Organization (WHO) European region. To date, no studies have addressed these associations in nationally representative samples of primary school children from such a large geographical area including 19 countries spread across Europe and Asia.

2. Materials and Methods

2.1. World Health Organization (WHO) European Childhood Obesity Surveillance Initiative (COSI)

The WHO European Childhood Obesity Surveillance Initiative (COSI) is a collaborative study that was initiated in 2008 by the WHO Regional Office for Europe with 13 member states. Currently, COSI is carried out in 37 European countries that co-operate in relation to survey content, methodology and timing using a common European protocol [19–21]. The study routinely measures overweight and obesity prevalence of primary schoolchildren aged 6 to 9 years old to monitor the progress of the obesity epidemic in this population group, allow between-country comparisons within the WHO European Region and inform action to reverse the trend [22]. The COSI is a unique system that provides a large dataset based on nationally representative samples and standardized weight and height measurements. A total of four rounds have been conducted to date: Round 1 in 2008, Round 2 in 2009/2010, Round 3 in 2012/2013, and Round 4 in 2015/2017.

In addition to the mandatory anthropometric examinations, data on simple indicators of dietary intake, physical activity, screen time use and parental education, amongst others, are collected through an optional family questionnaire [23]. The present study focuses on children from 19 countries (Albania, Bulgaria, Croatia, Czech Republic, Denmark, Georgia, Ireland, Kazakhstan, Latvia, Lithuania, Malta, Montenegro, Poland, Portugal, Romania, Russia (only Moscow), Spain, Tajikistan, and Turkmenistan) who participated in the study in Round 4 (2015/2017) and who had complete information on age, sex, weight, and height and had completed the family questionnaire.

The COSI study is conducted according to the guidelines laid down in the Declaration of Helsinki and all procedures involving human subjects were approved by the local ethics committee at each study site. Parents were fully informed about the study procedures. In some countries, parents had to provide written signed consent to allow their children to participate in the study (opt-in consent approach) whereas other countries adopted the opt-out consent approach. On the measurement day, verbal consent from the child to participate in the study was obtained.

Countries chose the most appropriate professionals to take the anthropometric measurements (e.g., physical education teachers, nationally- or regionally-based health professionals such as nutritionists, physicians, health care nurses, etc.) based on the local arrangements and available budgets. Paper and online versions of the family questionnaire were available for completion to collect information on the child's EBRB and household sociodemographic characteristics. The paper version was either presented to the parent and child during the measurements, sent home with the child, mailed directly to the household, or filled out during parents' meetings in the school. Parents were emailed the link to fill in the online version and completed the questionnaire jointly with their child. More details about the implementation characteristics of COSI rounds can be found elsewhere [23,24].

2.2. Sampling of Children

Main characteristics of study design including the sampling strategy, targeted age range, sample size and participation rates within each country are presented as Supplementary Material in Table S1. Two-stage cluster sampling was applied in most of the countries with the school as primary sampling unit and school classes as the secondary sampling unit to draw nationally representative samples of children. Poland and Bulgaria applied four-stage (region, sub-region, school, class), and three-stage (school, class, 7-year-old children) cluster sampling, respectively, while one-stage cluster sampling was adopted by Croatia (sampling unit = class), Denmark and Latvia (school for both). Primary schools/classes were selected randomly from the list of all primary schools available in each country through the ministry of education or at the national school registry. Bulgaria, Ireland and Lithuania followed a sentinel approach; therefore, the same schools measured in previous rounds were included and classes were randomly selected at each sentinel site. Lithuania followed a sentinel approach combined with the selection of new schools by region and by degree of urbanization. As an exception, the primary sampling unit in Czech Republic was composed of pediatric clinics which were randomly selected from the national list of primary care pediatricians following a cluster sampling design stratified by region and size of residential location. As for other countries, 11 of them stratified their sample: many considered a geographical or administrative division of the national territory (9 countries) and, to a lesser extent, the degree of urbanization of the child's place of residence or school location (4 countries). No specific sampling strategy was used in Malta as all 7-year-old children in the country were included in the study.

COSI targets children aged 6, 7, 8 and 9 years and countries can focus on one or more of these four age groups [21]. Spain targeted children aged 6 to 9 years old, Albania, Croatia, and Poland targeted 8-year-old children, Romania measured children aged 8 and 9 years, Kazakhstan only included those aged 9 years, and the 13 remaining countries targeted 7-year-old children. One class per school was drawn within a grade level when the targeted age group was in the same grade. On the other hand, all grades where children from this age group were present could be sampled if the targeted age group was spread across grades. All children registered in the sampled classes were invited to take part in the study and those who returned a signed parental consent (opt-in consent approach) or did not refuse to take part in the study (opt-out consent approach) and were present on the survey day were examined and received the family questionnaire. Further details about the sampling characteristics have been described elsewhere [23,24].

2.3. Measurements

2.3.1. Anthropometry

Weight and height measurements were carried out by trained fieldworkers following a standardized protocol on anthropometric procedures and data collection drawn up by the WHO [21]. Information on children's age and sex was also collected. Children were asked to wear normal, light, indoor clothing and remove their shoes. Body weight was measured in kilograms, to the nearest 0.1 kg, with portable electronic (digital) scales and was adjusted for the weight of the clothes worn. Children's height was measured in centimeters with stadiometers and the reading taken to the last completed 0.1 cm. Body mass index (BMI) was calculated from the formula: weight (kg) divided by height squared (m^2). The specific equipment used in each country can be found as Supplementary Material (Table S2). The 2007 WHO BMI-for-age (BMI/A) growth charts were used to compute BMI/A *z*-scores. Children were classified into two weight status categories: underweight/healthy weight and overweight/obese according to the WHO 2007 [25] and the International Obesity Task Force [26,27] and the sex- and age-specific cut-offs.

2.3.2. Energy Balanced-Related Behaviors

The specific questions asked on the EBRB through the family questionnaire are shown as Supplementary Material—Table S3.

Physical Activity

The number of hours per day the child played actively/vigorously (e.g., running, jumping outside or moving and fitness games indoors) in their free time was assessed for both weekdays and weekend days. Numeric answers were assigned to the five answer categories available in the form to convert the variables to a numerical scale: 'never' = 0; '<1 h/day' = 0.5; '1 h/day' = 1; '2 h/day' = 2; '$\geq$3 h/day' = 3. The average hours per day playing actively was computed as [(week days $\times$ 5) + (weekend days $\times$ 2)]/7.

Screen Time

Usual screen time was described in all countries by the time (hours/day) spent watching television (TV) and/or videos or using electronic devices such as computer, tablet, smartphone or other electronic devices (excluding moving or fitness games) either at home or outside home. Responses were provided separately for weekdays and weekend days. In Ireland, Lithuania and Spain, responses included five categories split into weekdays and weekend days. These categories were converted to a numerical scale: 'never' = 0; '<1 h/day' = 0.5; '1 h/day' = 1; '2 h/day' = 2; '$\geq$3 h/day' = 3. Usual screen time (hours/day) was computed as [(week days × 5) + (weekend days × 2)]/7.

Fruit, Vegetable and Sugared Soft Drinks Intake

Fruit, vegetable and sugared soft drinks (SSD) intake during a normal week was obtained through a qualitative food frequency questionnaire. Responses included four frequency categories of consumption: 'never /<once a week', 'some days (1–3 days)', 'most days (4–6 days)', 'every day'. Frequencies were converted into times per week ranging from 0 to 7. Fruit and vegetable responses were grouped into one group.

2.3.3. Parental Education Level

Data was collected separately for the mother and the father using five answer options and regrouped into four categories: 'primary school', 'secondary school/vocational school', 'undergraduate/Bachelor's degree', and 'Master's degree or higher'. One of the parents reported the education level of both parents. The highest level of education attained in the household by either the mother or the father was used for adjustment in multivariable models.

2.4. Statistical Analysis

Following data cleaning, which was performed locally by each country, all country datasets were reviewed in a standard manner for inconsistencies and incompleteness at the WHO Regional Office for Europe before being merged for the intercountry analyses. Children younger than 6 years (n = 6) and older than 9 years (n = 723) as well as children with biologically implausible BMI/A z-scores below −5 or above +5 z-scores (n = 124) were excluded from the analyses, as recommended by the WHO [28].

Cluster analyses were performed using the statistical software SPSS version 24.0 (SPSS Inc., IBM Corp., Armonk, NY, USA). Countries were grouped into four groups according to their geographical location and/or cultural similarities as follows: North Europe (Denmark and Ireland), East Europe (Albania, Bulgaria, Czech Republic, Lithuania, Latvia, Montenegro, Poland, Romania and Russia), South Europe/Mediterranean countries (Croatia, Malta, Portugal and Spain) and West-Central Asia (Georgia, Kazakhstan, Tajikistan and Turkmenistan). Clusters were computed specifically for each of the four groups. PA, screen time, F&V and SSD intake were the four EBRB indicators included in the analyses. Variables were standardized prior to data analyses given the variation in means, variances and units among them [29].

Cluster analysis was carried out in two steps applying a combination of hierarchical and non-hierarchical clustering methods [30]. Ward's method based on Euclidean distances [31] was applied in the first step as hierarchical cluster analysis. The high sensitivity of Ward's method to outliers was reduced by removing univariate outliers (z-values > ±3 standard deviation (SD)) and multivariate outliers (those with high values of the Mahalanobis distance) for any of the four variables tested (n = 383). In the second step, an iterative on-hierarchical K-means clustering procedure was carried out. Initial cluster centers based on Ward's hierarchical method were used as non-random starting points.

The third step consisted of testing the stability of the cluster solutions. The sample was randomly split into two sub-samples and the clustering procedure was repeated. The agreement between the main sample and two sub-samples was compared with Cohen's kappa (κ). Agreement ranged from 0.985 (North Europe) to 0.932 (South Europe) [32].

Descriptive statistics included mean (SD) values of weight, height, BMI, PA, screen time, and F&V and SSD intake, prevalence estimates for anthropometric indicators, and percentages of sex, parental education level and season of completion of the questionnaire separately per group of countries and per cluster solution.

Mixed-effects regression models with country as the grouping variable were used to investigate the associations between the clusters (independent variables) and anthropometric indicators and the prevalence of overweight/obesity (dependent variables). Univariate and multivariate mixed linear regression models were carried out to examine associations with the continuous dependent variable BMI/A z-score. Univariate and multivariate logistic regression models were conducted between the prevalence of overweight/obesity (dependent variables) and the obtained clusters. Multivariate models were adjusted for sex, age, parental education level and season of completion of the questionnaire. Country was entered as random intercept in all the mixed-effects models. The threshold for statistical significance was set at $p \leq 0.05$. The Stata version 13.0 (StataCorp LP, College Station, TX, USA) was used to perform these analyses.

3. Results

3.1. Sample Characteristics

The final dataset consisted of 63,215 children (49.9% girls) from 19 countries with complete data on age, sex, weight, height and with information on all four EBRB indicators. The main sample characteristics in terms of age, sex, weight, height, BMI, BMI/A, parental education, season of completion of the questionnaire, PA, screen time, F&V intake, and SSD intake are displayed in Table 1 separately for each group of countries. Mean age was around 8 years in all groups except in North Europe where children were younger (mean age = 7.2 years). North Europe had the highest educated sample as nearly 40% of the families were undergraduate or held a Bachelor's degree. The most common highest education level attained in East Europe, South Europe/Mediterranean countries and West-Central Asia was secondary/vocational school with 42.1%, 49.3% and 62.4% of the parents in this category, respectively. The lowest prevalence of overweight/obesity was observed in North Europe (16.6% WHO, 11.3% IOTF) and West-Central Asia (16.4% WHO, 11.5% IOTF) whereas the countries in the South European/Mediterranean group had the highest prevalence (35.3% WHO, 27.5% IOTF).

Table 1. Baseline characteristics of participants in the fourth round of the WHO European Childhood Obesity Surveillance Initiative (COSI), separately by group of countries.

	North Europe		East Europe		South Europe/ Mediterranean Countries		West-Central Asia	
	Mean	SD	Mean	SD	Mean	SD	Mean	SD
Age (years)	7.2	0.4	8.1	0.8	7.9	0.9	8.0	0.9
Weight (kg)	24.9	4.3	28.7	6.7	28.9	7.2	25.5	5.6
Height (cm)	125.1	5.8	130.7	7.4	128.6	8.1	125.4	7.8
BMI (kg/m^2)	15.9	1.8	16.7	2.7	17.3	2.8	16.1	2.4
BMI/A	0.10	1.0	0.29	1.3	0.62	1.3	−0.01	1.16
Physical activity (hours/day)	1.5	0.7	2.0	0.7	1.6	0.8	1.6	0.8
Screen time (hours/day)	1.9	0.9	1.7	1.0	1.4	0.8	1.6	1.1
Fruit and vegetable intake (times/week)	11.0	3.5	8.5	3.8	8.3	3.8	9.2	4.0
Soft drinks (times/week)	0.9	1.1	1.7	2.1	1.3	1.9	2.6	2.6
	n	%	*n*	%	*n*	%	*n*	%
Sex								
Boys	908	51.7	13,975	49.9	10,807	50.1	5966	50.3
Girls	850	48.3	14,018	50.1	10,785	49.9	5906	49.7
Parental education level								
Primary school	11	0.6	1937	7.2	1126	5.4	87	0.8
Secondary and vocational school	517	29.7	11,294	42.1	10,361	49.3	7098	62.4
Undergraduate/Bachelor degree	693	39.9	6223	23.2	7122	33.8	2603	22.9
Master degree or higher	519	29.8	7357	27.5	2419	11.5	1586	13.9
Season questionnaire completion								
Winter	605	34.4	915	3.3	8017	37.1	2681	22.6
Spring	180	10.2	16,596	59.3	7955	36.8	3047	25.7
Summer	252	14.4	1688	6.0	1232	5.7	1	0.01
Autumn	721	41.0	8794	31.4	4388	20.3	6143	51.7
Overweight/obese (WHO 2007)	291	16.6	7644	27.5	7611	35.3	1927	16.4
Overweight/obese (IOTF)	198	11.3	5824	20.9	5929	27.5	1346	11.5

BMI, body mass index; BMI/A, BMI-for-age; IOTF, International Obesity Task Force; WHO, World Health Organization. North Europe: Denmark and Ireland. East Europe: Albania, Bulgaria, Czech Republic, Latvia, Lithuania, Montenegro, Poland, Romania and Russia. South Europe: Malta, Croatia, Portugal and Spain. West-Central Asia: Georgia, Kazakhstan, Tajikistan and Turkmenistan.

PA levels were the highest in East Europe (2.0 h/day) and the lowest in North Europe (1.5 h/day). North Europe had the highest screen time (1.9 h/day) whereas the lowest amount of time spent on this behavior was observed in South Europe/Mediterranean countries (1.4 h/day). The highest and lowest intakes of F&V were observed in North Europe (11.0 times/week) and in South European/Mediterranean countries (8.3 times/week), respectively. West-Central Asia had the highest SSD intake (2.6 times/week) whereas the North European countries had the lowest intake (0.9 times/week).

3.2. Clusters Characteristics

Cluster analyses turned out in a seven-cluster solution as the most adequate, reliable, and stable representation of the clustering of EBRB in the four groups of countries. Figure 1 shows the specific characteristics of each cluster. Cluster labels are based on distinguishing features defined by high or low mean *z*-scores relative to other clusters. Clusters that were common across groups were given the same cluster number; therefore, a total of 13 distinctive clusters were identified across the four groups.

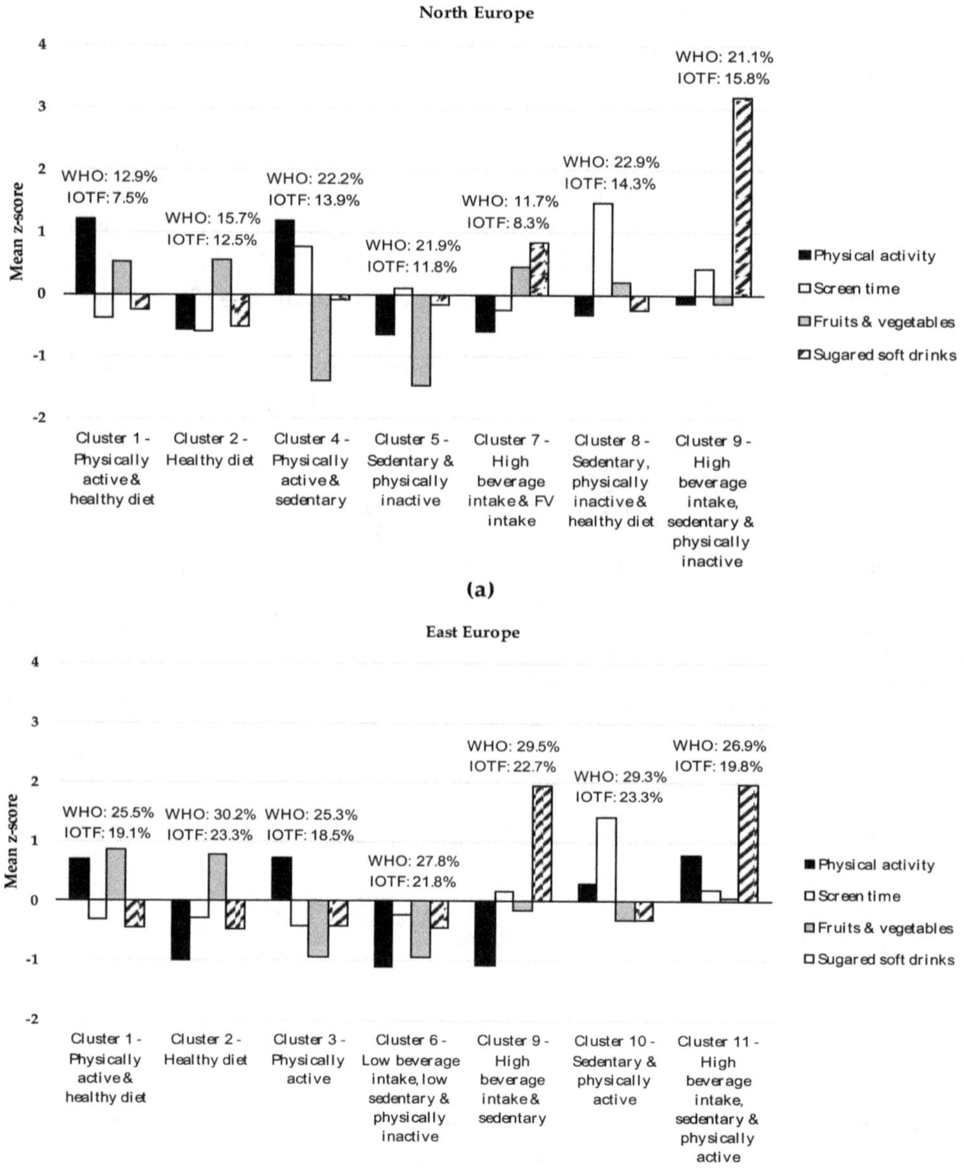

Figure 1. *Cont.*

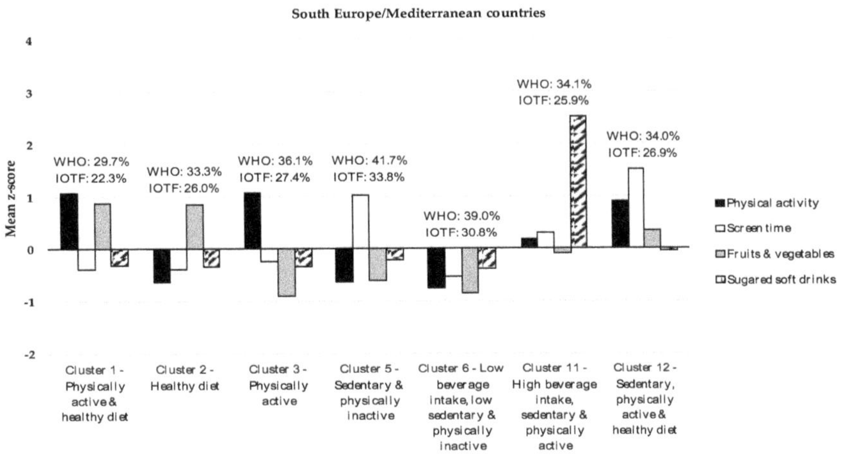

(c)

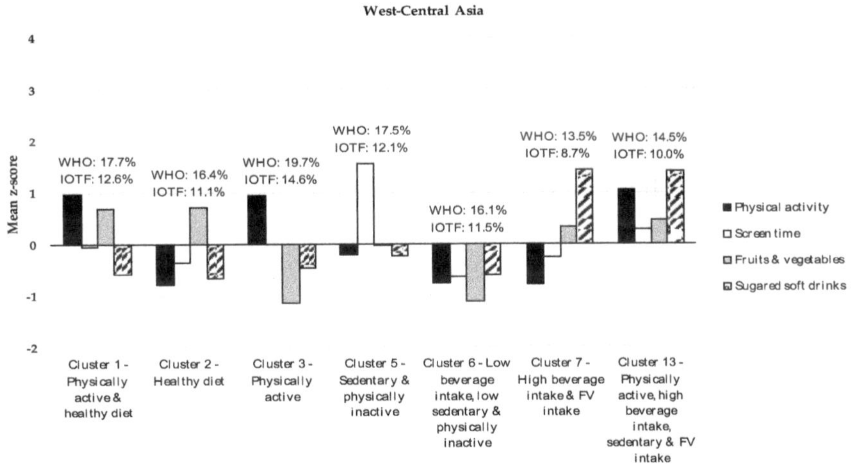

(d)

Figure 1. Group-specific cluster solutions (mean z-scores) of the four energy balance-related behaviors (EBRB) patterns among children participating in the fourth round of the World Health Organization European Childhood Obesity Surveillance Initiative: (**a**) Cluster solutions (mean z-scores) of the four EBRB patterns in North Europe; (**b**) Cluster solutions (mean z-scores) of the four EBRB patterns in East Europe; (**c**) Cluster solutions (mean z-scores) of the four EBRB patterns in South Europe/Mediterranean countries; (**d**) Cluster solutions (mean z-scores) of the four EBRB patterns in West-Central Asia. Overweight/obesity prevalence (%) by cluster membership is shown above each cluster. IOTF, International Obesity Task Force; WHO, World Health Organization.

Table 2 shows descriptive data for EBRB indicators and prevalence of overweight/obesity by cluster membership. Cluster 1 (C1, 'Physically active and healthy diet') was characterized by high PA levels and high F&V intake coupled with low screen time use and low intake of SSD. Cluster 2 (C2, 'Healthy diet') comprised children with high F&V intake and low SSD intake. C1 and C2 were observed in all four groups. Cluster 3 (C3, 'Physically active') was observed in East Europe, South Europe/Mediterranean countries and West-Central Asia and was described by high levels of PA. The main features of Cluster 4 (C4, 'Physically active and sedentary'), which only emerged in the North European countries, were high PA levels together with high levels of screen time use. Cluster 5 (C5, 'Sedentary and physically inactive'), with high levels of screen time and low levels of PA, was observed in three groups of countries (North Europe, South Europe/Mediterranean countries and West-Central Asia). Cluster 6 (C6, 'Low beverage intake, low sedentary and physically inactive') was characterized by low levels of all EBRB indicators, that is, low PA levels, low screen time, low F&V intake and low SSD intake. C6 was present in all the groups except in North Europe. Cluster 7 (C7,

'High beverage intake and F&V intake'), described by high intakes of SSD and of F&V, emerged in North Europe and in West-Central Asia.

Cluster 8 (C8, 'Sedentary, physically inactive and healthy diet'), with high levels of screen time, high F&V intake, low PA levels and low SSD intake, was specific to the North European countries. Cluster 9 (C9, 'High beverage intake, sedentary and physically inactive') comprised those in the North European and East European countries with high intake of SSD, high screen time use and low PA levels. Cluster 10 (C10, 'Sedentary and physically active') was only observed in East Europe and was described by high screen time and relatively high PA levels. The main features of Cluster 11 (C11, 'High beverage intake, sedentary and physically active') were high intake of SSD and relatively high screen time and PA levels and emerged in both East Europe and in South Europe/Mediterranean countries. Cluster 12 (C12, 'Sedentary, physically active and healthy diet'), specific to South Europe/Mediterranean countries, was characterized by high screen time use, high PA levels, high intake of F&V and low SSD intake. Cluster 13 (C13, 'Physically active, high beverage intake, sedentary and high F&V intake') was only observed in West-Central Asia and comprised children with high levels of all four EBRB.

In terms of prevalence of overweight/obesity, C9 ('High beverage intake, sedentary and physically inactive') and C8 ('Sedentary, physically inactive and healthy diet') showed, respectively, the highest prevalence with the WHO 2007 definition (22.9%) and with the IOTF definition (15.8%) in the North European countries. The lowest prevalence was observed for C1 ('Physically active and healthy diet', 12.9% WHO, 7.5% IOTF,) and for C7 ('High beverage intake and F&V intake', 11.7% WHO, 8.3% IOTF). C1 also had the lowest overweight/obesity prevalence in East Europe and South Europe/Mediterranean countries regardless of the obesity definition applied. C2 ('Healthy diet'), C9 ('High beverage intake, sedentary and physically inactive') and C10 ('Sedentary and physically active') had very similar high prevalence of overweight/obesity. The highest overweight/obesity prevalence in South Europe/Mediterranean countries was observed for C5 ('Sedentary and physically inactive', 41.7% WHO, 33.8% IOTF). As in the North European countries, C7 ('High beverage intake and F&V intake') in West-Central Asia had the lowest prevalence of overweight/obesity (13.5% WHO, 8.7% IOTF) whereas C3 ('Physically active') had the highest prevalence (19.7% WHO, 14.6% IOFT) regardless of the obesity definition used.

3.3. Associations between Cluster Membership and Anthropometric Indicators

Results from the mixed-effects regression models are shown in Table 3, separately by groups of countries. C1 ('Physically active and healthy diet') was chosen as the reference cluster in all groups as it showed lower overweight/obesity prevalence in most of the groups and it can be considered as the healthiest cluster. After adjusting for confounding factors, all the clusters in South Europe/Mediterranean countries, except C3 ('Physically active') with the IOTF definition, were significantly associated with higher BMI/A and higher odds of overweight/obesity, regardless of the obesity definition applied. In East Europe, a positive significant association was observed between C2 ('Healthy diet') (β = 0.17, 95% CI = 0.12–0.22), C6 ('Low beverage intake, low sedentary and physically inactive) (β = 0.13, 95% CI = 0.07–0.18), C9 ('High beverage intake, sedentary and physically inactive') (β = 0.08, 95% CI = 0.01–0.15) and C10 ('Sedentary and physically active') (β = 0.16, 95% CI = 0.10–0.22) and BMI/A. Likewise, those children in these clusters (C2, C6, C9 and C10) were at higher risk of overweight/obesity than their peers in C1. In the North European countries, BMI/A was significantly associated with the 'Sedentary, physically inactive and healthy diet' cluster (C8) (β = 0.25, 95% CI = 0.07–0.42). Children in C8 were also more likely to be overweight/obese (WHO: OR = 1.92, 95% CI = 1.21–3.05; IOTF: OR = 2.15, 95% CI = 1.22–3.77) than those in the 'Physically active and healthy diet' cluster (C1). Moreover, higher odds of being overweight/obese was observed among those in C2 ('Healhty diet') (IOTF: OR = 1.85, 95% CI = 1.15–2.97), C4 ('Physically active and sedentary') (WHO: OR = 1.68, 95% CI = 1.02–2.76), and C5 ('Sedentary and physically inactive') (WHO: OR = 1.63, 95% CI = 1.04–2.54). No significant associations were observed in the West-Central Asian countries between the clusters and BMI/A and the prevalence of overweight/obesity.

Table 2. Descriptive data of energy balance-related behaviors indicators and overweight/obesity prevalence by cluster membership among the participants in the fourth round of the WHO European Childhood Obesity Surveillance Initiative, by groups of countries.

	n	%	Sex				Physical Activity (Hours/Day)		Screen Time (Hours/Day)		Fruit and Vegetables (Times/Week)		Soft Drinks (Times/Week)		Overweight/ Obesity (WHO 2007)		Overweight/ Obesity (IOTF)	
			Boys		Girls													
			n	%	*n*	%	Mean	SD	Mean	SD	Mean	SD	Mean	SD	*n*	%	*n*	%
North Europe (*n* = 1758)																		
C1	374	21.3	195	52.1	179	47.9	2.3	0.3	1.6	0.6	12.8	1.7	0.6	0.7	48	12.9	28	7.5
C2	522	29.7	230	44.1	292	55.9	1.1	0.4	1.4	0.5	12.9	1.6	0.3	0.2	82	15.7	65	12.5
C4	158	9.0	86	54.4	72	45.6	2.3	0.4	2.6	0.9	6.0	3.0	0.9	0.8	35	22.2	22	13.9
C5	246	14.0	125	50.8	121	49.2	1.1	0.4	2.0	0.7	5.7	2.5	0.7	0.8	43	21.9	29	11.8
C7	205	11.7	112	54.6	93	45.4	1.1	0.4	1.7	0.6	12.5	1.7	2.0	0.0	24	11.7	17	8.3
C8	196	11.1	125	63.8	71	36.2	1.3	0.6	3.2	0.6	11.7	2.2	0.6	0.7	43	22.9	28	14.3
C9	57	3.2	35	61.4	22	38.6	1.4	0.7	2,3	0.8	10.5	3.1	5.0	0.0	12	21.1	9	15.8
East Europe (*n* = 27,993)																		
C1	6555	23.4	3174	48.4	3381	51.6	2.5	0.4	1.4	0.7	11.8	1.9	0.8	0.8	1662	25.5	1248	19.1
C2	4798	17.1	2170	45.2	2628	57.8	1.2	0.3	1.4	0.7	11.5	1.9	0.8	0.8	1443	30.2	1113	23.3
C3	4548	16.3	2357	51.8	2191	48.2	2.5	0.4	1.3	0.7	4.9	2.1	0.9	0.8	1146	25.3	837	18.5
C6	4028	14.4	1957	48.6	2071	51.4	1.2	0.4	1.5	0.8	4.9	2.1	0.8	0.8	1117	27.8	876	21.8
C9	1795	6.4	911	50.8	884	49.2	1.2	0.4	1.9	1.0	8.0	3.9	5.9	1.0	527	29.5	406	22.7
C10	3205	11.5	1726	53.9	1479	46.1	2.2	0.6	3.3	0.8	7.4	3.1	1.1	1.0	932	29.3	742	23.3
C11	3064	11.0	1680	54.8	1384	45.2	2.6	0.4	2.0	1.0	8.8	3.8	5.9	1.0	817	26.9	602	19.8
South Europe/Mediterranean countries (*n* = 21,592)																		
C1	2946	13.6	1556	52.8	1390	47.2	2.4	0.3	1.1	0.5	11.6	1.9	0.7	0.8	874	29.7	657	22.3
C2	5366	24.9	2488	46.4	2878	53.6	1.1	0.4	1.1	0.5	11.5	1.9	0.6	0.8	1789	33.3	1396	26.0
C3	2754	12.8	1501	54.5	1253	45.5	2.4	0.4	1.2	0.6	4.8	2.1	0.6	0.8	993	36.1	754	27.4
C5	2121	9.8	1059	49.9	1032	50.1	1.1	0.4	2.4	0.5	5.9	2.8	0.9	0.9	885	41.7	716	33.8
C6	4244	19.7	2018	47.6	2226	52.4	1.0	0.4	1.0	0.4	5.0	2.1	0.6	0.8	1654	39.0	1306	30.8
C12	1821	8.4	947	52.0	874	48.0	2.3	0.5	2.8	0.6	9.5	3.2	1.2	1.0	621	34.1	472	25.9
C11	2340	10.8	1238	52.9	1102	47.1	1.7	0.8	1.7	0.8	7.8	3.9	6.0	1.0	795	34.0	628	26.9
West-Central Asia (*n* = 11,872)																		
C1	1787	15.0	875	49.0	912	51.0	2.4	0.4	1.6	0.8	11.9	1.9	1.1	0.8	314	17.7	223	12.6
C2	2086	17.6	993	47.6	1093	52.4	1.0	0.4	1.2	0.7	12.1	1.9	0.9	0.8	339	16.4	230	11.1
C3	1511	12.7	794	52.6	717	47.4	2.4	0.4	1.6	0.9	4.6	2.2	1.4	1.6	296	19.7	220	14.6
C5	1270	10.7	697	54.9	573	45.1	1.5	0.6	3.4	0.8	9.1	3.5	2.0	2.0	220	17.5	152	12.1
C6	1911	16.1	917	48.0	994	52.0	1.0	0.4	0.9	0.7	4.6	2.2	1.0	1.3	303	16.1	217	11.5
C7	1728	14.6	839	48.6	889	51.4	1.0	0.4	1.4	0.9	10.6	3.6	6.3	1.0	230	13.5	149	8.7
C13	1579	13.3	851	53.9	728	46.1	2.5	0.4	2.0	1.0	11.0	3.1	6.2	1.0	225	14.5	155	10.0

Cluster 1 "Physically active and healthy diet"; Cluster 2 "Healthy diet"; Cluster 3 "Physically active"; Cluster 4 "Physically active and sedentary"; Cluster 5 "Sedentary and physically inactive"; Cluster 6 "Low beverage intake, low sedentary and physically inactive"; Cluster 7 "High beverage intake and F&V intake"; Cluster 8 "Sedentary, physically inactive and healthy diet"; Cluster 9 "High beverage intake, sedentary and physically inactive"; Cluster 10 "Sedentary and physically active"; Cluster 11 "High beverage intake, sedentary and physically active"; Cluster 12 "Sedentary, physically active and healthy diet"; Cluster 13 "Physically active, high beverage intake, sedentary and high F&V intake". IOTF, International Obesity Task Force; WHO, World Health Organization. North Europe: Denmark and Ireland. East Europe: Albania, Bulgaria, Czech Republic, Latvia, Lithuania, Montenegro, Poland, Romania and Russia. South Europe: Malta, Croatia, Portugal and Spain. West-Central Asia: Georgia, Kazakhstan, Tajikistan and Turkmenistan.

Table 3. Associations between cluster membership and anthropometric indicators among the participants in the fourth round of the WHO European Childhood Obesity Surveillance Initiative, by groups of countries.

	BMI/A				Overweight/Obesity (WHO 2007)				Overweight/Obesity (IOTF)			
	Crude Model		Adjusted Model [a]		Crude Model		Adjusted Model [a]		Crude Model		Adjusted Model [a]	
	β	95% CI	β	95% CI	OR	95% CI	OR	95% CI	OR	95% CI	OR	95% CI
North Europe (n = 1758)												
C1	ref.		ref.		ref.		ref.		ref.		ref.	
C2	0.07	−0.06–0.21	0.08	−0.05–0.22	1.32	0.89–1.94	1.35	0.91–2.00	1.83	1.15–2.92 *	1.85	1.15–2.97 *
C4	0.12	−0.07–0.31	0.07	−0.12–0.26	1.85	1.14–3.01 *	1.68	1.02–2.76 *	1.92	1.06–3.47 *	1.60	0.86–2.96
C5	0.12	−0.04–0.28	0.11	−0.05–0.27	1.67	1.07–2.60 *	1.63	1.04–2.54 *	1.71	0.99–2.97	1.63	0.94–2.83
C7	0.03	−0.15–0.21	0.04	−0.14–0.21	1.13	0.65–1.95	1.09	0.63–1.87	1.39	0.72–2.69	1.37	0.72–2.63
C8	0.22	0.05–0.40 *	0.25	0.07–0.42 **	1.93	1.22–3.05 **	1.92	1.21–3.05 **	2.08	1.19–3.63 *	2.15	1.22–3.77 **
C9	0.24	−0.05–0.52	0.18	−0.11–0.46	2.18	1.06–4.48 *	1.78	0.85–3.73	2.78	1.22–6.36 *	2.22	0.94–5.26
East Europe (n = 27,993)												
C1	ref.		ref.		ref.		ref.		ref.		ref.	
C2	0.16	0.11–0.21 ***	0.17	0.12–0.22 ***	1.30	1.20–1.42 ***	1.32	1.21–1.44 ***	1.34	1.22–1.47 ***	1.35	1.23–1.49 ***
C3	0.02	−0.04–0.07	0.03	−0.03–0.07	1.01	0.93–1.11	1.03	0.94–1.12	1.00	0.90–1.10	1.01	0.92–1.12
C6	0.12	0.07–0.17 ***	0.13	0.07–0.18 ***	1.17	1.07–1.28 **	1.18	1.08–1.30 ***	1.26	1.14–1.39 ***	1.28	1.15–1.41 ***
C9	0.06	−0.01–0.13	0.08	0.01–0.15 *	1.19	1.06–1.34 **	1.22	1.08–1.38 **	1.23	1.08–1.40 **	1.26	1.11–1.44 **
C10	0.16	0.10–0.21***	0.16	0.10–0.22 ***	1.22	1.11–1.34 ***	1.22	1.11–1.35 ***	1.30	1.17–1.45 ***	1.33	1.20–1.49 ***
C11	0.01	−0.05–0.07	0.03	−0.03–0.09	1.03	0.93–1.14	1.05	0.95–1.16	1.00	0.90–1.11	1.04	0.93–1.17
South Europe/Mediterranean countries (n = 21,592)												
C1	ref.		ref.		ref.		ref.		ref.		ref.	
C2	0.08	0.03–0.14 **	0.10	0.04–0.16 **	1.15	1.04–1.26 **	1.14	1.06–1.30 **	1.18	1.06–1.31 **	1.18	1.06–1.32 **
C3	0.11	0.05–0.18 **	0.08	0.01–0.14 *	1.21	1.08–1.35 **	1.17	1.04–1.31 **	1.19	1.05–1.34 **	1.12	0.99–1.27
C5	0.32	0.25–0.39 ***	0.30	0.23–0.37 ***	1.61	1.43–1.81 ***	1.59	1.40–1.79 ***	1.67	1.47–1.90 ***	1.61	1.42–1.84 ***
C6	0.17	0.11–0.23 ***	0.15	0.09–0.21 ***	1.35	1.21–1.49 ***	1.31	1.18–1.46 ***	1.37	1.23–1.54 ***	1.29	1.15–1.45 ***
C11	0.16	0.09–0.23 ***	0.11	0.04–0.18 **	1.29	1.15–1.46 ***	1.21	1.07–1.37 **	1.34	1.18–1.53 ***	1.23	1.08–1.40 **
C12	0.13	0.06–0.21 ***	0.10	0.03–0.18 **	1.26	1.11–1.44 ***	1.22	1.07–1.39 **	1.24	1.08–1.43 **	1.19	1.03–1.37 *
West-Central Asia (n = 11,872)												
C1	ref.		ref.		ref.		ref.		ref.		ref.	
C2	0.04	−0.03–0.12	0.05	−0.02–0.13	0.97	0.81–1.15	0.99	0.73–1.18	0.92	0.76–1.13	0.93	0.76–1.14
C3	−0.01	−0.09–0.07	0.01	−0.08–0.09	0.89	0.75–1.07	0.95	0.79–1.14	0.92	0.75–1.13	0.98	0.79–1.20
C5	0.06	−0.03–0.14	0.06	−0.02–0.15	1.03	0.85–1.25	1.04	0.85–1.26	1.00	0.80–1.25	1.02	0.81–1.28
C6	−0.03	−0.10–0.05	0.01	−0.07–0.08	0.87	0.73–1.04	0.92	0.76–1.10	0.88	0.71–1.08	0.93	0.76–1.15
C7	−0.03	−0.11–0.05	-0.02	−0.10–0.06	0.95	0.78–1.14	0.98	0.81–1.20	0.90	0.72–1.12	0.93	0.74–1.17
C13	0.01	−0.07–0.08	0.02	−0.06–0.10	0.90	0.74–1.08	0.94	0.78–1.14	0.89	0.72–1.11	0.95	0.76–1.19

[a] Adjusted for age, sex, parental education level, season of questionnaire completion. * $p < 0.05$, ** $p < 0.01$, *** $p < 0.001$. Cluster 1 "Physically active and healthy diet"; Cluster 2 "Healthy diet"; Cluster 3 "Physically active"; Cluster 4 "Physically active and sedentary"; Cluster 5 "Sedentary and physically inactive"; Cluster 6 "Low beverage intake, low sedentary and physically inactive"; Cluster 7 "High beverage intake and F&V intake"; Cluster 8 "Sedentary, physically inactive and healthy diet"; Cluster 9 "High beverage intake, sedentary and physically inactive"; Cluster 10 "Sedentary and physically active"; Cluster 11 "High beverage intake, sedentary and physically active"; Cluster 12 "Sedentary, physically active and healthy diet"; Cluster 13 "Physically active, high beverage intake, sedentary and high F&V intake". BMI/A, BMI-for-age; IOTF, International Obesity Task Force; WHO, World Health Organization. North Europe: Denmark and Ireland. East Europe: Albania, Bulgaria, Czech Republic, Latvia, Lithuania, Montenegro, Poland, Romania and Russia. South Europe: Malta, Croatia, Portugal and Spain. West-Central Asia: Georgia, Kazakhstan, Tajikistan and Turkmenistan.

4. Discussion

This study investigated the clustering of F&V and SSD intake patterns, physical activity and sedentary behavior and their cross-sectional associations with anthropometric indicators in a large sample of children in the WHO European region. Our findings showed that (1) some behaviors cluster in the same manner and are common across groups whereas others are specific to the geographical area, and (2) the associations of the clustering of the EBRB and the obesity indicators depend on the group of countries. To the best of our knowledge, this is the first study to examine the clustering of these EBRB and its association with obesity indicators in a large and geographically spread sample of school-aged children.

4.1. Clusters Characteristics

A 7-cluster solution was retained as the best solution within the four groups. While the clustering of some behaviors was common across groups, other behaviors clustered in a unique manner specific to each country grouping. This highlights the complexity of diet, PA and sedentary behavior and their relationships. The current globalization of EBRB [33] could explain the similarity of clusters across groups. On the other hand, group differences in the clustering of these behaviors seem to reflect group-specific EBRB patterns that persist regardless of such globalization, although to a lesser extent as these clusters tended to be less prevalent than the common ones.

4.2. Healthy and Unhealthy Energy Balance-Related Behaviors (EBRB) Clustering

C1 'Physically active and healthy diet' and C2 'Healthy diet', the clusters that represent healthier EBRB, were common across all groups. C3, the 'Physically active' cluster, was common in three groups however (East Europe, South Europe/Mediterranean countries, West-Central Asia). C1, considered as the 'healthy' cluster was characterized by high PA levels and high F&V intake and low levels of screen time and SSD intake. This cluster comprised most of the children in East Europe (23.4%) and was the second most prevalent cluster in North Europe (21.3%). C2 'Healthy diet', with high levels of F&V intake and low SSD intake, was the most prevalent cluster in North Europe (29.7%), South Europe/Mediterranean countries (24.9%) and West-Central Asia (17.6%), and the second that comprised most children in East Europe (17.1%). The healthy clustering of diet and PA in school-aged children has not consistently been observed in the literature. While some studies failed to observe a distinct healthy cluster among children [11,13,34], others reported one cluster in which healthy behaviors co-existed, in line with our results. Sánchez-Oliva et al. [14] identified a 'Healthy Lifestyle' cluster among children aged 8–11 years that was characterized by low levels of screen time and of total sedentary time, high levels of moderate-to-vigorous PA, and average levels of adherence to the Mediterranean diet. Likewise, a 'Healthier lifestyle' cluster with high PA, low sedentary behavior, longer sleep duration and healthier diet was reported in a sample of 9- to 12-year-old Spanish children [16]. In contrast to our findings, this cluster was not the most prevalent in neither of the studies. Another matter is whether children in these healthy clusters met the recommendations for these behaviors. An 'all-round healthy behavior' cluster was observed by Cameron et al. [35] in which children aged 5–12 years met the daily recommendations for moderate-to-vigorous PA, screen time, F&V intake and energy-dense food intake. Our results showed that children in C1 achieved >1 h/day of PA [36], screen time use was below the recommended 2 h/day [37] and SSD consumption was very low (≤once a week). F&V intake was also high; however, due to the nature of the questionnaire, it is very likely that the intake of F&V was underestimated as daily intakes were not available; therefore, it is unknown whether children met the guidelines in this regard.

Consistent with previous literature [14,16–18,34,35], we found clustering of unhealthy behaviors which comprised children with high levels of screen use and high SSD intake. In a review of cross-sectional and longitudinal studies, Pearson and Biddle [38] already reported a positive association between sedentary behaviors and elements of a less healthy diet in children such as energy-dense drinks, snacks and fast food. Nevertheless, this clustering of unhealthy behaviors was the least prevalent in the two groups of countries where it was observed (3.2% North Europe, 6.4% East Europe).

4.3. Co-Occurrence of Healthy and Unhealthy EBRB

As already highlighted by previous studies [11,13,18,34,35], healthy and unhealthy levels of EBRB co-occurred in some regions in all groups, but not in others. Most of these clusters were characterized by high levels of screen time coupled with high levels of PA (C4, C10) and/or high F&V intake (C8, C12). A cluster (C7) combining high F&V intake with high SSD intake was observed in North Europe and West-Central Asia. It is noteworthy that a cluster with high levels of all four behaviors (C13) emerged in West-Central Asia. We found no studies that had already reported such a clustering of EBRB in which individuals had high levels of all healthy and unhealthy behaviors simultaneously. We hypothesized that the co-existence of healthy and unhealthy behaviors in the same cluster could suggest a conscious compensation, by the parents, of the unhealthy behavior by adhering to a healthy one. Parents could engage their children in a particular healthy behavior such as PA performance and/or healthy eating to compensate for engaging in other practices such as high screen time use and/or unhealthier dietary patterns. Although this behavior has only been investigated in adults [39], it may be plausible in our study as data were reported by the parents.

It should be noted that several clusters were characterized by high levels of screen time. In three groups, a sedentary cluster (C5) coupled with low levels of PA emerged comprising children with high screen time use above the recommendations, especially in West-Central Asia (3.4 h/day). Leech et al. [10] already reported in their review a common pattern among several studies in which many clusters were defined by high levels of sedentary behaviors. These findings seem to reflect the current high levels of screen time associated with the use of new technologies and the negative impact that they can already have on the lifestyle of those at still early ages.

4.4. Low EBRB Levels

By contrast, all groups except North Europe had a cluster characterized by low levels of PA, screen time, F&V intake and SSD intake. Likewise, three studies conducted in European children aged 2–9 years [11,13] and 10–12 years [17] found a clustering of low levels on all behaviors. Co-occurrence of low consumption of SSD and low screen time use levels, despite the low PA levels and low F&V intake, could be regarded as positive in terms of health promotion and disease prevention. In fact, the findings in the study from Bel-Serrat et al. [11] suggested that the cardiovascular profile of children with low levels of TV/video/DVD viewing together with low SSD intake was healthier than for those physically active or with high F&V intake. This cluster was considered by the authors as the healthiest cluster solution given that they failed to find a ´healthy´ cluster, which could have been associated with an even healthier cardiovascular profile.

Future research should focus on investigating how clusters track over time in this age group. The longitudinal stability of cluster membership was examined among Australian 10–12-year-old children over a 3-year period and was observed to be moderate [12]. While the 'most healthy' clusters showed the lowest stability over time, tracking was highest for the 'high sedentary behavior/low moderate and vigorous PA'. According to the authors, further investigation is still needed to figure out the reason why some clusters tracked better than others [12].

4.5. Associations between Cluster Membership and Anthropometric Indicators

4.5.1. Differences across Groups of Countries

Associations between the clustering of EBRB and anthropometric indicators notably varied per group of countries. All clusters except two were associated with higher BMI/A *z*-score and higher risk of overweight/obesity regardless of the obesity definition used in South Europe/Mediterranean countries and in East Europe, respectively. Only a small number of associations was observed in North Europe and no associations were observed in West-Central Asia. Although we cannot compare group-specific clusters because they are unique to each area, common clusters were not associated with obesity indicators in the same manner across groups. These differences may represent different stages of evolution of the obesity epidemic in different countries and populations groups, with variable responses in terms of behaviors, norms, and different physical, social, cultural and economic environments. We also hypothesized that countries could be at a different stage of the diffusion of innovation theory from Rogers [40] in terms of obesity prevention strategies and their adoption by the population. Briefly, the diffusion of innovation theory explains how, an idea, behavior or product spreads through a specific population and it is adopted by this population. Adoption, however, does not occur simultaneously within the target population and, there are, indeed, five adopter categories: innovators, early adopters, early majority, late majority and laggards [40]. While in North Europe most of the population may have adopted these strategies in terms of EBRB, in South Europe/Mediterranean countries and in East Europe, the adoption of EBRB strategies is still at earlier stages, which is also reflected by the remarkably higher mean BMI/A and overweight/obesity prevalence observed in these countries.

Nevertheless, it should be kept in mind that the education level in the North European countries was higher than in the other three groups, which could also have an impact on the observed findings as it could imply a healthier cohort of children. In West-Central Asia, however, children could still follow a quite traditional behavior pattern that prevents them from being overweight/obese, even considering that obesity prevention strategies focusing on EBRB in these countries may not be as developed as in Europe given their relatively low overweight/obesity rates as compared with the other countries. Examining the associations between cluster membership and sociodemographic factors in this specific age group deserves more attention and future research. Fernández-Alvira et al. [17] observed that children from seven European countries aged 10–12 years old with lower educated parents were more likely to have unhealthier clustering of EBRB, i.e., low activity/sedentary pattern and sedentary and sugared drinks consumers. Likewise, the 'energy-dense consumers who watch TV' cluster comprised more children with lower educated mothers among Australian 5–6- and 10–12-year-old children [34].

Differences in the observed associations between the clustering of EBRB and overweight/obesity across regions could also be explained by other factors not examined in this study and that have also been shown to play a role in the development of overweight/obesity such as sleep duration, well-being and/or genetic variations, amongst others. Findings from a meta-analysis reported that short sleep duration increased the risk of childhood obesity [41]; however, we did not observe much variation on average sleep time among regions: 11 h/day in the North European countries and 10 h/day in the other three groups of countries. Moreover, obesity has a pronounced genetic component as genetic factors account for between 30–70% of variation in BMI between individuals [42]. The prevalence of obesity also differs between ethnic groups [42]. This could partially explain the low prevalence of overweight/obesity observed in the West-Central Asian countries as opposed to the higher prevalence in the South Europe/Mediterranean countries. On the other hand, the nature of the methodology applied may have a role in explaining the lack of consistent results across regions. A key limitation of self-reported measures is their validity. For that reason, the presence of misclassification bias needs to be considered given that parentally reported measures are subject to possible misreporting of PA, sedentary behaviors and diet.

4.5.2. Synergies among Multiple EBRB and Overweight/Obesity

The synergistic effect of having high levels of PA and high intake of F&V combined with low screen time use and low SSD intake was associated with children being less likely to be overweight/obese. Having only a diet rich in F&V or being physically active did not seem to be associated with children being less overweight/obese as compared with their peers who were engaged in both EBRB simultaneously, even when screen time use and SSD intake were low. The fact that C6 ('Low beverage intake, low sedentary and physically inactive') was also associated with higher odds of overweight/obesity supports this hypothesis. Unlike our findings, Bel-Serrat et al. [11] and Santaliestra-Pasías et al. [13] found that the clustering of low levels of all EBRB was associated with reduced levels of body fat. However, both studies failed to observe a healthy cluster to compare this cluster with. Nevertheless, the evidence on the potential cumulative effect of these behaviors in children is still inconsistent. In the review by Leech et al. [10], five studies found evidence of a possible synergistic effect of multiple EBRB on overweight/obesity whereas seven studies found no association. Differences in the EBRB indicators used, the statistical methods applied to compute the clusters, the culture and/or the specific population studied, amongst others, limit the comparability among studies and could partially explain the lack of agreement.

4.5.3. Measures of EBRB

The low z-scores observed in C6 for all the EBRB could suggest that there might be other underlying factors associated with overweight/obesity that were not captured by either these EBRB measures, i.e., engagement in other eating and/or movement behaviors like light PA, or beyond these EBRB, as mentioned earlier. Therefore, future studies in children may need to target more comprehensive measures of EBRB. In terms of PA, this could include light PA in addition to moderate and vigorous PA, structured and unstructured PA, and PA performance during school time and outside school hours. Assessment of both multiple sedentary behaviors (e.g., screen use (TV, videos, computer, table, smartphone, etc.), reading, socializing) and of domain-specific behaviors (e.g., sitting at school or at home, motorized travel) should be considered [43] in future research. Furthermore, the dietary assessment methodologies applied should provide information not only on the individual foods consumed but on the overall diet to obtain a better understanding of the dietary factors that are related to health outcomes. The combination of several dietary assessment methods, such as food frequency questionnaires and 24-h dietary recalls, is frequently used to fulfill this need. However, the nature of information to be collected and the methodology should be specified by the survey itself. For instance, while accelerometry offers a convenient and accurate measurement of PA, it should be kept in mind that questionnaires are cost-effective, readily accessible to most of the population and have a relatively low participant burden [43]. These aspects are crucial in surveillance where data are collected in an ongoing and systematic basis.

4.5.4. Role of Sedentary Behaviors

Our findings showed that most of the clusters that were associated with an increased risk of overweight/obesity were characterized by high levels of screen time use, regardless of being combined with other healthy/unhealthy behaviors or not. This suggests that high screen time use could mask the potential positive role of PA and of a healthy diet on reducing the obesogenic risk. This 'outweighing' effect of one particular behavior over another has been reported previously [10,18]. In agreement with our results, four studies in the review by Leech et al. [10] found a positive association between overweight and high sedentary behavior. Similarly, Dumuid et al. [18] and Sánchez-Oliva [14] observed that membership of the high sedentary time cluster was associated with higher BMI and higher risk of overweight/obesity and with higher body fat percentage, respectively.

4.5.5. Role of Sedentary Behaviors and Sugared Soft Drinks (SSD) Consumption

It deserves attention the fact that clusters that combined both high levels of screen time use and high consumption of SSD comprised children who were more likely to be overweight/obese. Leech et al. [12] already showed that TV viewing in combination with energy-dense food and drinks consumption predicted overweight and obesity among Australian children. Evidence form cross-sectional, longitudinal, interventional studies carried out in children supports the link between SSD intake and not only unhealthy weight gain, but other adverse health outcomes such as dental caries, high blood pressure, earlier timing of puberty, poor sleep and hyperactivity/inattention [44]. This is a matter of concern given that children in these clusters are simultaneously engaged in two unhealthy behaviors and, therefore, could be at an increased risk of developing health issues linked to these behaviors not only during childhood, but also during adolescence and adulthood.

4.6. Strengths

The main strengths of this study include the application of standardized data collection procedures across countries, the large sample size of more than 60,000 children from diverse geographical areas of Europe and Asia, and the country-based sampling strategies designed to yield nationally representative samples. The inclusion of important obesity-related EBRB, the use of objectively measured height and weight, and the adjustment of regression models for important confounders can also be regarded as study strengths. Furthermore, cluster analysis, a data-driven approach, is able to identify clusters of EBRB patterns, which offers certain superiority as opposed to a priori methods such as indexes [34].

4.7. Limitations

These findings should be interpreted in the context of several limitations. The cross-sectional design of this study does not allow us to make any causal inferences. Differences in sampling methods and target age group(s) across countries should be regarded as a study limitation. Despite the large sample size and the fact that countries selected nationally representative samples, the survey nature of the data and the differences in each country contribution to both the groups sample and population were not considered in the analyses. Therefore, it should be kept in mind when interpreting these findings that they refer to the study sample rather than to any population. Moreover, some degree of selection bias cannot be precluded given the low levels of participation observed in some countries.

Further limitations include the parentally reported EBRB variables which are subject to measurement error, recall bias and socially desirable answers. Therefore, a certain degree of differential misreporting, i.e., over-reporting of healthier behaviors and under-reporting of those regarded as less healthy, cannot be precluded. Also, the parental estimates of their children's behavior patterns may be error-prone, especially when these behaviors took place out of home or in the child's bedroom. School-based PA was not captured by the questionnaire and, therefore, estimates rely only on PA during free time. One of the major challenges in nutritional epidemiology is the measurement error in dietary intake data and, therefore, misreporting cannot be ruled out, especially among parents with overweight/obese children [45]. Furthermore, the nature of the questionnaire could lead to an underestimation of those food items that were consumed several times a day such as F&V intake. Therefore, intakes of F&V in this sample could be higher than those observed in these analyses. The fact that the reliability of the questionnaire has not been examined yet should be regarded as another study limitation. Nevertheless, the COSI food frequency consumption list was designed as an easily applicable monitoring tool to get an overall indication of the children's usual consumption frequencies of a food group, but it did not include portion sizes. Besides, the low cost and ease of administration of the questionnaires makes them the most common tool used in large epidemiological and surveillance studies, despite their methodological limitations.

It should be acknowledged that the grouping of the countries was not perfect and that the use of another grouping system could have resulted in a more accurate grouping. For example, Georgia is not an Asian country as it is located between Western Asia and Eastern Europe. However, the grouping of the countries was limited by the number of countries with available data. Furthermore, the clustering of EBRB and the prevalence of overweight and obesity observed within each group do not represent the current picture of the entire region as many countries were not included in the analyses. Therefore, no attempts should be made to compare data across regions/groups of countries. Nevertheless, it was preferred to group the countries rather than following a country by country approach given the advantages of the former approach in terms of data analysis and reporting and interpretation of the results.

The data-driven and person-centered nature of the cluster analysis approach is also subject to several limitations such as a high degree of subjectivity and lack of generalization of findings to other populations. This implies the need for caution when comparing our results with other studies. Furthermore, there is no agreement on how to best minimize subjectivity when determining the optimal number of clusters [46]. Several clusters were common across groups with similar characteristics;

however, they did not necessarily have the same exact characteristics such as identical levels of a given EBRB indicator. Furthermore, data was collected across all four seasons and, therefore, cluster membership could be different between seasons.

5. Conclusions

Our study identified clustering patterns of diet, PA and screen time in children, and across European and Asian countries. These findings showed the importance of following a healthy lifestyle to prevent overweight/obesity and support the hypothesis that unfavorable weight status is associated with a particular combination of EBRB patterns. However, associations differed by group of countries and cluster characteristics. These discrepancies might suggest that more behaviors beyond these four may need to be targeted. Obesity prevention strategies need to consider the synergistic effect of these behaviors, and future public health initiatives should target a reduction in screen time use and SSD intake coupled with increased levels of PA and F&V intake. Examining the stability or evolution of the clusters over time in this age group and the associations between cluster membership and sociodemographic factors are potential areas of further research.

Supplementary Materials:
Table S1: Main characteristics of study design within each country participating in the fourth round of the WHO Europe Childhood Obesity Surveillance Initiative (2015/2017); Table S2: Measuring equipment used within each country participating in the fourth round of the WHO Europe Childhood Obesity Surveillance Initiative (2015/2017); Table S3: Questions on energy balance-related behaviors asked through the family survey questionnaire in the fourth round of the WHO Europe Childhood Obesity Surveillance Initiative (2015/2017).

Author Contributions: S.B.-S. conceptualized the manuscript and conducted all analyses; S.B.-S. and A.O.-R drafted the manuscript; C.C.K., M.M.H. and C.M.M. made substantial contributions to the conception, interpretation of the results and drafts of the manuscript; M.M.H., M.B., S.A., V.D., V.F.S.A., A.F., T.H., C.H., J.H., E.K., S.M.M., G.O., N.P.-F., A.P., A.I.R., L.S., R.T.B., H.R., C.M.M., C.C.K. and J.B. contributed with data collection and data cleaning, and critically reviewed the manuscript. All authors contributed to and approved the final manuscript.

Acknowledgments: We gratefully acknowledge all participating children, their parents, and school teachers and principals for kindly volunteering to participate in the study. We also thank the researchers who collected data in each country.

Disclaimer: The authors alone are responsible for the views expressed in this article and they do not necessarily represent the views, decisions or policies of the institutions they are affiliated with. Dr João Breda, Dr Marta Buoncristiano and Mrs Guljemal Ovezmyradova are staff members of the WHO Regional Office for Europe. The World Health Organization is not liable for any use that may be made of the information contained therein.

References

1. Commision on Ending Childhood Obesity. Facts and Figures on Childhood Obesity. Available online: http://www.who.int/end-childhood-obesity/facts/en/ (accessed on 8 December 2018).
2. Abarca-Gómez, L.; Abdeen, Z.A.; Hamid, Z.A.; Abu-Rmeileh, N.M.; Acosta-Cazares, B.; Acuin, C.; Adams, R.J.; Aekplakorn, W.; Afsana, K.; Aguilar-Salinas, C.A.; et al. Worldwide trends in body-mass index, underweight, overweight, and obesity from 1975 to 2016: A pooled analysis of 2416 population-based measurement studies in 128.9 million children, adolescents, and adults. *Lancet* **2017**, *390*, 2627–2642. [CrossRef]

3. Bischoff, S.C.; Boirie, Y.; Cederholm, T.; Chourdakis, M.; Cuerda, C.; Delzenne, N.M.; Deutz, N.E.; Fouque, D.; Genton, L.; Gil, C.; et al. Towards a multidisciplinary approach to understand and manage obesity and related diseases. *Clin. Nutr.* **2017**, *36*, 917–938. [CrossRef] [PubMed]
4. Bradlee, M.L.; Singer, M.R.; Qureshi, M.M.; Moore, L.L. Food group intake and central obesity among children and adolescents in the Third National Health and Nutrition Examination Survey (NHANES III). *Public Health Nutr.* **2010**, *13*, 797–805. [CrossRef] [PubMed]
5. Mellendick, K.; Shanahan, L.; Wideman, L.; Calkins, S.; Keane, S.; Lovelady, C. Diets Rich in Fruits and Vegetables Are Associated with Lower Cardiovascular Disease Risk in Adolescents. *Nutrients* **2018**, *10*, 136. [CrossRef] [PubMed]
6. DeBoer, M.D.; Scharf, R.J.; Demmer, R.T. Sugar-sweetened beverages and weight gain in 2- to 5-year-old children. *Pediatrics* **2013**, *132*, 413–420. [CrossRef] [PubMed]
7. Malik, V.S.; Pan, A.; Willett, W.C.; Hu, F.B. Sugar-sweetened beverages and weight gain in children and adults: A systematic review and meta-analysis. *Am. J. Clin. Nutr.* **2013**, *98*, 1084–1102. [CrossRef] [PubMed]
8. Wei, X.; Zang, Y.; Jia, X.; He, X.; Zou, S.; Wang, H.; Shen, M.; Zang, J. Age, period and cohort effects and the predictors of physical activity and sedentary behaviour among Chinese children, from 2004 to 2011. *BMC Public Health* **2017**, *17*, 353. [CrossRef] [PubMed]
9. Falbe, J.; Rosner, B.; Willett, W.C.; Sonneville, K.R.; Hu, F.B.; Field, A.E. Adiposity and different types of screen time. *Pediatrics* **2013**, *132*, e1497–e1505. [CrossRef] [PubMed]
10. Leech, R.M.; McNaughton, S.A.; Timperio, A. The clustering of diet, physical activity and sedentary behavior in children and adolescents: A review. *Int. J. Behav. Nutr. Phys. Act.* **2014**, *11*, 4. [CrossRef] [PubMed]
11. Bel-Serrat, S.; Mouratidou, T.; Santaliestra-Pasias, A.M.; Iacoviello, L.; Kourides, Y.A.; Marild, S.; Molnar, D.; Reisch, L.; Siani, A.; Stomfai, S.; et al. Clustering of multiple lifestyle behaviours and its association to cardiovascular risk factors in children: The IDEFICS study. *Eur. J. Clin. Nutr.* **2013**, *67*, 848–854. [CrossRef] [PubMed]
12. Leech, R.M.; McNaughton, S.A.; Timperio, A. Clustering of diet, physical activity and sedentary behaviour among Australian children: Cross-sectional and longitudinal associations with overweight and obesity. *Int. J. Obes.* **2015**, *39*, 1079–1085. [CrossRef] [PubMed]
13. Santaliestra-Pasias, A.M.; Mouratidou, T.; Reisch, L.; Pigeot, I.; Ahrens, W.; Marild, S.; Molnar, D.; Siani, A.; Sieri, S.; Tornatiris, M.; et al. Clustering of lifestyle behaviours and relation to body composition in European children. The IDEFICS study. *Eur. J. Clin. Nutr.* **2015**, *69*, 811–816. [CrossRef] [PubMed]
14. Sanchez-Oliva, D.; Grao-Cruces, A.; Carbonell-Baeza, A.; Cabanas-Sanchez, V.; Veiga, O.L.; Castro-Pinero, J. Lifestyle Clusters in School-Aged Youth and Longitudinal Associations with Fatness: The UP & DOWN Study. *J. Pediatr.* **2018**, *203*, 317–324. [CrossRef] [PubMed]
15. Seghers, J.; Rutten, C. Clustering of multiple lifestyle behaviours and its relationship with weight status and cardiorespiratory fitness in a sample of Flemish 11- to 12-year-olds. *Public Health Nutr.* **2010**, *13*, 1838–1846. [CrossRef] [PubMed]
16. Perez-Rodrigo, C.; Gil, A.; Gonzalez-Gross, M.; Ortega, R.M.; Serra-Majem, L.; Varela-Moreiras, G.; Aranceta-Bartrina, J. Clustering of Dietary Patterns, Lifestyles, and Overweight among Spanish Children and Adolescents in the ANIBES Study. *Nutrients* **2016**, *8*, 11. [CrossRef] [PubMed]
17. Fernandez-Alvira, J.M.; De Bourdeaudhuij, I.; Singh, A.S.; Vik, F.N.; Manios, Y.; Kovacs, E.; Jan, N.; Brug, J.; Moreno, L.A. Clustering of energy balance-related behaviors and parental education in European children: The ENERGY-project. *Int. J. Behav. Nutr. Phys. Act.* **2013**, *10*, 5. [CrossRef] [PubMed]
18. Dumuid, D.; Olds, T.; Lewis, L.K.; Martin-Fernandez, J.A.; Barreira, T.; Broyles, S.; Chaput, J.P.; Fogelholm, M.; Hu, G.; Kuriyan, R.; et al. The adiposity of children is associated with their lifestyle behaviours: A cluster analysis of school-aged children from 12 nations. *Pediatr. Obes.* **2018**, *13*, 111–119. [CrossRef] [PubMed]
19. Wijnhoven, T.; Branca, F.; WHO European Childhood Obesity Surveillance Initiative. *Protocol, Version January 2008*; WHO Regional Office for Europe: Copenhagen, Denmark, 2008.
20. WHO European Childhood Obesity Surveillance Initiative. *Protocol, Version October 2012*; WHO Regional Office for Europe: Copenhagen, Denmark, 2012.

21. WHO European Childhood Obesity Surveillance Initiative. *Protocol, Version October 2016*; World Health Organization Regional Office for Europe: Copenhagen, Denmark, 2016. Available online: http://www.euro.who.int/__data/assets/pdf_file/0018/333900/COSI-protocol-en.pdf?ua=1 (accessed on 8 December 2018).
22. Wijnhoven, T.M.; van Raaij, J.M.; Spinelli, A.; Starc, G.; Hassapidou, M.; Spiroski, I.; Rutter, H.; Martos, E.; Rito, A.I.; Hovengen, R.; et al. WHO European Childhood Obesity Surveillance Initiative: Body mass index and level of overweight among 6–9-year-old children from school year 2007/2008 to school year 2009/2010. *BMC Public Health* **2014**, *14*, 806. [CrossRef] [PubMed]
23. WHO European Childhood Obesity Surveillance Initiative. *Overweight and Obesity among 6-to-9-Year-Old Children. Results of the Third Round of Data Collection 2012–2013*; World Health Organisation: Copenhagen, Denmark, 2018. Available online: http://www.euro.who.int/__data/assets/pdf_file/0010/378865/COSI-3.pdf?ua=1 (accessed on 8 December 2018).
24. Wijnhoven, T.; van Raaij, J.; Breda, J. *WHO European Childhood Obesity Surveillance Initiative: Implementation of Round 1 (2007/2008) and Round 2 (2009/2010)*; WHO Regional Office for Europe: Conpenhagen, Denmark, 2014. Available online: http://www.euro.who.int/__data/assets/pdf_file/0004/258781/COSI-report-round-1-and-2_final-for-web.pdf?ua=1 (accessed on 8 December 2018).
25. de Onis, M.; Onyango, A.W.; Borghi, E.; Siyam, A.; Nishida, C.; Siekmann, J. Development of a WHO growth reference for school-aged children and adolescents. *Bull. World Health Organ.* **2007**, *85*, 660–667. [CrossRef] [PubMed]
26. Cole, T.J.; Bellizzi, M.C.; Flegal, K.M.; Dietz, W.H. Establishing a standard definition for child overweight and obesity worldwide: International survey. *BMJ* **2000**, *320*, 1240–1243. [CrossRef] [PubMed]
27. Cole, T.J.; Flegal, K.M.; Nicholls, D.; Jackson, A.A. Body mass index cut offs to define thinness in children and adolescents: International survey. *BMJ* **2007**, *335*, 194. [CrossRef] [PubMed]
28. World Health Organization (WHO). *AnthroPlus for Personal Computers Manual: Software for Assessing Growth of the World's Children and Adolescents*; World Health Organization: Geneva, Switzerland, 2009. Available online: http://www.who.int/entity/growthref/tools/who_anthroplus_manual.pdf (accessed on 8 December 2018).
29. Milligan, C.W.; Cooper, M.C. Methodology review: Clustering methods. *Appl. Psychol. Meas.* **1987**, *11*, 329–354. [CrossRef]
30. Gore, P.A. Cluster analysis. In *Handbook of Applied Multivariate Statistics and Mathematical Modeling*, 1st ed.; Tinsley, H.E.A., Brown, S.D., Eds.; Academic Press: San Diego, CA, USA, 2000; pp. 297–321.
31. Everitt, B. *Cluster Analysis*; Heinemann Educational Books: London, UK, 1980.
32. Viera, A.J.; Garrett, J.M. Understanding interobserver agreement: The kappa statistic. *Fam. Med.* **2005**, *37*, 360–363. [PubMed]
33. Popkin, B.M.; Adair, L.S.; Ng, S.W. Global nutrition transition and the pandemic of obesity in developing countries. *Nutr. Rev.* **2012**, *70*, 3–21. [CrossRef] [PubMed]
34. Leech, R.M.; McNaughton, S.A.; Timperio, A. Clustering of children's obesity-related behaviours: Associations with sociodemographic indicators. *Eur. J. Clin. Nutr.* **2014**, *68*, 623–628. [CrossRef] [PubMed]
35. Cameron, A.J.; Crawford, D.A.; Salmon, J.; Campbell, K.; McNaughton, S.A.; Mishra, G.D.; Ball, K. Clustering of obesity-related risk behaviors in children and their mothers. *Ann. Epidemiol.* **2011**, *21*, 95–102. [CrossRef] [PubMed]
36. Physical Activity and Young People. Recommended Levels of Physical Activity for Children Aged 5–17 Years. Available online: https://www.who.int/dietphysicalactivity/factsheet_young_people/en/ (accessed on 8 December 2018).
37. Strasburger, V.C.; Hogan, M.J.; Mulligan, D.A.; Ameenuddin, N.; Christakis, D.A.; Cross, C.; Fagbuyi, D.B.; Hill, D.L.; Levine, A.E.; McCarthy, C.; et al. Children, Adolescents, and the Media. *Pediatrics* **2013**, *132*, 958–961. [CrossRef]
38. Pearson, N.; Biddle, S.J. Sedentary behavior and dietary intake in children, adolescents, and adults. A systematic review. *Am. J. Prev. Med.* **2011**, *41*, 178–188. [CrossRef] [PubMed]
39. Vingerhoets, A.M.; Croon, M.; Jeninga, A.; Menges, L. Personality and health habits. *Psychol. Health* **1990**, *4*, 333–342. [CrossRef]
40. Rogers, E.M. *Diffussion of Innovations*; Free Press of Glencoe: New York, NY, USA, 1962.

41. Li, L.; Zhang, S.; Huang, Y.; Chen, K. Sleep duration and obesity in children: A systematic review and meta-analysis of prospective cohort studies. *J. Pediatr. Child Health* **2017**, *53*, 378–385. [CrossRef] [PubMed]
42. Chesi, A.; Grant, S.F.A. The Genetics of Pediatric Obesity. *Trends Endocrinol. Metab.* **2015**, *26*, 711–721. [CrossRef] [PubMed]
43. Atkin, A.J.; Gorely, T.; Clemes, S.A.; Yates, T.; Edwardson, C.; Brage, S.; Salmon, J.; Marshall, S.J.; Biddle, S.J. Methods of measurement in epidemiology: Sedentary behaviour. *Int. J. Epidemiol.* **2012**, *41*, 1460–1471. [CrossRef] [PubMed]
44. Scharf, R.J.; DeBoer, M.D. Sugar-Sweetened Beverages and Children's Health. *Annu. Rev. Public Health* **2016**, *37*, 273–293. [CrossRef] [PubMed]
45. Collins, C.E.; Watson, J.; Burrows, T. Measuring dietary intake in children and adolescents in the context of overweight and obesity. *Int. J. Obes.* **2010**, *34*, 1103–1115. [CrossRef] [PubMed]
46. Everitt, B.S.; Landau, S.; Leese, M.; Stahl, D. *Cluster Analysis*, 5th ed.; John Wiley & Sons Ltd.: West Sussex, UK, 2011.

12

Melanocortin-4 Receptor and Lipocalin 2 Gene Variants in Spanish Children with Abdominal Obesity: Effects on BMI-SDS after a Lifestyle Intervention

Lydia Morell-Azanza [1,2], Ana Ojeda-Rodríguez [1,2], Johanna Giuranna [3], Mª Cristina Azcona-SanJulián [2,4], Johannes Hebebrand [3], Amelia Marti [1,2,5,*] and Anke Hinney [3]

1 Department of Nutrition, Food Sciences and Physiology, University of Navarra, c/Irunlarrea, 1. 31008 Pamplona, Spain; lmorell.1@alumni.unav.es (L.M.-A.); aojeda.5@alumni.unav.es (A.O.-R.)
2 IdiSNA, Instituto de Investigación Sanitaria de Navarra, c/Irunlarrea, 3. 31008 Pamplona, Spain; cazcona@unav.es
3 Department of Child and Adolescent Psychiatry, Psychosomatics and Psychotherapy, University Hospital Essen, University of Duisburg-Essen, Virchowstr. 174, D-45147 Essen, Germany; johanna.giuranna@uni-due.de (J.G.); johannes.hebebrand@uni-duisburg-essen.de (J.H.); anke.hinney@uni-due.de (A.H.)
4 Department of Paediatrics, Clínica Universidad de Navarra, Paediatric Endocrinology Unit, c/Piío XII, 36. 31008 Pamplona, Spain
5 Biomedical Research Centre Network on Obesity and Nutrition (CIBERobn), Physiopathology of Obesity and Nutrition, Institute of Health Carlos III, Av. Monforte de Lemos, 3-5. 28029 Madrid, Spain
* Correspondence: amarti@unav.es

Abstract: Mutations leading to a reduced function of the melanocortin-4 receptor (MC4R) exert a major gene effect on extreme obesity. Recently it was shown that the bone derived hormone lipocalin 2 (LCN2) binds to the MC4R and activates a MC4R dependent anorexigenic pathway. We identified mutations in both genes and screened the effects of *MC4R* and *LCN2* mutations on eating behavior and weight change after a lifestyle intervention. One hundred and twelve children (11.24 ± 2.6 years, BMI-SDS 2.91 ± 1.07) with abdominal obesity participated in a lifestyle intervention. *MC4R* and *LCN2* coding regions were screened by Sanger sequencing. Eating behavior was assessed at baseline with the Children Eating Behavior Questionnaire (CEBQ). We detected three previously described non-synonymous *MC4R* variants (Glu42Lys, Thr150Ile, and Arg305Gln) and one non-synonymous polymorphism (Ile251Leu). Regarding *LCN2*, one known non-synonymous variant (Thr124Met) was detected. Eating behavior was described in carriers of the *MC4R* and *LCN2* mutation and in non-carriers. *MC4R* and *LCN2* mutations were detected in 2.42% and 0.84%, respectively, of Spanish children with abdominal obesity. A number of subjects with functional mutation variants in *MC4R* and *LCN2* were able to achieve a reduction in BMI-SDS after a lifestyle intervention.

Keywords: childhood obesity; CEBQ; eating behavior and Ile251Leu

---

1. Introduction

Obesity has been defined by the World Health Organization (WHO) as an abnormal or excessive body fat accumulation that may impair health [1]. Both environmental and genetic factors have an influence on weight gain [2]. The impact of genetics on obesity is heterogeneous. For a small number of subjects obesity is caused by mutations in single genes, for the majority of the population obesity has a polygenic nature [2,3].

One of the most common single genes harboring variants associated with obesity is the melanocortin-4 receptor gene (*MC4R*) [4,5]. It is known as a regulator of energy homeostasis due to its effect on food intake and energy expenditure via neuronal melanocortinergic pathways [6]. More than 369 mutations including non-synonymous, nonsense, and frameshift mutations have been identified mainly in obese individuals [7,8]. Most of the non-synonymous mutations lead to partial or complete loss of function of the *MC4R* [9]. The polymorphism Ile251Leu leads to an increased function of MC4R and is associated with a reduced BMI [7].

The protein lipocalin 2 has been associated with obesity [10,11] and was thought to be secreted from adipose tissue as an adipokine [12]. However recent studies discovered a ten-fold higher expression in osteoblasts than in adipose tissue. In this line, recent studies have shown that lipocalin 2 (LCN2) binds to the MC4R to activate MC4R-dependent anorexigenic pathways [13]. It has also been observed that obese participants heterozygous for *MC4R* mutations leading to impaired function have higher levels of plasma LCN2 than BMI-matched MC4R wild-type controls [13].

Our aim was to screen for mutations in the *MC4R* and *LCN2* genes in a Spanish pediatric population with abdominal obesity. Moreover, we investigated the effects on eating behavior and weight change after participating in a one-year lifestyle intervention for carriers versus non-carriers of *MC4R* and *LCN2* variants.

2. Materials and Methods

2.1. Subjects

For this study, a total of 112 children between 7 to 16 years of age and with abdominal obesity defined as a waist circumference higher than the 90th percentile [14] participate in a lifestyle intervention. The IGENOI study is a 2-year lifestyle intervention program for children with abdominal obesity carried out by GENOI group *("Grupo de Estudio Navarro de la Obesidad infantil")*. This study is a randomized control trial (NCT03147261) conducted in Pamplona, Spain. Children were recruited from the Pediatric Endocrinology at "Clinica Universidad de Navarra" and "Complejo hospitalario de Navarra", and from health care centers around Pamplona and its neighborhoods.

Participants with previous diabetes, presence of other diseases beside obesity, major psychiatric illness including bulimia nervosa, pharmacological treatment, food intolerance, or treatment with special diets, or frequent alcohol or drug consumption were excluded. Children and their parents signed a written informed consent in the screening visit. The study protocol was performed in accordance with the ethical standards of the Declaration of Helsinki (Fortaleza, Brasil, October 2013), and was approved by the ethics committee of the University of Navarra (Reference number 044/2014).

2.2. Experimental Design

The lifestyle intervention comprises an 8-week intensive phase ($N = 104$ subjects) and a follow-up period of 10 months ($N = 85$ subjects, 1 year). The dropout rate was 7% at week 8 and 24% at 1 year of follow up.

A multidisciplinary team conformed by dietitians, pediatricians, nurses, physical activity experts, and laboratory technicians were involved in the development of the study protocol. Participants were randomly assigned into two different groups: intensive care and usual care group, following a 3:1 ratio. The first one was given a moderate hypocaloric Mediterranean diet, as previously described [15], while the usual care group received usual pediatric advice with healthy diet recommendations [16]. Specifically, intensive care participants were prescribed with a moderate hypocaloric diet based on a fixed full-day meal plan. The restriction, not to interfere with growth, was calculated depending on the degree of obesity (from −10% to −40% of total energy intake). A Mediterranean-style diet based consists of high consumption of fruit, vegetables, whole grains, legumes, nuts, seeds, and olive oil, minimally processed foods; moderate consumption of dairy products, fish, and poultry; and low consumption of red meat [15]. Both groups were encouraged to increase their physical activity to at least 200 minutes per week as recommended by The American College of Sports Medicine to prevent weight gain [17].

The intervention group participants had 30-minute individual sessions with the dietitian every two weeks during the 8-week treatment phase. In these sessions a follow-up about the accomplishment of the diet and anthropometric measurements was performed. In addition, the parents or legal guardians had one parallel group session where they received education about their role in the study and obesity related problems, while intensive care participants were encouraged to make healthy lifestyle decisions about food choices, eating behavior, sedentary activities, and physical activity. On the other hand, usual care participants and their parents received one 30-min individual session with the dietitian and five monitoring visits to assess anthropometric parameters.

During the follow-up period, participants had monitoring visits at 3, 4,5,6,9, and 12 months from the baseline visit.

2.3. *Anthropometric, Clinical and Biochemical Measurements*

All anthropometric measurements were performed at baseline, after 8 weeks, and at 1 year of follow up according to standard procedures and calibrated tools in the paediatric population [18]. Measurements were performed by trained personnel in a wide space, while the participants were asked to stand barefoot and wore light clothing, without hair ornaments or jewels.

Body weight and body fat were determined using a digital scale BC-418 Segmental Body Composition Analyzer according to manufacturer instructions (Tanita, Tokyo, Japan). To measure height, participants were asked to stand on stadiometer with the feet placed parallel and slightly apart, and heels, buttocks, scapula, and occipital head area touching the vertical board at the same time. A non-stretchable measuring tape (type SECA 200) was used for measuring waist circumference (WC) and hip circumference (HC) by standard procedures (Type SECA 200). The waist-to-hip and waist-to-height ratios were also calculated.

Body mass index was calculated as weight divided by squared height (Kg/m^2). BMI-standard deviation (BMI-SDS) is BMI values converted into standard deviation using age and specific cut-points according to Spanish reference growth charts [19]. Pubertal status was determined using Tanner stage and was evaluated by a paediatrician. The presence of *Acanthosis Nigricans* was diagnosed by pediatricians of the team at baseline. Blood pressure was measured following standard procedures, as described elsewhere [20].

Venous blood samples were obtained by specialized trained nurses at the Hospital after an overnight fast. Glucose, insulin leptin, and lipid profiles were determined by standard autoanalyzer techniques at baseline. Insulin resistance was calculated from the homeostasis model assessment of insulin resistance (HOMA-IR).

2.4. *Physical Activity*

Moderate-to-vigorous physical activity was assessed at baseline using triaxial accelerometry (Actigraph wGT3X-BT, Actigraph LLC, Penascola, FL, USA). Briefly, participants wore the accelerometer around the non-dominant waist for four days, including, at least, two weekend days, as described elsewhere [21]. Accelerometry data were analysed using ActiLife 6.0 software (Actigraph LLC, Penascola, FL, USA) as describe elsewhere [22].

2.5. *Children Eating Behavior Questionnaire (CEBQ)*

The Children Eating Behaviour Questionnaire (CEBQ) is a multidimensional parent-reported questionnaire about their children's eating behaviour [23]. It includes 35 items regarding eating styles that are clustered into eight subscales. The eight subscales are classified into two dimensions: food approach or food avoidance. The food approach dimension comprises the following subscales: "Emotional overeating", "Enjoyment of food", "Desire for drink", and "Food responsiveness". Food avoidance is represented by the following: "Slowness in eating", "Satiety responsiveness", "and Emotional undereating", and "Food fussiness". It was fulfilled by parents or legal guardians at baseline.

For each behaviour subscale parents report their children's behaviour on a five-point Likert Scale, that ranges from never, rarely, sometimes, often, or always (1 to 5). A ratio was calculated between the sums of the food approach vs. the sum of the food avoidance subscales.

2.6. DNA Extraction

Venous blood samples were obtained on ethylendiaminetetraacetic acid (EDTA) tubes, which were centrifuged 30 minutes after the extraction at 3500 rpm for 15 minutes at 4 °C. DNA was extracted from the buffy coat fraction using a commercial kit MasterPure DNA purification kit for Blood Version II (Epicenter Biotechnologies, Madison, WI, USA). Its quality and quantity were determined with a Nanodrop spectrometer ND-1000 (Nanodrop Technologies, Wilmington, Delware, USA) and it was stored at −80 °C until processing.

2.7. Mutation Screen

MC4R and *LCN2* genes were screened for mutations. All subjects were heterozygous for the mutations. *MC4R* was analyzed with one PCR fragment, while *LCN2* was divided into four PCR fragments. Methodological details can be obtained from the authors.

All samples were commercially Sanger sequenced by LGC Genomics (Berlin, Germany). Analyses of the sequences were performed by two experienced individuals in Essen (Germany). Samples with discrepancies were re-sequenced by Seqlab laboratories (Göttingen, Germany).

2.8. Statistical Analysis

Statistical analyses were performed using STATA version 12 (StataCorp, College Station, TX, USA). Normality was assessed by Shapiro-Wilk. All the tests were two-sided and the significance level was set at $\alpha = 0.05$. We did not correct for multiple testing.

We used Wilcoxon rank-sum test for the comparison between subjects with Ile 251Leu MC4R mutation and without MC4R mutation for the variables studied at baseline.

Paired t-test was applied for assessing changes in BMI-SDS between baseline vs. week 8, and baseline vs. 1 year. Furthermore, we performed a comparison between subjects with Ile 251Leu MC4R mutation and without MC4R mutation for changes in BMI-SDS (week 8 and one year, Wilcoxon rank-sum test).

3. Results

One hundred and twelve children with abdominal obesity (mean age 11.24 years, males 38%, BMI-SDS 2.93) participated in the study.

3.1. Description of Identified Variants

Mutation screen of the coding region of MC4R identified a total of four variants, three known nonsynonymous variants, rs776051881 (Glu42Lys), rs766665118 (Thr150Ile), and rs775382722 (Arg305Gln), and one nonsynonymous polymorphism rs52820871 (Ile251Leu) (Table 1). First, we classified variants as leading to reduced receptor function or similar to the wild type MC4R function. Three previously reported variants (Glu42Lys, Thr150Ileu, and Arg305Gln) lead to a reduced MC4R function as classified by in-silico predictors [24] that claim them to be disease causing. Furthermore, some in-vitro analyses had described reduced function for the mutations Thr150Ileu and Arg305Gln [9,25,26]. Our study shows a frequency of 2.52% of MC4R mutations leading to a reduced function in our sample of Spanish of children with abdominal obesity.

Table 1. MC4R and LCN2 genetic variants in Spanish children with abdominal obesity.

Gene Subject	N° of Subjects	Aminoacid Exchange	rs Number	In-silico Prediction*	Function	Reference of Functional Analysis
MC4R Mutations						
Glu42Lys	1	p.Glu42Lys	rs776051881	Disease causing	Not known	-
Thr150Ile	1	p.Thr150Ile	rs766665118	Disease causing	Reduced	[9,25]
Arg305Gln	1	p.Arg305Gln	rs775382722	Disease causing	Reduced	[26]
Polymorphisms						
Ile251Leu	5	p.Ile251Leu	rs52820871	Disease causing	Like wild type	[27–31]
LCN2 Mutations						
Thr124Met	1	p.Thr124Met	rs79993583	Probably harmless	-	-

Abdominal obesity was defined as waist circumference (WC) above the sex and age-specific 90th percentile. * In-silico prediction was performed by mutation taster www.mutationtaster.org.

The mutation screen of the coding region of LCN2 identified a total of twelve variants, eleven are located in intronic regions (rs2232632, rs202024127, rs11794980, rs2232629, rs2232625, rs2232626, rs116745581, rs2232628, rs568419305, rs2232631, rs2232632) and one is a known nonsynonymous variant: rs79993583 (Thr124Met). The analysis of all detected variants by in-silico predictors show that three of them could be disease causing (Supplementary Table S1).

3.2. Phenotypic Description of Mutation Carriers

In Table 2 phenotypic characteristics of participants with mutations at MC4R and LCN2 genes at baseline are described in detail. We also provide data from obese participants of IGENOI study without mutations in the coding regions of these genes.

For 103 children (37.8% males) with a mean age of 11.32 years no mutations in MC4R and LCN2 genes were found, they are wild type carriers. Mutated subjects are compared with them in the subsequent analyses. All wild type carriers were also obese (BMI-SDS: 2.92 ± 1.10) and 41.7% showed clinical evidence for insulin resistance in the presence of Acanthosis Nigricans that was accompanied by a HOMA-IR of 4.03 ± 3.17.

A 14 year-old girl was heterozygous for the Glu42Lys mutation at the MC4R gene. She suffers from severe-obesity (BMI-SDS:4.04) reflected in a fat mass of 40.8%. The main clinical features of this participant were leptin levels higher than expected for the BMI [32], and the presence of insulin resistance observed as hyperinsulinemia, increased HOMA-IR (4.23), and Acanthosis Nigricans.

Mutation Thr150Ileu at the MC4R gene was observed in an eight year-old boy with a BMI-SDS of +3.5. Biochemical parameters were normal and the participant was physically active (50.65 min/day). One participant carries two variants at the MC4R gene: Arg305Gln and the polymorphism Ile251Leu. She is a 12 year-old girl with a BMI-SDS of 2.91, and a fat mass of 43.2% (measured by bioimpedance). Five independent children also carried the polymorphism Ile251Leu. They had a mean age of nine years and a mean BMI-SDS of 2.69. In comparison with the participants with the wild type receptor, none of the participants carrying this polymorphism showed Acanthosis Nigricans.

The polymorphism Ile251Leu of MC4R was observed in five participants with a mean age of nine years old. We found increased levels of total cholesterol and LDL-cholesterol in comparison to participants without MC4R mutation ($p = 0.004$ and $p = 0.013$; Wilcoxon rank-sum test). These differences persist when subjects with the Ile251Leu MC4R mutation were compared to age and sex matched subjects without MC4R mutation (Supplementary Table S2).

One male 15 year-old heterozygously carried the mutation Thr124Met at the LCN2 gene. Clinical characteristics of this participant included severe obesity (BMI-SDS = +4.01) accompanied by an elevated percentage of fat mass (38.7%). Also, a remarkable difference of higher levels of MVPA was detected in comparison with the wild type population. The carrier of this mutation was much more active than the wild-type controls (120.92 min/day vs. 44.82 min/day, $p = 0.088$). We also evaluated the siblings (three girls) of the index patient, all of them were obese. Two of them were also carriers of Thr124Met (BMI-SDS: 3.47 and BMI-SDS: 3.76). The MAF for this variant in the LCN2 gene in the study population is 0.44%.

Table 2. Baseline characteristics of heterozygous MC4R and LCN2 variant carriers and wild type Spanish children with abdominal obesity.

		MC4R Mutations				LCN2 Mutation
	Wt Population	Glu42Lys	Thr150Ile	Arg305Gln+Ile251Leu	Ile251Leu	Thr124Met
N	103	1	1	1	5	1
Age (years)	11.32 (2.46)	14	8	12	9 (1)	15
Sex (Male/Female)	39/64	Female	Male	Female	2/3	Male
Tanner (I/II/III/IV/V)	31/17/18/6/24	V	I	II	4/-/1/-/-	V
Height (cm)	151.23 (12.72)	168	137.8	151	137.3 (13.86)	175.9
Weight (Kg)	66.71 (18.77)	97	49.1	67.2	49.94 (17.87)	112.9
BMI (Kg/m^2)	28.55 (4.51)	34.4	25.85	29.5	25.64 (3.53)	36.5
BMI-SDS	2.92 (1.10)	4.04	3.5	2.91	2.69 (1.05)	4.01
WHR	0.88 (0.06)	0.90	0.89	0.93	0.86 (0.04)	0.82
% fat mass	37.22 (6.33)	40.8	32.1	43.2	33.98 (9.28)	38.7
Acantosis nigricans (+/-)	43/52	+	-	-	0/5	+
Glucose (mg/dL)	89.04 (6.58)	85	88	78	88.25 (6.84)	87
Insulin (µu/mL)	17.92 (13.29)	20.2	7	13.5	11.87 (6.43)	11.4
HOMA-IR	4.03 (3.17)	4.23	1.52	2.6	2.66 (1.68)	2.44
Total Colesterol (mg/dL)	162.65 (24.97)	116	162	157	198.75 (14.88)*	160
HDL-colesterol (mg/dL)	46.70 (9.96)	42	53	46	56.75 (12.25)	41
LDL-colesterol (mg/dL)	97.67 (21.15)	64	96	97	125.75 (16.82)*	99
Triglycerides (mg/dL)	94.48 (44.73)	49	64	68	81.25 (41.65)	98
Leptin (ng/mL)	36.41 (18.60)	90.8	14	NA	33.52 (13.11)	8.1
MVPA (min/day)	44.88 (23.69)	37.5	50.65	30.93	44.55 (18.37)	120.92
CEBQ ratio	1.22 (0.42)	0.82	1.25	NA	1.01 (0.12)	0.85

Data are expressed as mean (SD), * $p < 0.05$ for the comparison between Ile 251Leu MC4R mutation subjects and subjects without MC4R mutation, Wilcoxon rank-sum test was applied Abdominal obesity was defined as WC above the sex and age-specific 90th percentile. BMI-SDS, standard deviation score for body mass index; CEBQ, Children Eating Behavior Questionnaire Ratio; MVPA, moderate to vigorous physical activity; WHR: waist to height ratio.

3.3. Children Eating Behavior

The eating behavior scores with four dimension charts of children with abdominal obesity at baseline is described in Figure 1. Wild type subjects (no mutations in MC4R and LCN2 genes) had a score of 1.19. Carriers of the MC4R Thr150Ileu and LCN2 Thr124Met variants had nominally higher scores than wild type subjects, while participants with Ile251Leu polymorphism have lower score.

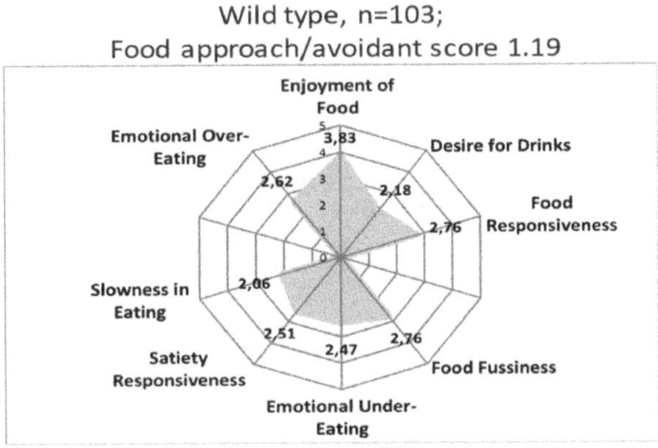

Figure 1. *Cont.*

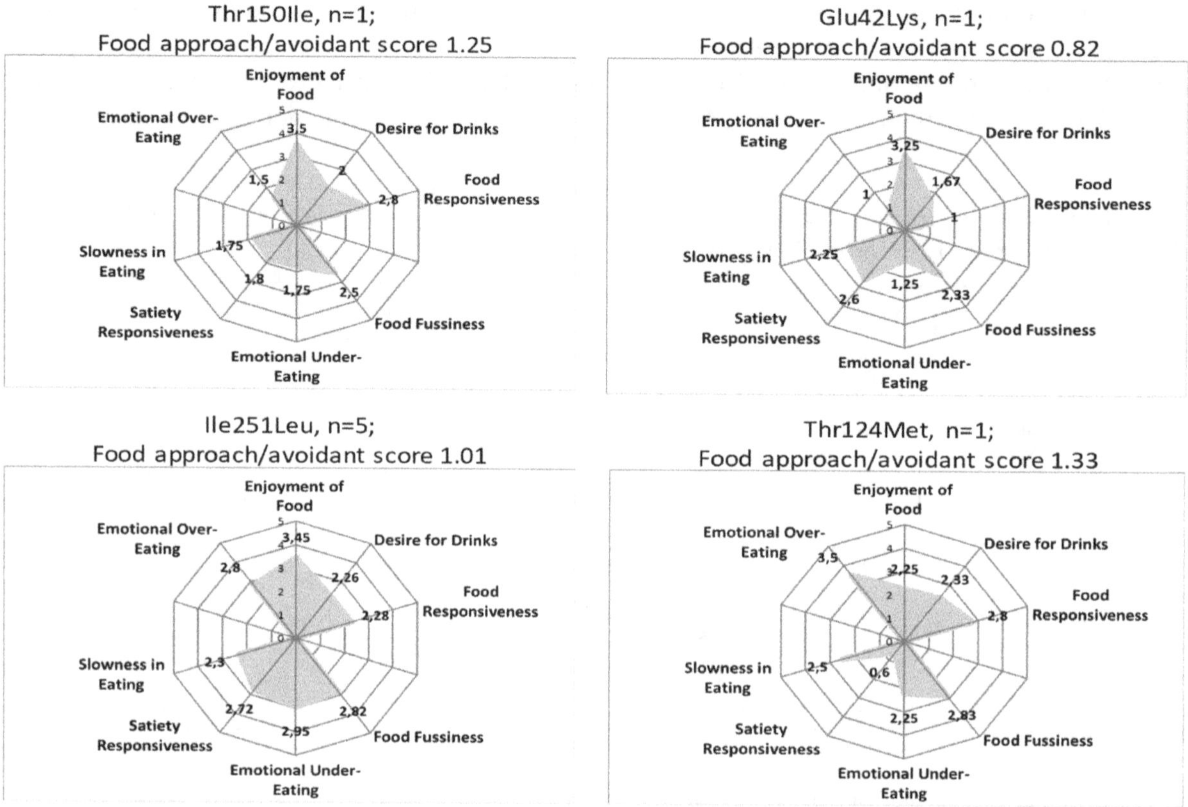

Figure 1. Childhood Eating Behavior Score (CEBQ) in Spanish children with abdominal obesity. The Food approach/avoidant score refers to the quotient between the sums of scores of the "food approach" subscales divided by the sum of the scores of the "food avoidant" subscales. Subjects with mutations in MC4R (Thr124Met, Thr150Ileu) and LCN2 (Thr124Met) genes were evaluated.

3.4. *Change in BMI-SDS and Mutations in MC4R and LCN2 After 8-Week and 1-Year of Follow Up*

Carriers of mutations that lead to a reduced function in MC4R and LCN2 genes showed a disparity of responses to the lifestyle intervention (Table 3). Changes in BMI-SDS of the five subject carriers of the Ile251Leu polymorphism are quite variable with two of them not showing any improvement at 1 year. Moreover, no significant differences in BMI-SDS changes were found after eight weeks or one-year of follow up in mutated carriers vs. non carriers subjects in analysis conducted in matched age and sex subjects with and without a functional mutation in MC4R (Supplementary Table S3).

Table 3. Changes in BMI-SDS according to MC4R and LCN2 variants after an 8-week and 1-year lifestyle intervention.

		ΔBMI-SDS			
		8 Week		**1 Year**	
		Mutation Carriers	**Non Carriers**	**Mutation Carriers**	**Non Carriers**
Usual Care Group			$n = 27$ −0.44 (0.66)***		$n = 22$ −0.47 (0.52)***
MC4R: Glu42Lys		− 0.51		Drop out	
MC4R: Thr150Ile		−0.67		−0.90	
Intensive Care group			$n = 68$ −0.51 (0.38)***		$n = 56$ −0.60 (0.72)***
MC4R: Arg305Gln + Ile251Leu		−0.13		−0.81	
MC4R: Ile251Leu	Mean ($n = 5$)	−0.74 (0.41)**		−1.02 (1.21)	
	Carrier 1	−0.95		−1.47	
	Carrier 2	−0.10		0.07	
	Carrier 3	−0.56		0.38	
	Carrier 4	−1.14		−1.56	
	Carrier 5	−0.97		−2.53	
LCN2: Thr124Met		−0.59		Drop out	

Data are expressed as mean (SD). Paired t-test for changes between baseline vs. 8 week, and baseline vs. 1 year was applied (** < 0.010, *** < 0.001).

4. Discussion

To our knowledge, this is the first study evaluating *MC4R* and *LCN2* gene variants, in a population of children and adolescents with abdominal obesity. In addition, we measured the eating behavior in all participants with the CEBQ. Finally, we reported changes in BMI-SDS achieved after eight weeks and 1 year of follow-up according to the two different strategies (usual care or intensive care) and the presence of *MC4R* and *LCN2* gene variants.

The rate of participants carrying a *MC4R* mutation leading to a reduced function was 2.67 %. This frequency is in accordance with the reported values in Czech children with obesity being 2.4% [33]. Previously, a wide variability (ranging from 0.5 to 5.8%) in the frequency of *MC4R* mutations had been described in children and adolescents with obesity in different populations [33–36].

In our population, we found one extremely obese participant (BMI-SDS +4.04) carrying the *MC4R* mutation Glu42Lys. This mutation was previously reported in 5.6% of Turkish children with obesity [37]. In our case, the minor allele frequency (MAF) for this mutation was 0.89%.

Moreover, an eight year-old boy with a BMI-SDS of +3.5 was a heterozygous carrier of the *MC4R* Thr150Ileu variation. This mutation had previously been described in an obese Chilean child with a BMI-SDS of +2.79 [38]. In the Chilean population the MAF for this variant was 0.45% similar to the observed value in our Spanish population (0.84%).

Mutation Arg305Gln of the *MC4R* gene was characterized in functional studies as a variation that causes a decrease in MC4R constituently activity and in the response to the agonist [9]. We found this mutation in a 12 year-old girl with obesity (43.2% body fat mass and BMI-SDS +2.91). This participant also carries the Ile251Leu polymorphism. There is also a German obese boy harboring this Arg305Gln variation (BMI-SDS +2.5) [39]. The frequency of this variation in our population is 0.84% while in the German population was 0.19%.

Two polymorphisms in the *MC4R* (Val103Ileu and Ile251Leu) had been demonstrated to reduce the risk of obesity [40–42]. Val103Ileu was described in white Europeans with frequencies between 1–4% [2]. In our study, we did not observe carriers of this variation. In other independent studies in Spanish children the frequencies of this polymorphism were lower than in other European countries [43–45]. The frequency of the Ile251Leu variation in our studied sample was 5.04% (6 children with abdominal obesity), which is higher than the observed values in other Spanish and Polish pediatric populations [28,43,44]. Heterozygous subjects for the Ile251Leu SNP showed higher levels of total cholesterol and LDL-cholesterol. There are studies on the association between *MC4R* variants and other lipid markers in several populations [31,46].

To our knowledge this is the first study evaluating non-common variants in the *LCN2* gene in children with abdominal obesity. We found one heterozygous carrier of the Thr124Met variant that was severely obese (BMI-SDS: + 4.01) despite being physically active (more than 2 hours per day on moderate-to-vigorous physical activity).

It has been demonstrated that LCN2 suppresses appetite by signaling trough MC4R [13]. For this reason we evaluated eating behavior in our population with the children eating behavior questionnaire (CEBQ), for which solid reproducibility and high internal consistency had been reported [47]. In particular we represent graphically the multidimensionality of participants carrying *MC4R* and *LCN2* mutations. We observed that carriers of the Thr150Ile (*MC4R*) and Thr124Met (*LCN2*) variants showed slightly higher eating behavior scores than obese individuals without *MC4R* variants. This tentatively suggests an effect of these mutations on eating behavior, as mutation carriers showed lower scores on food avoidance subscales. However, as the number of mutation carriers is very low, meaningful statistical analyses are not possible.

Regarding the mutation Thr150Ile of the *MC4R* gene, an association between this variant and eating behavior in three Chilean obese carriers was reported. These participants had a cognitive restraint measured by the TFEQ-R18 questionnaire [48].

The participant carrying the *LCN2* Thr124Met allele showed lower satiety responsiveness (0.6 out of 5). This could be explained by a potential effect of LCN2 on appetite-suppressing activities [13]. Participants carrying the Ile251Leu polymorphism of the *MC4R* had lower scores in satiety responsiveness than the wild type population (1.01 vs. 1.19). Nevertheless, carrying the infrequent allele at *MC4R* Ile251Leu seems not to have an influence on eating behavior compared to children with obesity and variations in the *MC4R* gene. A previous study had described association between *MC4R* polymorphism rs17782313 (in the 3′ region of the gene) and childhood eating behavior. Satiety responsiveness dimension was decreased and enjoyment of food was increased in carriers of the CC allele [38]. However, the lack of significance in our results should be seen under the limited statistical power as we analyzed rare variants in a relatively small study group.

In our population, participants carrying mutations in *MC4R* and *LCN2* that lead to a reduced function were able to achieve similar or greater reduction in BMI-SDS than children without mutation in these genes after a lifestyle intervention. These results are in concordance with previous weight loss MC4R studies [4,39]. It had been demonstrated that children with mutations in *MC4R* had a significantly greater beneficial effect from the short lifestyle interventions than wild type carriers [49]. However, in our study one carrier of Arg305Gln only achieved a successful reduction in BMI-SDS after one year of intervention. When the polymorphism Ile251Leu of the *MC4R* gene was analyzed, some participants showed a reduction in BMI-SDS similar to that of wild type subjects after the intervention. Limitations of our study comprise of a relatively small sample size, the lack of a normal-weight study group, that no functional in vitro tests were performed, and also that we cannot exclude the presence of mutations in other genes involved in monogenic obesity.

5. Conclusions

In summary, *MC4R* and *LCN2* mutations were detected in 2.42% and 0.84%, respectively, of Spanish children with abdominal obesity. Our data suggests a putative association between profiles of eating behavior and functional mutations in *MC4R* gene. Specifically, *MC4R* and *LCN2* mutation carriers having abdominal obesity were able to reduce BMI-SDS after a lifestyle intervention.

Supplementary Materials:
Table S1: *LCN2* genetic variants in Spanish children with abdominal obesity. Table S2: Baseline characteristics from a subpopulation of matched age and sex subjects with the Ile251Leu MC4R mutations and without the mutation. Table S3: Changes in anthropometric and biochemical from a subpopulation of matched age and sex subjects with the Ile251Leu MC4R mutations and without the mutation.

Author Contributions: Conceptualization, M.C.A.-S., A.H. and A.M.; methodology, L.M.-A., A.O.-R. and J.G.; formal analysis, L.M.-A., J.G., A.O.-R. and A.H.; resources, M.C.A.-S., J.H., A.H., and A.M.; data curation, L.M.-A. and A.H.; writing—original draft preparation, L.M.-A.; writing—review and editing, A.O.-R., J.G., M.C.A.-S., J.H., A.H. and A.M.; supervision, A.H.; project administration, M.C.A.-S. and A.M.; funding acquisition, M.C.A.-S., J.H., A.H. and A.M.

Acknowledgments: We thank all the children and families in the trial for their enthusiastic and maintained collaboration, and other investigators of the IGENOI group for their participation in the recruitment process and the acquisition of the data. We are indebted to S. Düerkop and J. Andrä for technical support. L.M.-A. and A.O.-R. acknowledge their fellowships from the "la Caixa" Banking Foundation.

References

1. World Health Organization. Obesity and Overweight. Available online: https://www.who.int/news-room/fact-sheets/detail/obesity-and-overweight (accessed on 1 June 2018).
2. Loos, R.J.F. The genetic epidemiology of melanocortin 4 receptor variants. *Eur. J. Pharmacol.* **2011**, *660*, 156–164. [CrossRef] [PubMed]

3. Razquin, C.; Marti, A.; Martinez, J.A. Evidences on three relevant obesogenes: MC4R, FTO and PPARγ. Approaches for personalized nutrition. *Mol. Nutr. Food Res.* **2011**, *55*, 136–149. [CrossRef]
4. Koochakpoor, G.; Hosseini-Esfahani, F.; Daneshpour, M.S.; Hosseini, S.A.; Mirmiran, P. Effect of interactions of polymorphisms in the Melanocortin-4 receptor gene with dietary factors on the risk of obesity and Type 2 diabetes: A systematic review. *Diabet. Med.* **2016**, *33*, 1026–1034. [CrossRef] [PubMed]
5. Saeed, S.; Bonnefond, A.; Manzoor, J.; Shabir, F.; Ayesha, H.; Philippe, J.; Durand, E.; Crouch, H.; Sand, O.; Ali, M.; et al. Genetic variants in *LEP*, *LEPR*, and *MC4R* explain 30% of severe obesity in children from a consanguineous population. *Obesity* **2015**, *23*, 1687–1695. [CrossRef] [PubMed]
6. Zlatohlavek, L.; Hubacek, J.A.; Vrablik, M.; Pejsova, H.; Lanska, V.; Ceska, R. The Impact of Physical Activity and Dietary Measures on the Biochemical and Anthropometric Parameters in Obese Children. Is There Any Genetic Predisposition? *Cent. Eur. J. Public Health* **2015**, *23*. [CrossRef]
7. Hinney, A.; Volckmar, A.-L.; Knoll, N. Chapter Five - Melanocortin-4 Receptor in Energy Homeostasis and Obesity Pathogenesis. In *G Protein-Coupled Receptors in Energy Homeostasis and Obesity Pathogenesis*, 1st ed.; Elsevier Inc.: New York, NY, USA, 2013; Volume 114, pp. 147–191.
8. Collet, T.H.; Dubern, B.; Mokrosinski, J.; Connors, H.; Keogh, J.M.; Mendes de Oliveira, E.; Henning, E.; Poitou-Bernert, C.; Oppert, J.-M.; Tounian, P.; et al. Evaluation of a melanocortin-4 receptor (MC4R) agonist (Setmelanotide) in MC4R deficiency. *Mol. Metab.* **2017**, *6*, 1321–1329. [CrossRef]
9. Lubrano-Berthelier, C.; Dubern, B.; Lacorte, J.M.; Picard, F.; Shapiro, A.; Zhang, S.; Bertrais, S.; Hercberg, S.; Basdevant, A.; Clément, K.; et al. Melanocortin 4 receptor mutations in a large cohort of severely obese adults: Prevalence, functional classification, genotype-phenotype relationship, and lack of association with binge eating. *J. Clin. Endocrinol. Metab.* **2006**, *91*, 1811–1818. [CrossRef]
10. Catalán, V.; Gómez-Ambrosi, J.; Rodríguez, A.; Ramírez, B.; Valentí, V.; Moncada, R.; Silva, C.; Salvador, J.; Frühbeck, G. Peripheral mononuclear blood cells contribute to the obesity-associated inflammatory state independently of glycemic status: involvement of the novel proinflammatory adipokines chemerin, chitinase-3-like protein 1, lipocalin-2 and osteopontin. *Genes Nutr.* **2015**, *10*. [CrossRef]
11. Elkhidir, A.E.; Eltaher, H.B.; Mohamed, A.O. Association of lipocalin-2 level, glycemic status and obesity in type 2 diabetes mellitus. *BMC Res. Notes* **2017**, *10*, 1–6. [CrossRef] [PubMed]
12. Zhang, Y.; Foncea, R.; Deis, J.A.; Guo, H.; Bernlohr, D.A.; Chen, X. Lipocalin 2 expression and secretion is highly regulated by metabolic stress, cytokines, and nutrients in adipocytes. *PLoS ONE* **2014**, *9*, 1–9. [CrossRef] [PubMed]
13. Mosialou, I.; Shikhel, S.; Liu, J.M.; Maurizi, A.; Luo, N.; He, Z.; Huang, Y.R.; Zong, H.H.; Friedman, R.A.; Barasch, J. MC4R-dependent suppression of appetite by bone-derived lipocalin 2. *Nature* **2017**, *543*, 385–390. [CrossRef] [PubMed]
14. Serra Majem, L.; Aranceta Bartrina, J.; Ribas Barba, L.; Pérez Rodrigo, C.; García Closas, R. *Estudio enKid: objetivos y metodología. Crecimiento y desarrollo. Estudio enKid*; Masson S.A.: Barcelona, Spain, 2000; Volume 4.
15. Ojeda-Rodríguez, A.; Zazpe, I.; Morell-Azanza, L.; Chueca, M.J.; Azcona-Sanjulian, M.C.; Marti, A. Improved diet quality and nutrient adequacy in children and adolescents with abdominal obesity after a lifestyle intervention. *Nutrients* **2018**, *10*, 1500. [CrossRef]
16. Aranceta Batrina, J.; Arija Val, V.; Maíz Aldalur, E.; de Victoria Muñoz, E.M.; Ortega Anta, R.M.; Pérez Rodrigo, C.; Quiles Izquierdo, J.; Rodríguez Martín, A.; Román Viñas, B.; Salvador i Castell, G.; et al. Guías alimentarias para la población española (SENC, diciembre 2016); la nueva pirámide de la alimentación saludable. *Nutr. Hosp.* **2015**, *31*, 1–145. [CrossRef]
17. Donnelly, J.E.; Blair, S.N.; Jakicic, J.M.; Manore, M.M.; Rankin, J.W.; Smith, B.K. Appropriate physical activity intervention strategies for weight loss and prevention of weight regain for adults. *Med. Sci. Sports Exerc.* **2009**, *41*, 459–471. [CrossRef]
18. Morell-Azanza, L.; García-Calzón, S.; Rendo-Urteaga, T.; Martin-Calvo, N.; Chueca, M.; Martínez, J.A.; Azcona-Sanjulián, M.C.; Marti, A. Serum oxidized low-density lipoprotein levels are related to cardiometabolic risk and decreased after a weight loss treatment in obese children and adolescents. *Pediatr. Diabetes* **2017**, *18*, 18. [CrossRef]
19. Sobradillo, B.; Aguirre, A.; Uresti, U.; Bilbao, A.; Fernández-Ramos, C.; Lizarraga, A.; Lorenzo, H.; Madariag, L.; Rica, I.; Ruiz, I.; et al. Curvas y tablas de Crecimiento. Estudios Longitudinal y Transversal. Bilbao: Fundación Faustino Orbegozo Eizaguirre. 2004. Available online: https://www.fundacionorbegozo.com/wp-content/uploads/pdf/estudios_2004.pdf (accessed on 20 January 2015).

20. Pickering, T.G.; Hall, J.E.; Appel, L.J.; Falkner, B.E.; Graves, J.; Hill, M.N.; Jones, D.W.; Kurtz, T.; Sheps, S.G.; Roccella, E.J. Recommendations for blood pressure measurement in humans and experimental animals: Part 1: Blood pressure measurement in humans—A statement for professionals from the Subcommittee of Professional and Public Education of the American Heart Association Council on High Blood Pressure Research. *Circulation* **2005**, *111*, 697–716. [CrossRef]
21. Morell-Azanza, L.; Ojeda-Rodríguez, A.; Ochotorena-Elicegui, A.; Martín-Calvo, N.; Chueca, M.; Marti, A.; Azcona-San Julian, C. Changes in objectively measured physical activity after a multidisciplinary lifestyle intervention in children with abdominal obesity: A randomized control trial. *BMC Pediatr.* **2019**, 6–13. [CrossRef]
22. Konstabel, K.; Veidebaum, T.; Verbestel, V.; Moreno, L.A.; Bammann, K.; Tornaritis, M.; Eiben, G.; Molnár, D.; Siani, A.; Sprengeler, O.; et al. Objectively measured physical activity in European children: The IDEFICS study. *Int. J. Obes.* **2014**, *38*, S135–S143. [CrossRef]
23. González, A.; Martínez, J.L.S.; Santos-Martínez, J.L. Adaptación y aplicación del cuestionario de conducta de alimentación infantil CEBQ. Fundam Nutr y Dietética Bases Metod y Apl. 2011, pp. 339–344. Available online: https://dialnet.unirioja.es/servlet/articulo?codigo=6364656 (accessed on 2 March 2017).
24. MutationTaster. Available online: www.mutationtaster.org (accessed on 5 April 2017).
25. Xiang, Z.; Pogozheva, I.D.; Sorenson, N.B.; Wilczynski, A.M.; Holder, J.R.; Litherland, S.A.; Millard, W.J.; Mosberg, H.I.; Haskell-Luevano, C. Peptide and small molecules rescue the functional activity and agonist potency of dysfunctional human melanocortin-4 receptor polymorphisms. *Biochemistry* **2007**, *46*, 8273–8287. [CrossRef] [PubMed]
26. Calton, M.A.; Ersoy, B.A.; Zhang, S.; Kane, J.P.; Malloy, M.J.; Pullinger, C.R.; Bromberg, Y.; Pennacchio, L.A.; Dent, R.; McPherson, R.; et al. Association of functionally significant Melanocortin-4 but not Melanocortin-3 receptor mutations with severe adult obesity in a large North American case-control study. *Hum. Mol. Genet.* **2009**, *18*, 1140–1147. [CrossRef]
27. Thearle, M.S.; Muller, Y.L.; Hanson, R.L.; Mullins, M.; AbdusSamad, M.; Tran, J.; Knowler, W.C.; Bogardus, C.; Krakoff, J.; Baier, L.J. Greater impact of melanocortin-4 receptor deficiency on rates of growth and risk of type 2 diabetes during childhood compared with adulthood in Pima Indians. *Diabetes* **2012**, *61*, 250–257. [CrossRef] [PubMed]
28. Nowacka-Woszuk, J.; Cieslak, J.; Skowronska, B.; Majewska, K.A.; Stankiewicz, W.; Fichna, P.; Switonski, M. Missense mutations and polymorphisms of the MC4R gene in Polish obese children and adolescents in relation to the relative body mass index. *J. Appl. Genet.* **2011**, *52*, 319–323. [CrossRef] [PubMed]
29. Bonnefond, A.; Keller, R.; Meyre, D.; Stutzmann, F.; Thuillier, D.; Stefanov, D.G.; Froguel, P.; Horber, F.F.; Kral, J.G. Eating Behavior, Low-Frequency Functional Mutations in the Melanocortin-4 Receptor (MC4R) Gene, and Outcomes of Bariatric Operations: A 6-Year Prospective Study. *Diabetes Care* **2016**, *39*, 1384–1392. [CrossRef] [PubMed]
30. Rovite, V.; Petrovska, R.; Vaivade, I.; Kalnina, I.; Fridmanis, D.; Zaharenko, L.; Peculis, R.; Pirags, V.; Schioth, H.B.; Klovins, J. The role of common and rare MC4R variants and FTO polymorphisms in extreme form of obesity. *Mol. Biol. Rep.* **2014**, *41*, 1491–1500. [CrossRef]
31. Melchior, C.; Schulz, A.; Windholz, J.; Kiess, W.; Schneberg, T.; Krner, A. Clinical and functional relevance of melanocortin-4 receptor variants in obese german children. *Horm. Res. Paediatr.* **2012**, *78*, 237–246. [CrossRef] [PubMed]
32. Koester-Weber, T.; Valtuena, J.; Breidenassel, C.; Beghin, L.; Plada, M.; Moreno, S.; Huybrechts, I.; Palacios, G.; Gomez-Martinez, S.; Albers, U.; et al. Valores de referencia para leptina, Cortisol, Insulina y glucosa entre los adolescentes europeos y su asociaciÓn con adiposidad: Estudio helena. *Nutr. Hosp.* **2014**, *30*, 1181–1190. [CrossRef] [PubMed]
33. Hainerova, I.; Larsen, L.H.; Holst, B.; Finkova, M. Melanocortin 4 Receptor Mutations in Obese Czech Children: Studies of Prevalence, Phenotype Development, Weight Reduction Response, and Functional Analysis. *J. Clin. Endocrinol. Metab.* **2007**, *92*, 3689–3696. [CrossRef]
34. Hinney, A.; Bettecken, T.; Tarnow, P.; Brumm, H.; Reichwald, K.; Lichtner, P.; Scherag, A.; Nguyen, T.T.; Schlumberger, P.; Rief, W.; et al. Prevalence, spectrum, and functional characterization of melanocortin-4 receptor gene mutations in a representative population-based sample and obese adults from Germany. *J. Clin. Endocrinol. Metab.* **2006**, *91*, 1761–1769. [CrossRef] [PubMed]

35. Miraglia del Giudice, E.; Cirillo, G.; Nigro, V.; Santoro, N.; D'Urso, L.; Raimondo, P.; Cozzolino, D.; Scafato, D.; Perrone, L. Low frequency of melanocortin-4 receptor (MC4R) mutations in a Mediterranean population with early-onset obesity. *Int. J. Obes.* **2002**, *26*, 647–651. [CrossRef]
36. Stutzmann, F.; Tan, K.; Vatin, V.; Dina, C.; Jouret, B.; Tichet, J.; Balkau, B.; Potoczna, N.; Horber, F.; O'Rahilly, S.; et al. Prevalence of melanocortin-4 receptor deficiency in europeans and their age-dependent penetrance in multigenerational pedigrees. *Diabetes* **2008**, *57*, 2511–2518. [CrossRef]
37. Demiralp, D.O.; Berberoğlu, M.; Akar, N. Melanocortin-4 receptor polymorphisms in Turkish pediatric obese patients. *Clin. Appl. Thromb.* **2011**, *17*, 70–74. [CrossRef] [PubMed]
38. Valladares, M.; Domínguez-Vásquez, P.; Obregón, A.M.; Weisstaub, G.; Burrows, R.; Maiz, A.; Santos, J.L. Melanocortin-4 receptor gene variants in Chilean families: Association with childhood obesity and eating behavior. *Nutr. Neurosci.* **2010**, *13*, 71–78. [CrossRef]
39. Reinehr, T.; Hebebrand, J.; Friedel, S.; Toschke, A.M.; Brumm, H.; Biebermann, H.; Hinney, A. Lifestyle Intervention in Obese Children With Variations in the Melanocortin 4 Receptor Gene. *Obesity* **2009**, *17*, 382–389. [CrossRef] [PubMed]
40. Young, E.H.; Wareham, N.J.; Farooqi, S.; Hinney, A.; Hebebrand, J.; Scherag, A.; O'rahilly, S.; Barroso, I.; Sandhu, M.S. The V103I polymorphism of the MC4R gene and obesity: Population based studies and meta-analysis of 29 563 individuals. *Int. J. Obes.* **2007**, *31*, 1437–1441. [CrossRef] [PubMed]
41. Stutzmann, F.; Vatin, V.; Cauchi, S.; Morandi, A.; Jouret, B.; Landt, O.; Tounian, P.; Levy-Marchal, C.; Buzzetti, R.; Pinelli, L.; et al. Non-synonymous polymorphisms in melanocortin-4 receptor protect against obesity: The two facets of a Janus obesity gene. *Hum. Mol. Genet.* **2007**, *16*, 1837–1844. [CrossRef] [PubMed]
42. Wang, D.; Ma, J.; Zhang, S.; Hinney, A.; Hebebrand, J.; Wang, Y.; Wang, H.J. Association of the MC4R V103I polymorphism with obesity: A chinese case-control study and meta-analysis in 55,195 individuals. *Obesity* **2010**, *18*, 573–579. [CrossRef]
43. Ochoa, M.C.; Razquin, C.; Azcona, C.; García-Fuentes, M.; Martínez, J.A. Val103Ile and Ile251Leu polymorphisms in MC4R gene in Spanish children and adolescents. *Rev. Española Obes.* **2005**, *3*, 250–272.
44. Ochoa, M.C.; Azcona, C.; Biebermann, H.; Brumm, H.; Razquin, C.; Wermter, A.K.; Martínez, J.A.; Hebebrand, J.; Hinney, A.; Moreno-Aliaga, M.J.; et al. A novel mutation Thr162Arg of the melanocortin 4 receptor gene in a Spanish children and adolescent population. *Clin. Endocrinol. (Oxf).* **2007**, *66*, 652–658. [CrossRef]
45. Marti, A.; Corbala, M.S.; Forga, L.; Martinez, J.A.; Hinney, A.; Hebebrand, J. A novel nonsense mutation in the melanocortin-4 receptor associated with obesity in a Spanish population. *Int. J. Obes.* **2003**, *27*, 385–388. [CrossRef] [PubMed]
46. Fernandes, A.E.; de Melo, M.E.; Fujiwara, C.T.H.; Pioltine, M.B.; Matioli, S.R.; Santos, A.; Cercato, C.; Halpern, A.; Mancini, M.C. Associations between a common variant near the MC4R gene and serum triglyceride levels in an obese pediatric cohort. *Endocrine* **2015**, *49*, 653–658. [CrossRef]
47. Ashcroft, J.; Semmler, C.; Carnell, S.; van Jaarsveld, C.H.M.; Wardle, J. Continuity and stability of eating behaviour traits in children. *Eur. J. Clin. Nutr.* **2008**, *62*, 985–990. [CrossRef] [PubMed]
48. Santos, J.L.; Amador, P.; Valladares, M.; Albala, C.; Martinez, J.A.; Marti, A. Obesity and eating behaviour in a three-generation Chilean family with carriers of the Thr150Ile mutation in the melanocortin-4 receptor gene. *J. Physiol. Biochem.* **2008**, *64*, 205–210. [CrossRef] [PubMed]
49. Zlatohlavek, L.; Vrablik, M.; Motykova, E.; Ceska, R.; Vasickova, L.; Dlouha, D.; Hubacek, J.A. FTO and MC4R gene variants determine BMI changes in children after intensive lifestyle intervention. *Clin. Biochem.* **2013**, *46*, 313–316. [CrossRef] [PubMed]

13

Relationship between Long Chain *n*-3 Polyunsaturated Fatty Acids and Autism Spectrum Disorder

Hajar Mazahery [1], Welma Stonehouse [2], Maryam Delshad [1], Marlena C. Kruger [3], Cathryn A. Conlon [1], Kathryn L. Beck [1] and Pamela R. von Hurst [1,*]

[1] Massey Institute of Food Science and Technology, School of Food and Nutrition, Massey University, Auckland 0745, New Zealand; h.mazahery@massey.ac.nz (H.M.); delshad.maryam@yahoo.com (M.D.); c.conlon@massey.ac.nz (C.A.C.); k.l.beck@massey.ac.nz (K.L.B.)

[2] Commonwealth Scientific Industrial Research Organisation (CSIRO) Food, Nutrition and Bioproducts, Adelaide SA 5000, Australia; welma.stonehouse@csiro.au

[3] Massey Institute of Food Science and Technology, School of Food and Nutrition, Massey University, Palmerston North 4410, New Zealand; m.c.kruger@massey.ac.nz

* Correspondence: p.r.vonhurst@massey.ac.nz

Abstract: Omega-3 long chain polyunsaturated fatty acid supplementation (*n*-3 LCPUFA) for treatment of Autism Spectrum Disorder (ASD) is popular. The results of previous systematic reviews and meta-analyses of *n*-3 LCPUFA supplementation on ASD outcomes were inconclusive. Two meta-analyses were conducted; meta-analysis 1 compared blood levels of LCPUFA and their ratios arachidonic acid (ARA) to docosahexaenoic acid (DHA), ARA to eicosapentaenoic acid (EPA), or total *n*-6 to total *n*-3 LCPUFA in ASD to those of typically developing individuals (with no neurodevelopmental disorders), and meta-analysis 2 compared the effects of *n*-3 LCPUFA supplementation to placebo on symptoms of ASD. Case-control studies and randomised controlled trials (RCTs) were identified searching electronic databases up to May, 2016. Mean differences were pooled and analysed using inverse variance models. Heterogeneity was assessed using I^2 statistic. Fifteen case-control studies (n = 1193) were reviewed. Compared with typically developed, ASD populations had lower DHA (−2.14 [95% CI −3.22 to −1.07]; $p < 0.0001$; $I^2 = 97\%$), EPA (−0.72 [95% CI −1.25 to −0.18]; $p = 0.008$; $I^2 = 88\%$), and ARA (−0.83 [95% CI, −1.48 to −0.17]; $p = 0.01$; $I^2 = 96\%$) and higher total *n*-6 LCPUFA to *n*-3 LCPUFA ratio (0.42 [95% CI 0.06 to 0.78]; $p = 0.02$; $I^2 = 74\%$). Four RCTs were included in meta-analysis 2 (n = 107). Compared with placebo, *n*-3 LCPUFA improved social interaction (−1.96 [95% CI −3.5 to −0.34]; $p = 0.02$; $I^2 = 0$) and repetitive and restricted interests and behaviours (−1.08 [95% CI −2.17 to −0.01]; $p = 0.05$; $I^2 = 0$). Populations with ASD have lower *n*-3 LCPUFA status and *n*-3 LCPUFA supplementation can potentially improve some ASD symptoms. Further research with large sample size and adequate study duration is warranted to confirm the efficacy of *n*-3 LCPUFA.

Keywords: meta-analysis; omega-3; long chain polyunsaturated fatty acids; concentration; intervention; autism; symptoms

---

1. Introduction

The prevalence of Autism Spectrum Disorder (ASD) has dramatically increased over the past few years. While previous prevalence studies of ASD identified less than 10 in 10,000 individuals [1], recent estimates suggest rates of 90 to 250 in 10,000 individuals [2–5]. ASD is a life-long neurodevelopment disorder that appears during the first years of life [6]. Depending on the child's predominant symptomatology, children with ASD exhibit difficulties with expressing and understanding certain emotions, understanding others' mood, expressive language, and maintaining normal eye contact, as well as preference for minimal changes to routine, restricted ways of using toys and isolated play, all of which make it difficult for individuals to establish relationships with others, to act in an appropriate way and to live independently [6]. In addition, children with ASD frequently experience behaviour problems and medical conditions, including inflammation, oxidative stress, and autoimmune disorders [7–12], and altered brain structure and function (in a subset of individuals) [13,14]. The rising ASD rates are ascribed, in part, to a complex interaction between multiple genes and environmental risk factors [15], among which omega-3 long chain polyunsaturated fatty acids (*n*-3 LCPUFAs) is a strong candidate. LCPUFAs and their metabolic products have been implicated in ASD via their roles in brain structure and function, neurotransmission, cell membrane structure and microdomain organisation, inflammation, immunity and oxidative stress [16–20].

Blood polyunsaturated fatty acids (plasma, serum, red blood cell (RBC), and whole blood) levels are considered reliable biomarkers of their status [21]. Abnormality in blood levels of *n*-3 LCPUFA has been reported in psychiatric disorders including, but not limited to, attention deficit hyperactivity disorder (ADHD) and ASD [22–24]. Explanations for such abnormalities have been suggested to be lower dietary intake of *n*-3 LCPUFAs, and disturbances in fatty acid metabolism and incorporation of these fatty acids into cellular membranes in autistic populations compared to healthy controls [24–26]. A smattering of reports indicate differences in *n*-3 LCPUFAs, *n*-6 LCPUFAs and/or *n*-6 to *n*-3 LCPUFA ratios between populations with autism and healthy controls [14,26], but a few also failed to show any differences [27,28]. The reason for such discrepancies is not well examined, and there have been no attempts to systematically compare these studies. Hence, systematic analysis and synthesis of the evidence are warranted to determine if there are any differences in these blood fatty acids levels among healthy and individuals with ASD, and if so, whether *n*-3 LCPUFA supplementation may be beneficial in reducing symptoms in ASD.

To our knowledge, the efficacy of *n*-3 LCPUFA supplementation in ASD has been investigated by six open-label trials [29–34] and one case study [35], the majority of which (six out of seven studies) showed significant improvement in symptoms of ASD (Table S1). Despite this promising evidence, randomised controlled trials (RCTs) examining the beneficial effect of *n*-3 LCPUFAs in reducing symptoms of ASD have yielded inconclusive results. For example, Amminger et al. (2007) showed that supplementation with *n*-3 LCPUFA (EPA + DHA) was superior over placebo in reducing stereotypy, inappropriate speech and hyperactivity [36], while Mankad et al. (2015) failed to show any effect of *n*-3 LCPUFA supplementation on autism severity symptoms, adaptive functioning, externalizing behaviour or verbal ability [37].

To date, two systematic reviews of interventions with *n*-3 LCPUFA in ASD have been published [38,39]. In the review by Bent et al., published in 2009, authors set broad inclusion criteria and included all intervention trials of *n*-3 LCPUFAs of any type, dose, and duration addressing core and associated symptoms of ASD [38]. They identified six studies; one randomised controlled trial, four open-label trials and one case-study and concluded that the evidence was insufficient to support clinical recommendations [38].

Two years later, James, Montgomery and Williams (2011) published a Cochrane review including only two RCTs and performing meta-analyses on three primary outcomes (social interaction, communication and stereotypy) and one secondary outcome (hyperactivity) [39]. The authors reached the same conclusion as the Bent et al. review [38], and identified four ongoing studies. At the time of writing this review, the findings of one trial was published [37], one was terminated in 2014 (NCT01248130), and no information was available regarding the recruitment status or the availability of data for two trials (NCT00467818 and NCT01260961).

An updated systematic review is timely; more studies are now available, the prevalence of ASD is increasing together with a greater interest in the medical community (health professionals) on the beneficial effect of n-3 LCPUFA in the treatment of neurodevelopment disorders, as well as an increasing interest in using complementary and alternative medication in this population [40]. We aimed to conduct a current examination of evidence. We designed two systematic reviews and meta-analyses;

- Meta-analysis 1: a meta-analysis of evidence regarding blood n-3 LCPUFA levels in populations with ASD compared to typically developing counterparts (with no neurodevelopmental disorders) of any age and sex. A secondary aim for meta-analysis 1 was to perform a priori subgroup analysis to investigate the influence of ASD on fatty acid composition across different age groups (studies including only young children vs. studies also including children, teenagers, and adults).
- Meta-analysis 2: a meta-analysis of randomised controlled trials of n-3 LCPUFA supplementation (of any type, dose and duration) in ASD populations (of any age and sex) to assess the clinical efficacy of n-3 LCPUFAs treatment in reducing core symptoms of ASD and co-existing conditions.

2. Materials and Methods

All study procedures for both meta-analyses were pre-defined, but have not been registered or published elsewhere.

2.1. Eligibility Criteria

For meta-analysis 1, we included case-control observational studies that examined the differences in blood fatty acid levels between populations with ASD and healthy typically developing controls (with no neurodevelopmental disorders) of any age and sex. Studies were excluded it they included non-typically developing controls, were non-English or unpublished. Because DHA, EPA and ARA are amongst the most reported fatty acids of n-3 LCPUFAs and n-6 LCPUFAs categories, respectively, and have been shown to be more biologically active in the brain and been linked to neurodevelopment disorders, we focused on these fatty acids as well as the ratio of ARA to EPA and DHA and the ratio of n-6 LCPUFA to n-3 LCPUFA [41,42]. We included studies that reported LCPUFA in various blood fractions expressed as either % of total fatty acids or in concentration units, including RBC, serum, plasma, plasma phospholipids and whole blood [21]. These fractions have been shown to be reliable markers for the general fatty acid pool [21].

For meta-analysis 2, we included RCTs of any dose, type, and duration of n-3 LCPUFAs in participants with ASD of any age and sex who were randomised to receive either intervention or placebo, and reporting one of the following outcome measures: core symptoms of ASD including social interaction, communication, and repetitive restrictive behaviours or interests (RRB), and symptoms or behaviours associated with ASD including hyperactivity, irritability, sensory issues, and gastrointestinal symptoms. Unpublished and non-English studies were excluded.

Meta-analyses were performed if at least two studies employed the same assessment tool to measure the outcome of interest. There is a large variability in outcome assessment methods in ASD studies [43]. This use of different tools not only compromises the validity of a study by increasing the likelihood of type 1 error [44], but also complicates an effective comparison across studies.

2.2. Search Methods for Identification of Studies

We searched PubMed, MEDLINE, Web of Science, CINAHL, PsycINFO, PsycARTICLES and PsycNET up to May, 2016 to identify relevant studies in English. We employed broad search terms to include all potential studies that may fall within each of the mentioned reviews. The search strategy used the following terms: ("omega 3" OR "omega3" OR "omega-3" OR "polyunsaturated fatty acids" OR "polyunsaturated fatty acid" OR "essential fatty acids" OR "essential fatty acid") AND ("autism" OR "autistic" OR "autism spectrum disorder" OR "Asperger"). We also reviewed the reference lists of all identified studies to identify additional studies. Results from each database were downloaded into EndNote (version X6, 2012, Thomson Reuters, Philadelphia, PA, USA). Duplicates were removed and abstracts were screened. When an abstract met the eligibility requirements, it was assigned to one of two meta-analyses and the full article was read to ensure the inclusion and exclusion criteria were met. The study identification was done by one investigator (H.M.).

2.3. Data Extraction, Management, and Quality Assessment

Two reviewers (H.M. and M.D.) independently performed data extraction from each study into pre-piloted extraction tables. Discrepancies in the data extraction were resolved by discussion and reaching consensus.

The following data were extracted for both meta-analyses: author, date of publication and setting, sources of funding, conflict of interest, aims, objectives and hypothesis, and population characteristics while extractions specific to each meta-analyses are described below.

For meta-analysis 1, the following data were also extracted: the mean and SD for blood *n*-3 LCPUFAs (DHA, EPA or total), *n*-6 LCPUFAs (ARA or total), and for *n*-6 to *n*-3 LCPUFA ratios (ARA to DHA, ARA to EPA, or total *n*-6 to total *n*-3 LCPUFA), fatty acid analysis method, the body tissue in which the fatty acid was measured, the unit of measure, and the significance value. If a study reported LCPUFA in two different blood tissues, the priority was given to RBC, followed by plasma phospholipids, serum/plasma, and whole blood. While RBC and plasma phospholipids LCPUFA reflects long-term fatty acid intake, serum/plasma or whole blood LCPUFA are influenced by recent intake of these fatty acids [21,45]. If a study reported both relative and absolute measures, the former measures were included in the meta-analysis to limit the methodological heterogeneity. The method by which blood fatty acid composition is expressed (relative vs. absolute) has been shown to modify the LCPUFA—disease relationship [46]. Inter-study variation in extraction and separation efficiencies in fatty acid analyses can be overcome by relative expression of fatty acids (expressed as a percentage of a fatty acid normalised to the total amount of all measured fatty acids in a sample) [46]. If more than two groups were included, only relevant groups were selected. A quality appraisal was performed in duplicate by two investigators (H.M. and M.D.) using the "Health Canada Quality Appraisal Tools for Observational Studies" [47]. A quality score of $\leq$6 was considered lower quality [47]. No studies were excluded based on quality scores, but sensitivity analysis was performed to assess the impact of these studies on the overall results.

For meta-analysis 2, study design, intervention (the dose of intervention was converted, where required, to gram from milligram for easy comparison), delivery method, compliance, intervention period, outcome measures, assessment tools, results, conclusion, potential confounders and assessment of bias risk following Cochrane bias risk assessment including selection, performance, detection, attrition, reporting and commercial bias were also extracted [48]. A further quality appraisal was performed in duplicate by two investigators (H.M. and M.D.) using the "Health Canada Quality Appraisal Tools for Randomised Controlled Trials" to assess the quality of the individual studies [47]. A quality score of $\leq$7 was considered lower quality [47].

2.4. Statistical Analysis

Both meta-analyses were performed using Review Manager (RevMan, version 5.3, The Nordic Cochrane Centre, Copenhagen, Denmark).

2.4.1. Meta-Analysis 1

For each outcome, the mean and SD for each study group (cases and controls) was entered into Review Manager. If *n*-3 to *n*-6 fatty acid (total *n*-3 to *n*-6 LCPUFA, EPA to ARA or DHA to ARA) was reported, the ratio was converted to *n*-6/*n*-3 (1/ratio). The Review Manager calculator (between group differences) was employed to calculate the SD for these reverse ratios. The reverse ratio and SD were calculated for five studies [49–53].

The primary meta-analysis compared mean differences (95% confidence intervals (CI)) in outcomes across study groups. Due to significant heterogeneity a random effects model was used to calculate the forest plots with standardised mean differences and 95% CI. Standardised mean differences were calculated because blood levels of LCPUFA were measured and reported in different ways. A combination of Chi^2-statistic ($p < 0.1$), I^2 statistics (I^2 0%–40%, low; 30%–60%, moderate; 50%–90%, substantial; 75%–100%, considerable heterogeneity), and considering the variation of point estimates and the overlap of CIs across different studies was performed to measure heterogeneity [48].

To avoid false positive or negative results, we limited the number of subgroup analyses to one (stratified by age) and sensitivity analyses to three (blood tissue type, study quality, and author's calculations). Then a priori subgroup analysis was performed using Chi^2-statistic with a p value of <0.05 taken to indicate statistical significance [48]. We could not conduct meta-regression to investigate the impact of the potential mediators (location, sex, and the way by which fatty acid composition is expressed) due to the limited study numbers. To include one mediator in the analysis, at least 10 studies are required [48]. These variables were however carefully examined when the results were interpreted. Publication bias was examined using funnel plots in which the SE of the studies were plotted against their corresponding effect sizes.

2.4.2. Meta-Analysis 2

For each outcome, the mean change and SD of change from baseline to endpoint for each intervention group (n-3 LCPUFA and placebo) was entered into Review Manager. If only baseline and end data were available the mean change was calculated by deducting the baseline from the end value, and the SD was then imputed from a mean correlation coefficient for an outcome from other studies in the meta-analysis. Standard deviations were calculated for one study [54]. Study authors were contacted for missing data, and if no response was received the data was not included in the meta-analysis. Data was unable to be retrieved for three studies [55–57].

The primary meta-analyses compared mean (95% CI) differences (net change in scores) in each domain between n-3 LCPUFA and control groups. Heterogeneity between studies was small hence a fixed-effects model was used to calculate forest plots with mean differences and 95% CI. Heterogeneity between studies was indicated using the same analyses employed in meta-analysis 1. No subgroup analyses or meta-regression were performed due to limited number of studies included in the meta-analysis. However, one sensitivity analysis was performed to evaluate the impact of calculations (SDs) and major methodological differences on heterogeneity and the overall results. Publication bias was not assessed due to the small number of studies included in this meta-analysis.

3. Results

From the initial searches, 510 articles and from the cross-reference check, five articles were retrieved. Titles and abstracts of 254 articles were screened after non-English and duplicates were removed. At this level, 216 were excluded as not relevant to the current topic. The remaining 38 articles were read and categorised into two groups; 24 articles into the case-control studies group and 15 into the intervention group (Figure 1, PRISMA Flow Diagram).

3.1. Systematic Review and Meta-Analysis 1

Of the 24 articles identified for meta-analysis 1, 15 were included in the meta-analysis. Reasons for exclusion were: not a case-control design [58,59], inappropriate control [25], the data not reported in a form suitable for analysis [26,60–62], and double-reporting [63,64]. Characteristics of included studies can be found in Table 1.

The majority of studies were conducted in the Middle East (n = 5; 2 Saudi Arabia (from one study group), 1 Oman, 2 Egypt) and Europe (n = 4; 2 UK, 1 Belgium, 1 Italy), with others conducted in the US (n = 2), Latin America (n = 1), Canada (n = 1), Asia (Japan, n = 1), and Australia (n = 1).

The 15 studies included 623 children and young people with ASD and 570 controls. Most studies included children under the age of 12, while a few included teenagers and adults also (n = 3) [24,49,53]. One study included adults up to age 22 years [49]. Cases and controls were matched on both age and sex ($n = 8$), two of which included other attributes such as IQ, home environment and dietary intake ($n = 1$) or geographical region ($n = 1$). Others matched two groups on either age ($n = 3$) or sex ($n = 1$), and one study included only males. Matching of cases and controls was not reported in two studies. In those studies including both sexes and reporting the sex distribution, the male/female ratio ranged from 2/1 to 12/1.

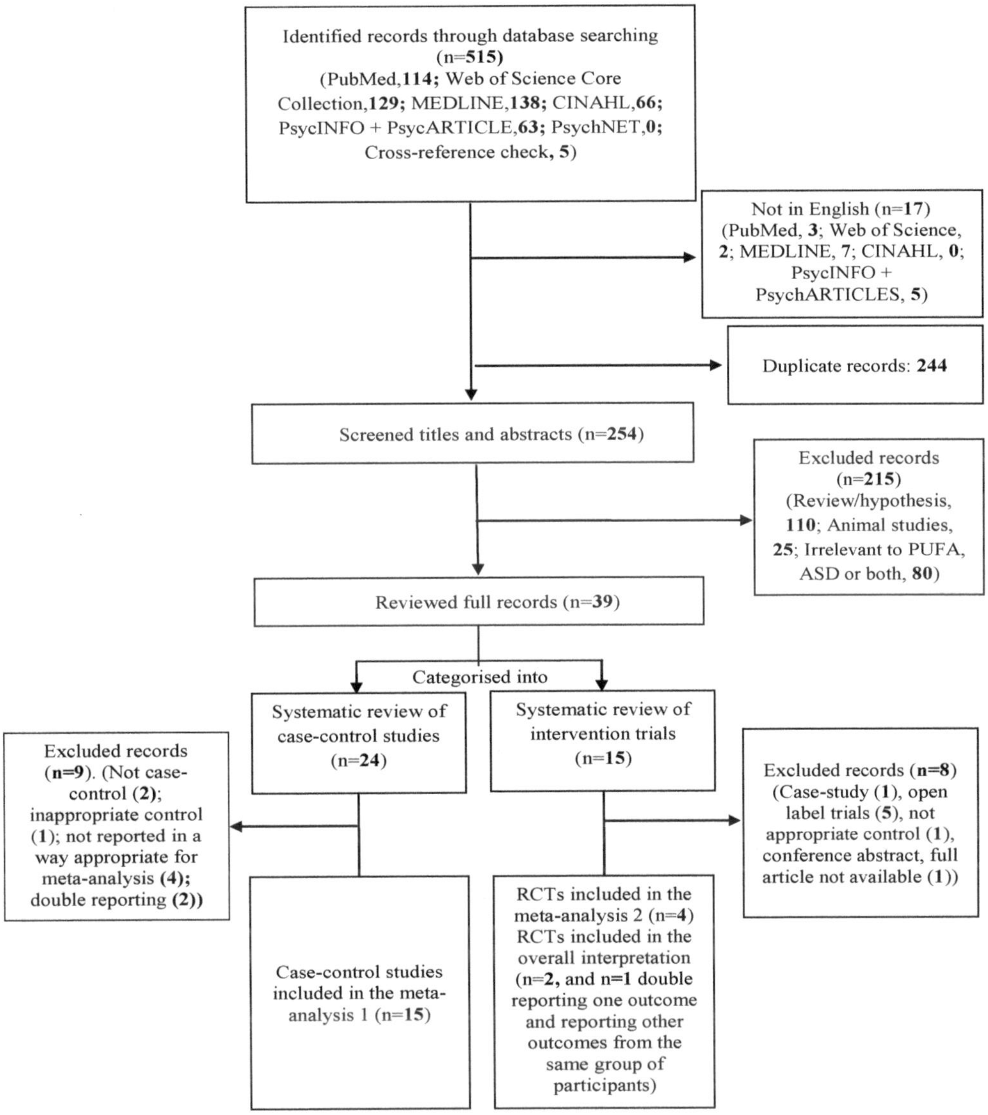

Figure 1. Flow diagram for selection of studies (PRISMA flow diagram).

Most studies did not report the fasting state of blood samples while one study analysed non-fasting blood samples, and five studies fasting blood sample (ranging from 2 h to overnight fasting) [28,49–51,65]. Fasting state is considered to affect fatty acid composition measured in plasma/serum but not in RBC [21,45]. While most studies reported serum/plasma fatty acid composition, four studies reported RBC levels [24,28,52,66] and two reported both [27,51]. Most studies reported relative levels while five studies reported absolute levels (all from the Middle East) [26,30,50,65,67], and one both levels [53]. Sensitivity analysis showed no impact of blood tissue type and the way by which fatty acid composition is expressed on the heterogeneity. However, the way by which fatty acid composition is expressed affected the overall effect size for some measures (Refer to the next section).

Table 1. Characteristics of case-control studies included in meta-analysis 1.

Reference and Setting	Cases Characteristics				Controls Characteristics				Matching	Outcome				Quality Score †
	N	Condition, Classification System, Tools $^{\delta}$	Age (Years) *	Sex (M, F)	*N*	Health Condition	Age (Years) *	Sex (M, F)		Blood Tissue Type	Fasting State (Length)	Values Reported as	FA and Ratios Compared and the Direction of Difference	
Al-Farsi (2013) [67] Oman	40	Autism, based on DSM-IV, NR	4.1 (0.9)	NR	40	Healthy and TD	4.1 (0.8)	NR	Age Sex	Serum	NR	µg/mL	DHA ↓	6
Bell (2004) [66] UK	29	11 classical autism and 18 regressive autism, NR, NR	NR	NR	55	Healthy and TD	NR	NR	None	RBC	NR	% of total FA	Total *n*3 ↓ DHA ↓ EPA ↓ Total ↔ ARA ↔ ARA/EPA ↑	4
Bell (2010) [27] UK	45	Autism, based on DSM-IV and ICD-10, ADI-R	7.5 (3.5)	39 M, 5 F	52	Healthy and TD	7.5 (3.6)	49 M, 3 F	Age Sex (45 pairs matched)	RBC Plasma	NR	% of total FA	Total *n*3 1 ↔ DHA ↔ EPA ↔ Total ↔ ARA ↔ Total *n*6/*n*3 2↑ ARA/EPA ↑	8
Brigandi (2015) [24] US	121	Autism (but not Asperger or PDD-NOS), based on DSM-IV, CARS	3–17 **	NR	110	Non autistic and developmentally delayed	3–17 **	NR	NR	RBC	No	% of total FA	Total *n*3 ↓ DHA ↓ EPA ↔ Total *n*6 ↓ ARA ↓ Total *n*6/*n*3 2↑	6
Bu (2006) [28] US	40	Autism and regressive autism, based on DSM-IV and ICD-10, ADI-R and ADOS	3.6 ***	37 M, 3 F	20	TD	3.5 ***	16 M, 4 F	Age Sex Geographical residential area	RBC	Yes (2 h)	% of total FA	Total *n*3 ↔ DHA ↔ EPA ↔ Total ↔ ARA ↔ ARA/EPA ↔	8
El-Ansari (2011a) [50] Saudi	25	Autism, NR, ADI-R, ADOS, 3di	4–12 **	NR	16	Healthy and TD	4–11 **	NR	Age	Plasma	Yes (10 h)	mmol/L	ARA/DHA ↓	7
El-Ansari (2011b) [65] Saudi Arabia	22	Autism, NR, ADI-R, ADOS, 3di	4–12 **	NR	26	Healthy and TD	4–11 **	NR	Age	Plasma	Yes (10 h)	mmol/L	DHA ↓ EPA ↔ ARA ↓	7
Ghezz (2013) [14] Italy	21	Autism, DSM-IV, ADOS and CARS	6.8 (2.2)	17 M, 4 F	20	Healthy and TD	7.6 (1.9)	14 M, 6 F	Age Sex	Serum	NR	% of total FA	DHA ↓ EPA ↓ ARA ↔ Total *n*6/*n*3 ↑	11
Jory (2016) [51] Canada	11	Autism, DSM (version NR), NR	3.9 (1.7)	8M, 3F	15	Healthy and TD	3.9 (1.1)	6 M, 9 F	Age	RBC Serum	Yes (NR)	% of total FA	DHA 1 ↓ EPA ↓ ARA ↓ Total *n*6/*n*3 ↑ ARA/DHA ↔ ARA/EPA ↔	7
Meguid (2008) [30] Egypt	30	Autism, DSM-IV, clinical evaluations and CARS	3–11 **	18 M, 12 F	30	Healthy and TD	NR	NR	Age Sex	Whole blood	NR	µg/mL	DHA ↓ ARA ↓ ARA/DHA ↓	7

Table 1. *Cont.*

Reference and Setting	Cases Characteristics				Controls Characteristics				Matching	Outcome				Quality Score †
	N	Condition, Classification System, Tools [δ]	Age (Years) *	Sex (M, F)	*N*	Health Condition	Age (Years) *	Sex (M, F)		Blood Tissue Type	Fasting State (Length)	Values Reported as	FA and Ratios Compared and the Direction of Difference	
Mostafa (2015) [26] Egypt	80	Autism, DSM-IV, clinical evaluation and CARS	7.4 (3.3)	66 M, 14 F	80	Healthy and TD	7.3 (3.1)	66 M, 14 F	Age Sex	Plasma	NR	mmol/L	DHA ↓ ARA ↓ ARA/DHA ↑	8
Parletta (2016) [52] Australia	85	Autism, clinical evaluation and CARS	5.3 (2.1) ^	68 M, 17 F	79	Healthy and TD	8.3 (2.5) ^	61 M, 18 F	Sex	RBC	NR	% of total FA	DHA ↓ EPA ↓ ARA ↓ Total $n6/n3$ ↑ ARA/EPA ↑	9
Sliwinski (2006) [49] Belgium	18	Autism with IQ > 55 and post pubertal, DSM-IV, ADI-R	12–20 **	Only male	22	TD post pubertal	12–22	Only male	None	Plasma	Yes (overnight)	% of total FA	Total $n3$ ↑ DHA ↑ EPA ↔ Total $n6$ ↔ ARA ↔ Total $n6/n3$ [2]↓	8
Tostes (2013) [68] Brazil	24	Autism, DSM-IV, clinical evaluation	7.4 (2.9)	18M, 6F	24	Healthy and TD	7.2 (1.8)	18 M, 6 F	Age sex	Plasma	NR	% of total FA	DHA ↓ EPA ↓ ARA ↑ ARA/DHA [3] ↑ ARA/EPA [3] ↑	9
Yui (2016) [53] Japan	28	Autism with IQ/70, DSM-IV, ADI-R	13.5 (4.7)	20M, 8F	21	Healthy and TD	13.9 (5.7)	15 M, 6 F	Age Sex IQ Eating habit Home environment	Plasma	NR	% of total FA and μg/mL	DHA [4] ↑ EPA ↑ ARA ↓ ARA/DHA ↓ ARA/EPA ↓	8

[δ] Psychological assessment tools used to confirm ASD diagnosis. * Reported as mean (SD) unless otherwise stated. † Health Canada Quality Appraisal Tool for Observational Studies; A quality score of ≥7 was considered higher quality [47]. ** Inclusion criteria. *** Median. ^ Significantly different. ↓ Cases had lower levels than controls ($p < 0.05$). ↑ Cases had higher levels than controls ($p < 0.05$). ↔ No difference across groups ($p > 0.05$). [1] RBC values are reported. [2] A borderline significance. [3] The significance was not reported. [4] % of total fatty acids is reported. ADI-R, Autism Diagnostic Interview-Revised; ADOS, Autism Diagnostic Observation Schedule; ARA, arachidonic acid; CARS, Childhood Autism Rating Scale; DHA, docosahexaenoic acid; DSM-IV, Diagnostic and Statistical Manual of Mental Disorder-Fourth Edition; EPA, eicosapentaenoic acid; F, female; FA, fatty acids; M, male; N, number of participants; NR, not reported; RBC, red blood cell; TD, typically developing; 3di, the Developmental, Dimensional, and Diagnostic Interview.

The majority of studies reported DHA, EPA and ARA levels while two studies did not report levels of EPA [26,67], and one ARA [67]. Five studies reported both total n-3 LCPUFA and total n-6 LCPUFA levels. One study did not report either of the mentioned measures but the ratio of ARA to DHA and ARA to EPA [50]. Total n-6/n-3 LCPUFA ratio was reported in six studies, of which two reported ARA/EPA ratio [27,52], and one reported both ARA/EPA and ARA/DHA also [51]. Of the remaining studies, two reported the ratio of ARA/EPA [28,66] and ARA/DHA each [26,30], one both [53], and three no ratios [65,67,68]. Reverse ratios and SDs were calculated in five studies ([50] (only the ARA to EPA) and [49,51–53]). With the exception of one study [50] (refer to the next section), sensitivity analysis showed no impact of calculation on the overall results.

All studies included in the review scored between four and nine points out of a possible 11 in our quality assessment tool, with three studies scoring ≤ 6 [24,66,67] (Table S2). It should be noted that the maximum score for the "Health Canada Quality Appraisal Tools for Observational Studies" is 12 [47] but because "measuring the exposure in duplicate or more" is of no relevance for case-control studies and all studies received a score of "0" for this criterion, the maximum score adds up to 11 for this review. Studies with scores of $\geq$7 are considered having higher quality. Sensitivity analysis showed no impact of removing studies with a quality score $\leq$6 on the heterogeneity or overall results.

The quality criteria failed by most studies were attrition and the reasons for attrition. Although attrition is not important for case-control studies, it could be of relevance to ASD clinical studies. Drop out of some populations with particular characteristics such as high anxiety levels or sensory issues (a distinct criterion under RRB domain in ASD diagnosis [6]) that are associated with fear of blood test and consequently inability to obtain a blood sample or withdrawal from a study could affect the external validity of a study. The most prevalent confounding factors that were not controlled for in statistical analysis were dietary intake of LCPUFA and medication use. No conflict of interest that may have affected study outcomes was apparent in any study.

3.1.1. Individual n-3 LCPUFA (DHA, EPA, and ARA) and Their Ratios (ARA to DHA and ARA to EPA)

Significant differences were seen between those studies that recruited children only vs. those that also included teenagers and adults for blood levels of DHA and EPA (Chi^2 = 11.78, p = 0.0006 and Chi^2 = 7.02, p = 0.008, respectively) but not ARA (Chi^2 = 1.49, p = 0.22) (Figure 2). Hence results for DHA and EPA for these subgroups were described separately. For ARA, the results described are from all studies combined.

Overall, in the younger age group studies, ASD children had significantly lower DHA and EPA levels than typically developing controls (standardised mean difference (95% CI) −2.14 [−3.22, −1.07], Z = 3.91, p < 0.0001 and −0.72 [−1.25, −0.18], Z = 2.64, p = 0.008, respectively). Considerable heterogeneity was seen for DHA (I^2 = 97%, p < 0.00001) and EPA (I^2 = 88%, p < 0.00001). Heterogeneity for DHA was not altered by removing any studies. Heterogeneity for EPA reduced slightly by removing the Parletta, 2016 study [52] (I^2 = 74%, p = 0.0008). Removal of this study together with the Tostes, 2013 study [68] significantly reduced heterogeneity for EPA (I^2 = 0%, p = 0.78) that was accompanied by a reduction in the difference between cases and controls (−0.30 [−0.51, −0.08], Z = 2.73, p = 0.006, n = 356). These two studies were different with respect to some characteristics that may affect outcomes compared to other studies; children with ASD were significantly younger than typically developing children in the Parletta, 2016 study [52], and 88% of children with ASD in the Tostes, 2013 study were on psychotropic drugs [68].

In studies including all age groups (children, teenagers, and adults), no significant differences were seen in DHA and EPA levels between cases and controls (0.28 [−0.59, 1.16] and 0.27 [−0.23, 0.76], respectively). Heterogeneity for DHA and EPA was substantial (I^2 = 90%, p = 0.0001 and I^2 = 68%, p = 0.04, respectively). Removal of the Brigandi, 2015 study [24] reduced the heterogeneity significantly for DHA (I^2 = 0%, p = 0.65) and slightly for EPA (I^2 = 64%, p = 0.10). Removal of this study resulted in children with ASD having significantly higher DHA (0.69 [0.26, 1.12], Z = 3.13, p = 0.002, n = 89) levels than typically developing controls but no impact on EPA. The Brigandi, 2015 study [24] was different from the other two studies in this subgroup in that both classic and regressive type ASD were included, cases and controls were not matched by any attributes, intellectual functioning of patients was not considered, and this study had a low quality appraisal score. The Sliwinski, 2006 [49] and Yui, 2016 [53] studies included ASD patients with a borderline or normal intellectual functioning (IQ > 70). The results should be interpreted with caution because the number of studies included is small ($n = 3$).

With regard to ARA, children with ASD had significantly lower ARA levels than typically developing controls (-0.83 [-1.48, -0.17], $Z = 2.48$, $p = 0.01$), but heterogeneity between studies was substantial ($I^2 = 96\%$, $p = 0.00001$). Heterogeneity was not reduced by excluding any single study. However, removing studies that reported absolute levels [26,30,65] resulted in a smaller overall effect estimate (-0.24 [-0.88, 0.41], $Z = 0.71$, $p = 0.48$, $n = 840$).

Only one study that included all age groups (children, teenagers, and adults) reported either ARA/DHA or ARA/EPA [53] thus the combined results of older and younger children are described (Figure 3). The ratio of ARA/DHA and ARA/EPA did not differ significantly between ASD populations and typically developing controls ($p = 0.94$ and $p = 0.09$, respectively). The heterogeneity was considerably high for both ratios. Heterogeneity was not reduced by excluding any studies (both ARA/DHA and ARA/EPA). With regard to ARA/EPA, however, the overall effect estimate changed considerably by the removal of El-Ansary, 2011a study [50] (0.99 [0.32, 1.67], $Z = 2.88$, $p = 0.004$, $I^2 = 91\%$). Cases and controls were not matched on sex in this study, the reverse ratio and SD was calculated, and the absolute level was reported.

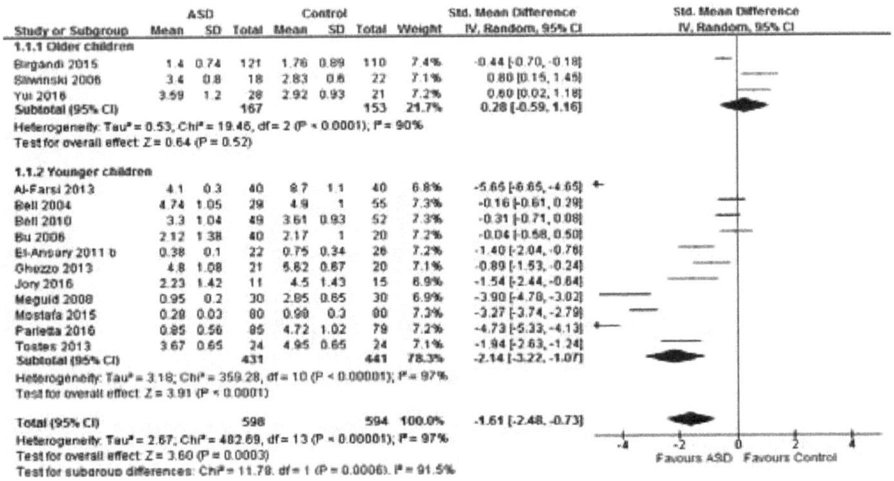

(A)

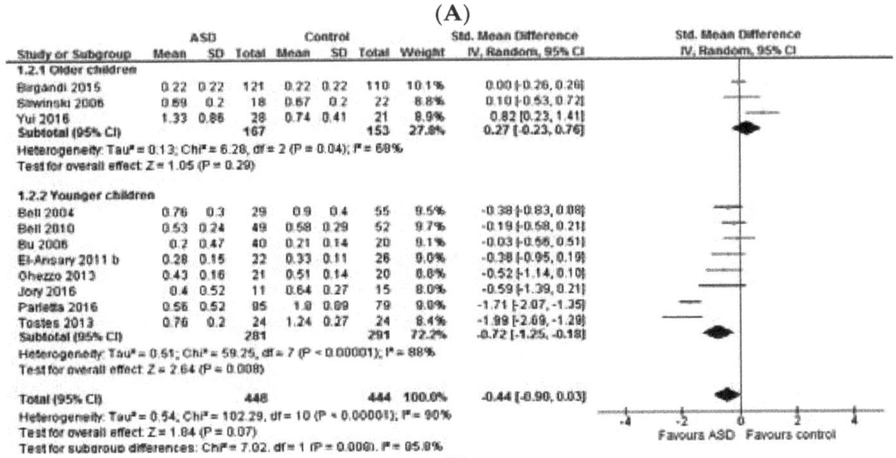

(B)

Figure 2. *Cont.*

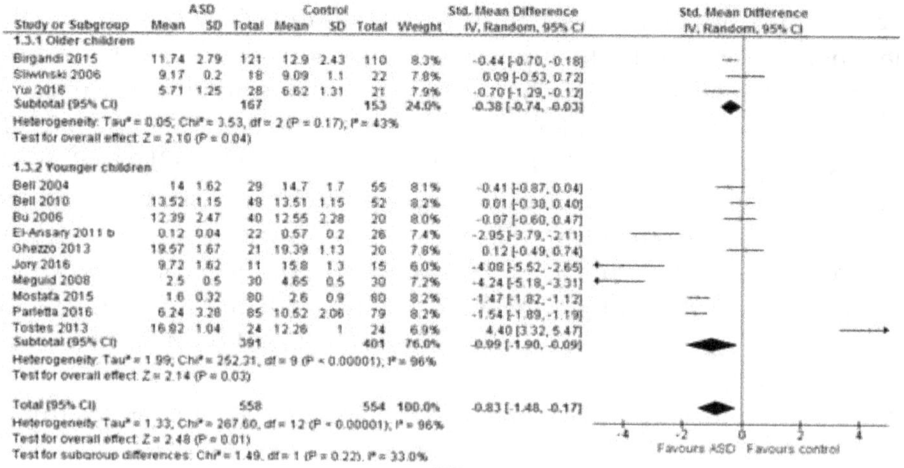

(C)

Figure 2. Forest plots of mean (95% confidence interval (CI)) weighted difference in blood levels of docosahexaenoic acid (DHA) (**A**); eicosapentaenoic acid (EPA) (**B**); and arachidonic acid (ARA) (**C**) between populations with Autism Spectrum Disorder (ASD) and typically developing controls stratified for subgroups with studies including all age groups (children, teenagers, and adults) vs. those including children only. Direction of effect (negative, lower mean in ASD group; positive, lower mean in control group; zero, no difference between groups).

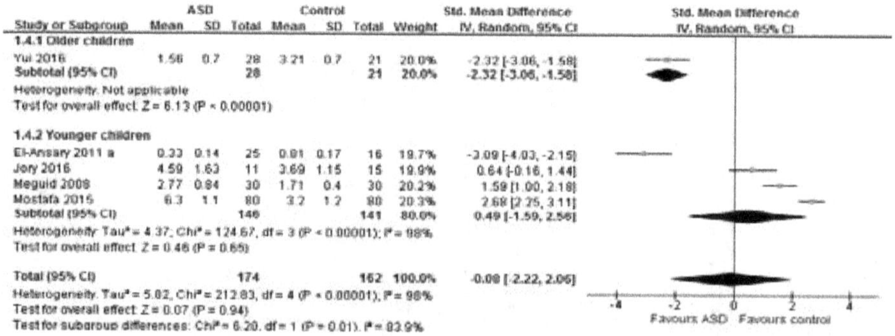

(A)

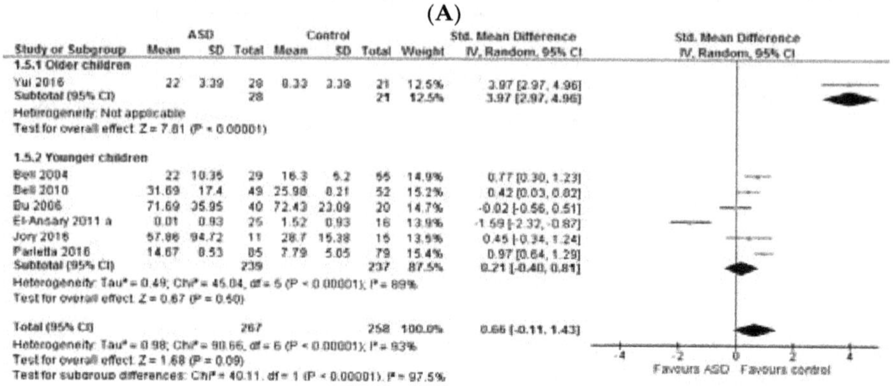

(B)

Figure 3. Forest plots of mean (95% confidence interval (CI)) weighted difference in the ratio of arachidonic acid (ARA) to docosahexaenoic acid (DHA) (**A**) and the ratio of ARA to eicosapentaenoic acid (EPA) (**B**) between populations with Autism Spectrum Disorder (ASD) and typically developing children stratified for subgroups with studies including all age groups (children, teenagers, and adults) vs. young children only. Direction of effect (negative, lower mean in ASD group; positive, lower mean in control group; zero, no difference between groups).

3.1.2. Total n-3 and n-6 LCPUFA and Their Ratios

No significant differences were observed in total n-3 and n-6 LCPUFA between studies including young children only and those including all age groups (children, teenagers, and adults) ($Chi^2 = 0.70$, $p = 0.40$ and $Chi^2 = 3.84$, $p = 0.05$, respectively) thus the results for the combined groups are described (Figure 4).

The pooled standard mean differences for the total n-3 LCPUFA and total n-6 LCPUFA between ASD and typically developing children were −0.16 [−0.54, 0.21] ($I^2 = 73\%$, substantial heterogeneity) and 0.57 [−0.19, 1.33] ($I^2 = 93\%$, considerable heterogeneity), respectively. Both were not statistically significant. Excluding comparisons that included teenagers and adults also [24,49] reduced heterogeneity in total n-3 LCPUA ($I^2 = 42\%$, $p = 0.18$) (−0.34 [−0.68, 0.01], $Z = 1.88$, $p = 0.06$, $n = 245$). Heterogeneity was reduced to an acceptable level when the Sliwinski, 2006 study [49] only was removed ($I^2 = 14\%$, $p = 0.32$) (−0.36 [−0.56, −0.15], $Z = 3.40$, $p = 0.0007$, $n = 472$). The Sliwinski, 2006 study [49] was different from other studies with respect to several characteristics; it included post pubertal youngsters up to age 22 years, it was a male-only study, and included those with an IQ > 55. Heterogeneity in total n-6 LCPUFA was not altered by the removal of any studies.

The ratio of total n-6 LCPUFA to n-3 LCPUFA did not differ significantly between studies including young children only and those including all age groups (children, teenagers, and adults) ($Chi^2 = 3.04$, $p = 0.08$) thus the overall results are described here (Figure 5). Children with ASD had a significantly higher n-6 LCPUFA to n-3 LCPUFA ratio (0.42 [0.06, 0.78], $Z = 2.27$, $p = 0.02$). The heterogeneity was substantial and was decreased by the exclusion of comparisons that also included teenagers and adults [24,49] ($I^2 = 29\%$, $p = 0.24$). The difference between cases and controls as well as the effect size increased considerably, 0.65 [0.36, 0.94], $Z = 4.43$, $p < 0.00001$, $n = 328$.

The funnel plots for DHA and ARA, indicated publication bias with a lack of smaller studies [studies with larger standard errors (SEs)] reporting negative results. Examination of funnel plot for EPA indicated no evidence of publication bias.

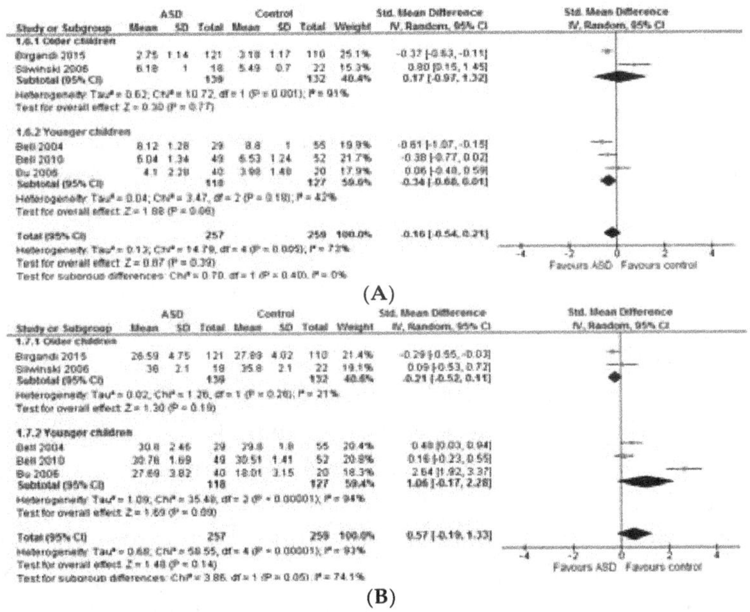

Figure 4. Forest plots of mean (95% confidence interval (CI)) weighted difference in the total n-3 long chain polyunsaturated fatty acids (n-3 LCPUFA) (**A**) and total n-6 long chain polyunsaturated fatty acids (n-6 LCPUFA) (**B**) between populations with Autism Spectrum Disorder (ASD) and typically developing children stratified for subgroups with studies including all age groups (children, teenagers, and adults) vs. young children only. Direction of effect (negative, lower mean in ASD group; positive, lower mean in control group; zero, no difference between groups).

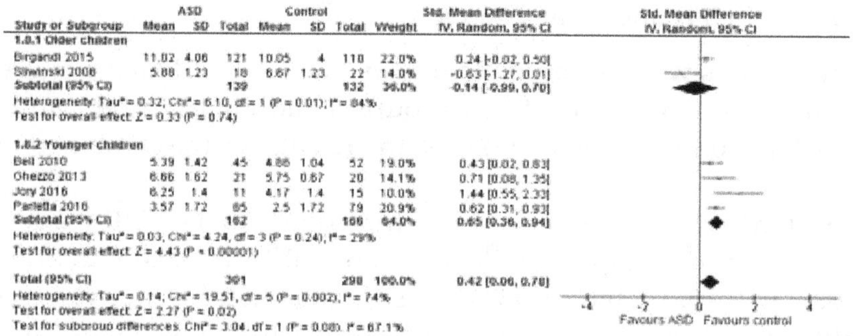

Figure 5. Forest plot of mean (95% confidence interval (CI)) weighted difference in the ratio of total n-6 long chain polyunsaturated fatty acids (n-6 LCPUFA) to total n-3 long chain polyunsaturated fatty acids (n-3 LCPUFA) between populations with Autism Spectrum Disorder (ASD) and typically developing children stratified for subgroups with studies including all age groups (children, teenagers, and adults) vs. young children only. Direction of effect (negative, lower mean in ASD group; positive, lower mean in control group; zero, no difference between groups).

3.2. Systematic Review and Meta-Analysis 2

Of the 15 RCTs identified for systematic review and meta-analysis 2, four were included in the meta-analysis [36,54,69,70], two were included in the overall interpretation but not included in the meta-analysis [37,55], one was a double-reporting of one outcome [54] and reporting other outcomes from the same group of participants [57], and eight were excluded (Figure 1). Reasons for not being included in the meta-analysis 2 but being included in the overall interpretation were: data not reported in a format suitable for analysis [55], and use of an assessment tool not used by others [37]. Reasons for complete exclusion were: a conference paper with unpublished results at the time of writing this review [56], one open label randomised parallel intervention trial including a low sugar healthy diet as the control [29], and not being a RCT (n = 6, one case-study and 5 open label trials [30–35]). Characteristics of included studies can be found in Table 2 and of excluded studies in Table S1.

Of those included in the meta-analysis 2, two were conducted in the US [69,70], one in Austria [36], and one in Japan [54]. In the four studies, 55 participants with ASD received n-3 LCPUFA supplements and 52 received placebo. The Bent, 2011 and 2014 studies included children under the age of 8 years [69,70], the Amminger, 2007 study included children under 17 years [36], and the Yui, 2011 study included children older than 6 years and adults up to 28 years [54].

Of the two studies that could not be included in the meta-analysis, one study was from the US [55] and one from Canada [37] together including 37 and 34 individuals in the intervention and placebo groups, respectively. Children under the age of 5 and 10 years were included in the Mankad, 2015 and Voigt, 2014 studies, respectively [37,55].

All but one (the Amminger, 2007 study included only males [36]) included both males and females. Study groups were not matched on sex in these trials. The male to female ratio ranged from 3/1 to 12/1.

Of the RCTs included in the meta-analysis 2, the severity of autism at baseline was not considered in two trials [36,70], and the other two included patients with pre-defined severity (moderate severity and ABC social withdrawal subscale of >10 in the Bent, 2011 and Yui, 2011 studies, respectively) and IQ level (>50 and >80 in the Bent, 2011 and Yui, 2011 studies, respectively [54,69]). Of those included in the overall interpretation, the Voigt, 2014 study included patients with pre-defined severity (CARS score of >30 [55] and the Mankad, 2015 study equally distributed the severity across groups [37]. Co-existing problem behaviour was an inclusion criteria in two trials entered the meta-analysis 2 (hyperactivity in the Amminger, 2007 [36] and Bent, 2014 studies [70]).

Study length ranged from 6–16 weeks in RCTs included in the meta-analysis 2 and was 26 weeks in RCTs included in the overall interpretation. The majority of participants were supplemented with both EPA and DHA. The Yui, study (2011 and 2012) [54,57] used a combination of DHA and AA and the Voigt, 2014 study used only DHA [55]. Intake of EPA and DHA ranged from 0.70 to 0.84 g/day and 0.24

to 0.70 g/day, respectively, with the Yui, 2011 (and 2012) and Voigt, 2014 studies having the lowest DHA dose [54,55,57]. The Mankad, 2015 study reported an initial total dose of EPA and DHA of 0.75 g/day for two weeks which was doubled when tolerability to that dose was determined [37]. Placebos used were olive oil [37,54,57], safflower oil [69,70], corn oil + soybean oil [55], and coconut oil [36].

Behaviours were assessed using a variety of assessment tools (ranging from one to six tools used in each study) including, Aberrant Behaviour Checklist (ABC) ([36,54,55,69,70] but the outcome was not reported), Social Responsiveness Scale (SRS) [57,69,70], Behaviour Assessment System for Children (BASC) [37,55,69], Clinical Global Impression (CGI) [37,55,69,70], and further several tools that were used in isolation. Of these, full data was available for only four studies using the same assessment tool (ABC) [36,54,69,70].

All studies included in the review were of good quality, scoring 11–14 points out of a possible 15 (Table S3). Studies with scores of >7 are considered as having higher quality.

The quality criteria failed by most studies were whether intention-to-treat or per-protocol analysis was conducted (though according to final sample size analysed—larger than the sample size with drop outs deducted—it was apparent that the majority employed intention-to-treat analysis), and controlling for potential confounders. The most prevalent potential confounding factors that were not reported or reported but not considered in statistical analysis were dietary intake of LCPUFA or baseline LCPUFA status (as a measure of LCPUFA status, either dietary intake or blood level of LCPUFA needs to be reported).With the exception of the Bent, 2011 study [69] which investigated the impact of baseline LCPUFA status on behavioural changes in response to supplementation, the majority of studies failed to examine such a relationship while assessing baseline LCPUFA status [37,54,55,57]. Further factors were compliance (not reported in most studies) and medical regimen (most studies recruited patients on a stable medical regimen but did not report the type of regimen and its distribution across groups). It is also worth noting that a small number of females were included in these studies (with a male/female ratio ranging from 1/3 to 1/12) which could be a limitation in terms of generalisability, though reflecting the gender distribution of ASD.

The risk of bias for each study is summarized in Figure S1. Participants in the Amminger, 2007 and Yui 2011 (and 2012) studies were reported to be randomised but no details were available for random sequence generation [36,54,57]. Other studies used computer generated number [69,70] and block randomisation stratified by attributes including severity [37] and sex [55]. With the exception of the Amminger, 2007 study [36], randomisation was prepared by a third party in all trials [37,54,55,57,69,70]. The Amminger, 2007 provided no details regarding who performed the randomization [36]. All studies were reported as double-blinded (both researchers/assessors and participants) [37,54,55,57,69,70]. However, in the Amminger, 2007 study it is unclear if the researchers/assessors were blinded [36]. It is also unclear when researchers/assessors and participants were unblinded in the Amminger, 2007, Yui, 2011 (and 2012), and Mankad, 2015 studies [36,37,54,57]. The blinding was kept for the entire study (including data analyses) in the Bent, 2011, Bent 2014, and Voigt, 2014 studies [55,69,70]. With the exception of the Yui, 2011 (and 2012, no drop outs) [54,57] and Bent, 2014 (all included in the final analyses) [70] studies, participants were lost to follow up in the Amminger, 2007 (one individual from control) [36], Mankad, 2015 (one individual from *n*-3 LCPUFA group) [37], Bent 2011 (two individuals; one from each arm) [69], and Voigt, 2014 (five from *n*-3 LCPUFA and nine from control) [55] studies. The reason for drop outs in the Voigt, 2014 study were difficulty with participation (four from *n*-3 LCPUFA and three from control), trouble taking the supplements (one from *n*-3 LCPUFA and three from control), and concerns about supplement side effects (three from control) [55]. Regarding the latter concern, it is not clear if participants withdrew due to worsening behaviour, not observing any improvement, or because of an actual side effect during the intervention. With the exception of the Voigt, 2014 study [55], all outcomes in all trials were reported. The Voigt, 2014 study examined 52 behavioural subscales but only three outcomes were reported [55]. It is worth noting that the primary outcome was the measure of CGI which was completely reported. Other sources of bias including commercial bias were not apparent in any study.

Table 2. Study characteristics of randomised controlled trials (RCTs) included in systematic literature review.

RCTs included in Meta-Analysis 2 (n = 4)									
Reference and Setting	Age (Years)	Sex Distribution (M, F)	Sample size	Intervention		Duration	Outcome Measure	Outcome	Quality Score †
				Active	Placebo				
Amminger (2007) [36] Austria Pilot	5–17	All male	Intervention (n = 7) Placebo (n = 6, 1 lost)	0.84 g/day EPA 0.7 g/day DHA	7 g/day coconut oil	6 weeks	ABC	No significant differences between groups at 6 weeks, but a greater change in hyperactivity and stereotypy subscale with a large effect size in the omega-3 group than placebo (7 and 2.4 units, effect size of 0.71 and 0.72, respectively). Well tolerated and safe.	10
Ben (2011) [69] US Pilot	3–8	24 M, 3 F	Intervention (n = 14, 1 lost and 4discontinued) Placebo (n = 13, 1 lost and 2 discontinued)	0.7 g/day EPA 0.46 g/day DHA	Orange flavoured pudding containing safflower oil	12 weeks	ABC PPVT EVT BASC SRS CGI-S	Significant increase in the percentage of serum omega-3 fatty acids. No significant differences in all measure across groups. Non-significant greater improvement in hyperactivity subscale in omega-3 group than placebo (2.7 vs. 0.3 units, effect size of 0.38). Decreases in some fatty acids correlated with decreased in hyperactivity. Well tolerated and safe.	13
Bent (2014) [70] US Internet-based	5–8	50 M, 7 F	Intervention (n = 29, 8 discontinued and 2 improper enrolment) Placebo (n = 28, 4 discontinued and 1 improper enrolment)	0.7 g/day EPA 0.46 g/day DHA	Orange flavoured pudding containing safflower oil	6 weeks	ABC-(parent and teacher) SRS CGI-I	No significant differences in changes in SRS and CGI-I between groups. Non-significant greater improvement in hyperactivity subscale in omega-3 group than placebo (−5.3 vs. −3.4, effect size of 0.26). Significantly greater improvements in stereotypy and lethargy subscales (p = 0.05 and 0.01, respectively). Well tolerated and safe.	13
Yui (2011 and 2012) * [54,57] Japan Pilot	6–28	12 M, 1 F	Intervention (n = 7) Placebo (n = 6)	0.24 g/day DHA 0.24 g/day AA	Olive oil	16 weeks	ABC ADI-R SRS	Significant increase in plasma AA. No differences in plasma DHA and EPA. Significant improvement in social withdrawal subscale of ABC (p = 0.04) and stereotyped and repetitive behaviours of ADI-R (p = 0.04). Significant improvement in communication subscale of SRS reported in both treatment and placebo groups, though the effect size was more favourable for the treatment group than placebo group (0.87 vs. 0.44, respectively). Safe.	10

Table 2. *Cont.*

RCTs Not included in the Meta-Analysis 2 but included in the Overall Interpretation (n = 2)									
Reference and Setting	Age (Years)	Sex Distribution (M, F)	Sample Size	Intervention		Duration	Outcome Measure	Outcome	Quality Score †
				Active	Placebo				
Mankad (2015) [37] Canada	2–5	27 M, 10 F	Intervention (n = 19, 4 drop outs) Placebo (n = 19, 2 drop outs) Stratified by severity	1.5 g/day EPA + DHA	Refined olive oil in medium chain triglyceride	6 months	PDDBI BASC-2 CGI-I VABS-II PLS-4	No significant differences between groups in all measures at 6 months, but mild improvement in BASC-2 externalising subscale in placebo but worsening in omega-3 group (−3 vs. 3, respectively, p = 0.02) Relatively well tolerated and safe.	13
Voigt (2014) [55] US	3–10	40 M, 8 F	Intervention (n = 24, 5 discontinued) Placebo (n = 24, 9 discontinued) Stratified by age	0.2 g/day DHA	0.25 g/day corn oil + 0.25 g/day soybean oil	6 months	CGI-I CDI ABC BASC	431% increase in plasma phospholipid DHA No significant differences in the percentage with a positive response (CGI-I) across groups and in all other measures across groups. Well tolerated and safe.	13

† Health Canada Quality Appraisal Tool for Experimental Studies; A quality score of ≥8 was considered higher quality [47]. * Different outcomes from the same group of participants were reported in two different papers. AA, arachidonic acid; ABC, Aberrant Behaviour Checklist; ADI-R, Autism Diagnostic Interview-Revised; BASC, Behaviour Assessment System for Children; CDI, Child Development Inventory; CGI-I, Clinical Global Impression-Improvement; CGI-S, Clinical Global Impression-Severity; DHA, docosahexanoic acid; EPA, eicosapentanoic acid; EVT, Expressive Vocabulary Test; F, Female; M, Male; n, Number; PDDBI, Pervasive Developmental Disorders Behavioural Inventory; PLS-4, Preschool Language Scale; PPVT, Peabody Picture Vocabulary Test; SRS, Social Responsiveness Scale; US, United States; VABS-II, Vineland Adaptive Behaviour Scale.

3.2.1. Effect of n-3 LCPUFA on Core Symptoms of ASD

Social interaction: The fixed mean difference for social interaction (assessed using ABC) significantly favoured n-3 LCPUFA with small effect (-1.96 [-3.5, -0.34], $Z = 2.37$, $p = 0.02$) and no heterogeneity ($I^2 = 0\%$, $p = 0.92$) (Figure 6A). Removing the Yui, 2011 study [54] did not change the results. The Yui, 2011 study [54] differs from others in that their sample included older participants (2–28 years) and those with IQ > 50, the daily dose of DHA was lower (0.24 g/day) and ARA (0.24 g/day) was added to the supplement, they used different dosing regimens for different age groups (half a dose for children aged 6–10 years) and SD was imputed resulting in a substantially greater SD in the n-3 LCPUFA group compared to the placebo group and other studies. Using SRS social interaction sub-domains (social motivation, social cognition, and social awareness), the Bent, 2014 study [70] found no effect of n-3 LCPUFA on social interaction (all domains > 0.05). Similarly, the Yui, 2012 study [57] did not find any effect of n-3 LCPUFA on any sub-domains of social interaction (measured by SRS, all $p > 0.05$). The social interaction in response to intervention did not differ across groups in the Mankad, 2015 study [37] where the authors used other assessment tools. The mean change scores decreased (showing an improvement) in both treatment groups in these studies. Voigt et al. (2014) found a significant difference in BASC social skills, favouring n-3 LCPUFA (-0.2 vs. 3.0, $p = 0.04$), which disappeared after correction for multiple comparisons [55].

Communication: Communication scores (assessed using ABC) did not differ between n-3 LCPUFA and placebo groups (-0.38 [-1.33, 0.56], $p = 0.42$) (Figure 6B). Moderate heterogeneity was seen in the meta-analysis for communication ($I^2 = 51\%$, $p = 0.11$). Removing the Yui, 2011 study [54] reduced the heterogeneity to 0% but had no impact on the overall result. Bent et al. (2011) and Bent et al. (2014) also used other tools including Peabody Picture Vocabulary Test (PPVT), Expressive Vocabulary Test (EVT) and the communication sub-domain of SRS, respectively [69,70]. Neither study found any effect of n-3 LCPUFA on communication. Similarly, the Mankad, 2015 study [37] did not find any differences across groups and the Voigt, 2014 study [55] reported worsened outcome (reported by teachers) in response to n-3 LCPUFA supplementation compared to placebo that showed improvement (1.4 vs. -4.5, $p = 0.02$). However, the Yui, 2012 study [57] found greater improvements in SRS communication sub-scale scores in n-3 LCPUFA group than the placebo group (-23.6 vs. -20.6, $p = 0.03$).

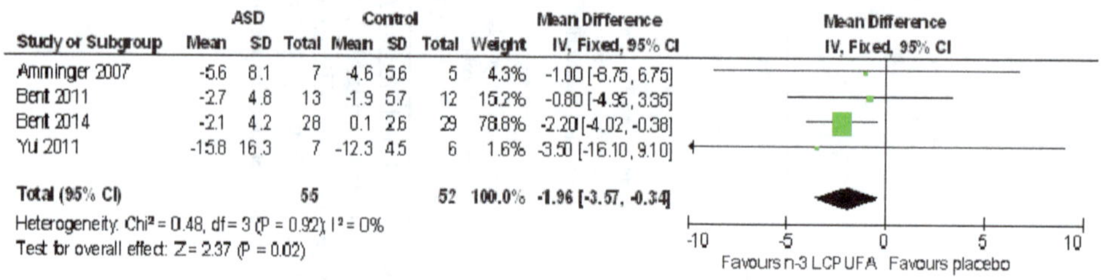

(A)

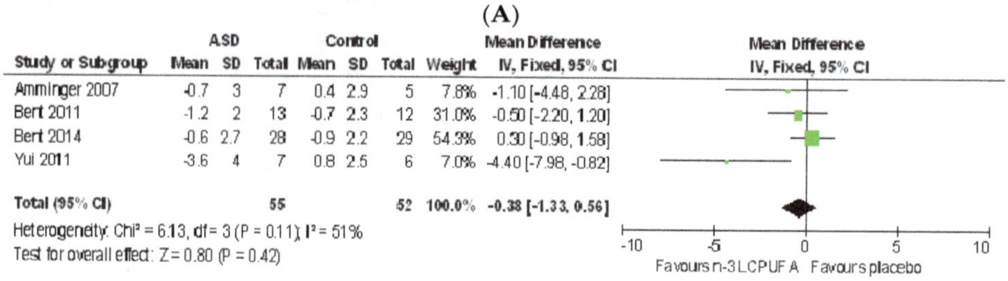

(B)

Figure 6. *Cont.*

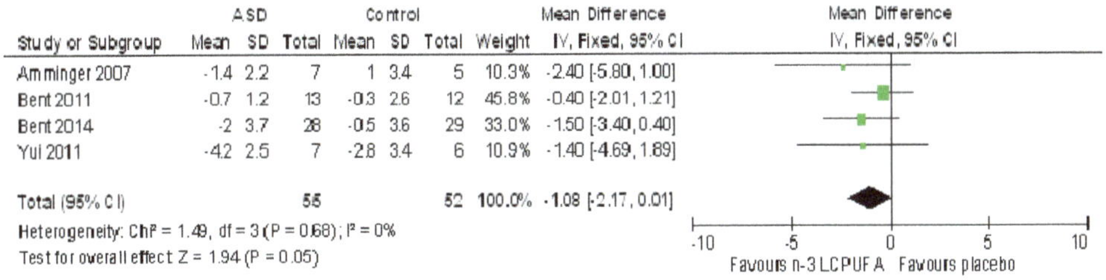

(C)

Figure 6. Forest plot of mean (95% confidence interval (CI)) fixed difference in change in social interaction (ABC) (**A**); communication (ABC) (**B**); and repetitive and restricted interests and behaviours (ABC) (**C**) in populations with Autism Spectrum Disorder (ASD) receiving *n*-3 long chain polyunsaturated fatty acid supplementation (LCPUFA) and placebo. Direction of effect (negative, more improvement in *n*-3 LCPUFA groups; positive, more improvement in placebo group; zero, no difference between groups).

Repetitive and restricted interests and behaviours: The fixed mean difference for RRB (assessed using ABC) favoured *n*-3 LCPUFA with small effect (−1.08 [−2.17, −0.01], $Z = 1.94$, $p = 0.05$) (Figure 6C) and nil heterogeneity ($I^2 = 0\%$, $p = 0.68$). Removing the Yui, 2011 study [54] removed the significance ($p = 0.08$) perhaps due to low statistical power. Using the Autism Diagnostic Interview-Revised (ADI-R) scale, Yui et al. (2011) also reported a significant improvement in one of four RRB sub-domains, stereotyped and repetitive motor movement (−1.7 vs. −0.7, $p = 0.04$). However, Bent et al. (2014), using the RRB sub-domain of SRS, reported a trend favouring placebo, -2.9 ± 12.0 (placebo) vs. -8.6 ± 11.4 (*n*-3 LCPUFA), $p = 0.08$ [70]. Neither Yui et al. (2012) (using SRS RRB subscale) nor Mankad et al. (using Pervasive Developmental Disorders Behavioural Inventory (PDDBI) resistance to change subscale) showed an effect of *n*-3 LCPUFA intervention on RRB ($p > 0.05$) [37,57]. The mean scores improved in both treatment groups in these studies.

3.2.2. Effect of LCPUFA on Co-Existing Conditions

Hyperactivity: Hyperactivity scores (assessed using ABC) did not differ between treatment groups (−2.13 [−4.89, 0.62], $p = 0.13$) (Figure 7A) and heterogeneity was nil ($I^2 = 0\%$, $p = 0.98$). Sensitivity analysis by removing studies including older participants [36,54] had no effect on the overall result. Similarly, using BASC hyperactivity sub-domain, the Bent, 2011 study [69] did not find any difference between groups ($p = 0.83$). Using the BASC externalizing behaviour scale, Mankad et al. (2015) reported a significantly worsened outcome in response to *n*-3 LCPUFA supplementation compared to placebo (3.2 vs. −3.0, $p = 0.02$) [37]. It should be noted that BASC externalizing behaviour is a composite measure of hyperactivity, aggression and conduct problem. The authors suggested that greater pre-existing gastrointestinal distress at baseline (8/19 vs. 1/19, in the *n*-3 LCPUFA group vs. placebo group) may have predisposed the *n*-3 LCPUFA group to higher externalizing behaviour.

Irritability: Irritability scores (assessed using ABC) did not differ between groups (0.13 [−2.08, 2.34], $p = 0.91$) (Figure 7B) and heterogeneity was nil ($I^2 = 0\%$, $p = 1.00$). Sensitivity analysis by removing studies including older participants [36,54] had no effect on the overall result.

Sensory issues: The Mankad, 2015 study [37] was the only study that assessed the effect of *n*-3 LCPUFA supplementation on sensory issues (using sensory/perceptual approach behaviour domain of PDDBI). Sensory symptoms comparably improved in both study groups. It should be noted that this domain has five clusters, all of which tap into a variety of repetitive behaviours.

Gastrointestinal symptoms: The Mankad, 2015 study [37] was the only study that assessed the effect of the intervention on gastrointestinal distress and found no differences across treatment groups ($p > 0.9$) (assessed using CGI-I).

Publication bias could not be determined for any outcome measures due to small number of studies included in the meta-analysis (n = 4).

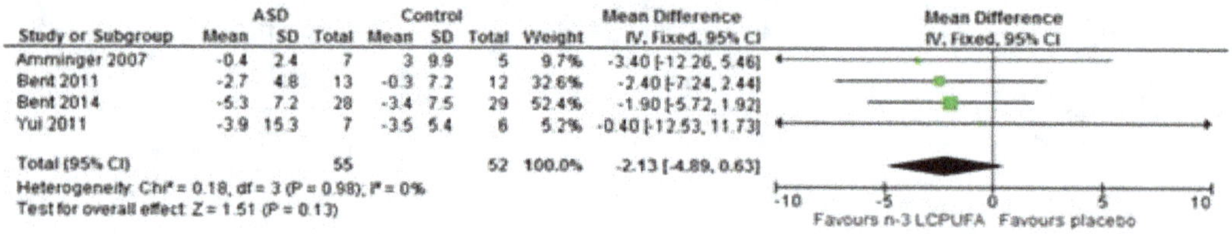

(A)

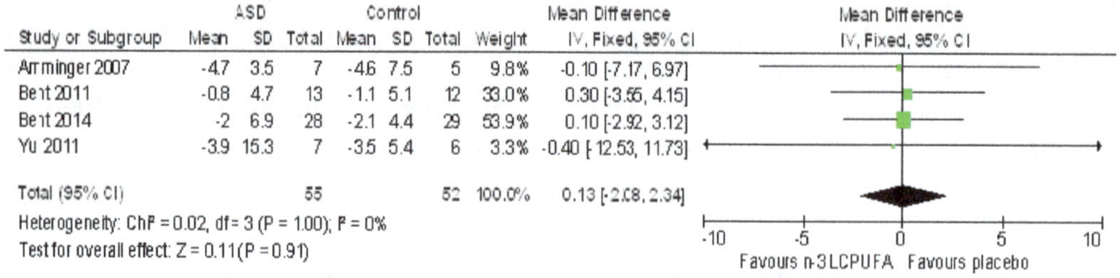

(B)

Figure 7. Forest plot of mean (95% confidence interval (CI)) fixed difference in change in hyperactivity (ABC) (**A**) and irritability (ABC) (**B**) in populations with Autism Spectrum Disorder (ASD) receiving n-3 long chain polyunsaturated fatty acid supplementation (n-3 LCPUFA) and placebo. Direction of effect (negative, more improvement in n-3 LCPUFA group; positive, more improvement in placebo group; zero, no difference between groups).

3.2.3. Tolerability and Safety of LCPUFA Supplementation

All RCTs included in this review concluded that LCPUFA supplementation was well tolerated and safe. Adverse effects reported were not serious and were comparable across treatment groups.

4. Discussion

The findings of each meta-analysis are individually discussed (starting with a discussion of findings of meta-analysis 1 and then meta-analysis 2) followed by a discussion on potential mechanistic pathways that might underlie the relationship between LCPUFA and ASD.

4.1. Systematic Review and Meta-Analysis 1

The current study (meta-analysis 1), to our knowledge, is the first meta-analysis of case control studies of blood fatty acid levels in populations with ASD. The findings of this study were that children with ASD had lower levels of DHA, EPA, and higher total n-6 LCPUFA to n-3 LCPUFA ratio, but not ARA to DHA and ARA to EPA ratios, compared to typically developing children. However, the differences were only evident in studies that included children only and not in studies with wide age ranges that also included adolescents and adults. One should be cautious to make conclusions regarding the modulating effect of age on the relationship since the number of studies including homogenous samples of adolescents and homogenous samples of adults are limited.

Herein we compare the findings of the current study with those of meta-analyses in ADHD because there is an overlap in symptoms between ASD and ADHD. Our results are in agreement with recently published meta-analyses showing lower n-3 LCPUFA levels, with larger effect size when DHA and EPA within each study were pooled than when these fatty acids were separately considered [71], and higher ratios of n-6 LCPUFA to n-3 LCPUFA [42] in patients with ADHD compared with healthy controls.

Another finding of the current study is that while the majority of included studies were of high quality, there was large methodological and clinical heterogeneity between studies, highlighting the importance of discussing the results in light of the study and population characteristics. The type of blood tissue in which the fatty acid composition is analysed has been suggested to affect the findings of case-control studies [27,51]. Bell et al. (2010) and Jory (2016) compared plasma/serum fatty acid composition with those of RBC [27,51]. The authors found significantly lower LA [27], ARA, DHA, and EPA [51] and higher *n*-6 LCPUFA to *n*-3 LCPUFA ratio [51] in RBC of autistic children compared with healthy controls. No polyunsaturated fatty acids in Bell et al.'s study [27] and only DHA in Jory's study [51] were found to be significantly different across groups when plasma/serum were compared. However, sensitivity analysis in the current study revealed no effect of removing studies that reported RBC fatty acids on heterogeneity.

The method by which blood fatty acid composition is expressed (relative vs. absolute) has also been shown to alter the findings of case-control studies investigating the fatty acid composition across groups and to modify the LCPUFA—disease relationship [46,53]. Yui et al. (2016) compared relative levels of plasma fatty acids with the same fatty acids expressed as absolute [53]. The authors found a significant difference in DHA, EPA, DPA, and arachidic acid, and the ratios of ARA to DHA and ARA to EPA (the reverse ratios were reported) across groups when relative levels were expressed. However, the significance disappeared for DHA and arachidic acid when absolute levels were compared. Although the removal of those studies reporting absolute levels had no impact on the heterogeneity, it resulted in the loss of significance across groups for ARA and in a significantly higher ARA to EPA in populations with ASD than typically developing controls. These findings highlight the importance of taking the method by which blood fatty acid composition is expressed into account when blood fatty acid profile is investigated. A potential explanation for such findings could be the inter-study variation in extraction and separation efficiencies in fatty acid analysis [46].

The high heterogeneity reported in this meta-analysis could also be explained by populations' characteristics. The role of age and sex on fatty acid status has been well documented [60,72,73]. Using a linear model, Wiest et al. (2009) demonstrated that ARA level was modified by sex; while ARA level did not differ between male autistic children and healthy controls, female autistic children had significantly lower ARA than healthy controls [60]. Thus, an uneven distribution of age (particularly if a wide age range is included) and sex across groups could alter the results in different ways; mask the difference, change the effect direction, or influence the effect size, all of which may contribute to heterogeneity seen in this study. Lack of effect in the Bell, 2004 study (EPA, DHA, and ARA) [66], change of direction in the El-Ansary, 2011a (ARA/EPA and ARA/DHA ratios) and 2011b (ARA), and Sliwinski, 2006 studies (total *n*-3 LCPUFA, DHA, and total *n*-6/*n*-3 LCPUFA ratio) [49,50,65], and the large effect size in the Parletta, 2016 study (EPA, DHA, ARA and their ratios) [52] may be explained by such characteristics.

The use of psychotropic medication can be another modifier. Psychotropic medications such as rispiradone may affect RBC fatty acid composition through their effect on oxidative stress and lipid peroxidation [23,74]. The Parletta, 2016 study [52] together with the Tostes, 2013 study [68] resulted in high levels of heterogeneity in EPA. ASD children in the former study were significantly younger than typically developing children [52], and approximately 88% of children with ASD in the Tostes, 2013 study were on psychotropic medication [68].

Location is another factor that may modify the fatty acid composition–autism relationship. With reference to those studies included in this meta-analysis, the Yui, 2016 [53] and Sliwinski, 2006 [49] were conducted in Japan and Belgium (among European countries) where the habitual dietary intake of fish and fish products are potentially high [75]. Both studies reported the autistic population having significantly higher DHA and EPA levels and lower *n*-6 to *n*-3 LCPUFA ratio than healthy controls, and both affected heterogeneity largely [49,53]. High consumption of *n*-3 LCPUFA rich foods can mask the difference, and in populations who are potentially prone to disturbances in fatty acid metabolism can alter the effect direction [49,53].

Altered fatty acid composition in ASD has been suggested to be, in part, due to low dietary intake of LCPUFA. Children with ASD have very limited food preferences that may result in these children having limited intake of LCPUFA rich foods [67]. Only three studies included in this meta-analysis assessed the dietary intake of fatty acids [14,53,67]. Al-Farsi, 2013 reported a lower intake of ALA, assessed using a semi-quantitative food frequency questionnaire, in children with ASD than healthy controls [0.8 (0.2) vs. 1.2 (0.4) g/day, $p = 0.001$] [67]. However, Ghezzo et al. (2013) [14] and Yui et al. (2016) [53] found no difference in LCPUFA intake across groups, pointing to the facts that these abnormalities could be due to disturbances in fatty acid metabolism rather than intake. For a brief discussion on the potential mechanistic pathways of LCPUFA in ASD refer to Section 4.3 (Potential mechanistic pathways).

4.2. Systematic Review and Meta-Analysis 2

Few RCTs have been completed and reported to date on *n*-3 LCPUFA supplementation for ASD; only six trials were included in this review (four included in the meta-analysis and two in the overall interpretation), with a total of 178 participants. In this meta-analysis, a small but significant benefit of *n*-3 LCPUFA supplementation was found for social interaction and RRB but not communication and co-existing behaviours and conditions. No evidence of significant heterogeneity between trials were found.

Four trials included in the present meta-analysis with a total of 107 participants are however insufficient to provide robust evidence. Furthermore, the findings cannot be generalised to all children on the autism spectrum because the included children predominantly comprised males, were of different age groups (less than eight years and up to 28 years), displayed moderate to severe symptoms [54,69] or high hyperactivity level [36,70].

The findings of this review to some extent contradict the results of previous systematic reviews and meta-analysis [38,39]. These reviews did not find any statistically significant improvement in behaviour, but reported a larger positive effect on hyperactivity [38,39] while the present review found a significant improvement in social interaction and no improvement in hyperactivity. Our results, however, are in line with those of previous reviews [38,39] in that no improvement was identified in communication and irritability. With respect to RRB, sensory issues and gastrointestinal symptoms, no comparison can be made because they were not considered by these reviews. It should be noted that the small number of RCTs included in the review by Bent et al. ($n = 1$) [38] and James et al. ($n = 2$) [39] could have compromised the statistical power to detect any difference across groups.

Although case-control and open label studies provided evidence for a role of *n*-3 LCPUFA in ASD, RCTs of supplementation with *n*-3 LCPUFA yielded mixed results. One reason for such inconsistencies between studies may result from inadequately controlling for age, trial duration, habitual dietary intake of *n*-3 LCPUFA and levels of these fatty acids in the circulation over the course of trial, participants' general health conditions at the baseline and over the course of study, and outcome tools assessing behaviour. Response to *n*-3 LCPUFA supplementation has been shown to be predicted by body weight adjusted dose, baseline omega-3 index (RBC DHA + EPA), sex, age, and physical activity level; with populations receiving larger doses, having lower starting omega-3 index, older population, females and those with higher physical activity level experiencing a greater increase in the omega-3 index in response to supplementation [76].

Dietary intake of *n*-3 LCPUFA rich foods in children with autism is low [67]. However, omega-3 fatty acid supplements are among the most commonly used complementary and alternative medication in ASD [40]. It is plausible to suggest that even though the mentioned trials excluded participants that used *n*-3 LCPUFA supplements on their own initiatives at baseline, participants may have had high habitual dietary intake of these fatty acids due to their popularity, therefore responding differently to supplements which leads to diminishing the differences across treatment groups. An example of such implication could be the Voigt, 2014 study [55]; all children in this study had baseline LCPUFA levels above paediatric reference ranges for nutritional deficiencies and metabolic disorders (established at the Mayo Clinic [77]), and despite an increase of 431% in plasma DHA level, no improvement in behaviour was reported. Bent et al. (2011), on the other hand, showed that higher baseline level of some *n*-6 and *n*-3 polyunsaturated fatty acids including eicosadienoic acid ($r = -0.79$, $p = 0.02$), docosadienoate acid ($r = -0.65$, $p = 0.03$), and ALA ($r = -0.64$, $p = 0.03$) were associated with reduction in hyperactivity [69]. In an open label trial of *n*-3 LCPUFA in 41 autistic children aged 7–18 years, Ooi et al. (2015) showed an inverse correlation between autism mannerism severity and change in RBC fatty acids after 12 weeks of intervention and the severity was associated with baseline EPA level [32]. Unfortunately, the number of trials included in this review was inadequate to provide data on the effect of baseline *n*-3 LCPUFA intake or status on behavioural changes in response to supplementation.

The sex differences in ASD might be partly explained by sex differences in fatty acid metabolism; males may be more vulnerable than females to deficiencies in LCPUFA because of hormonal reasons [78], and thus may respond poorly to supplements [76]. With the exception of one study [36], no trials included in this review stratified the randomisation by sex. Unfortunately, no analysis could be performed for subgroups stratified by sex in this review because far more males than females were included and no studies reported behavioural changes in response to supplementation for males and females separately. With regard to the potential effect of age, three out of six studies included a wide age range (children and young people up to 28 years) which may have resulted in greater response variability. Due to the small number of studies included in this review, we could not perform subgroup analysis for different age bands to examine the effect of age on behavioural change in response to omega-3 supplementation.

The trial duration varied widely in studies included in this review (6–26 weeks). Evidence suggests that PUFA erythrocyte membrane reaches a steady state after 6 months [79] and at least 4 months is needed to demonstrate an effect on cognitive performance [41]. It has also been suggested that longer study periods of one year might be needed to demonstrate behavioural changes in response to *n*-3 LCPUFA supplementation [80]. Furthermore, the majority of outcome assessment tools are retrospectively completed (and duration over which behaviour is assessed varies depending on the assessment tool used); for example, parents are required to consider the behaviour over the past four weeks when completing ABC questionnaire while the timeframe for SRS is the past six months. It is of importance to avoid assessing and considering behaviour when the LCPUFA erythrocyte membrane has not yet reached its steady state. Therefore, wide variation and insufficient trial duration could explain the inconsistencies. Due to the small number of studies included in this review, we could not perform subgroup analysis for different intervention lengths to examine the effect of duration on behavioural change in response to omega-3 supplementation.

Gastrointestinal symptoms are highly prevalent in populations with ASD [81–83]. Mazurek et al. (2013) reported that of 2973 children with ASD, 24.7% had at least one chronic gastrointestinal symptom [83]. Compared to typically developing children, developmentally delayed and ASD children were more likely to have at least one frequent gastrointestinal symptom [83]. ASD children with frequent abdominal pain, gaseousness, diarrhea, constipation or pain on stooling had worse scores in four (irritability, social withdrawal, stereotypy, and hyperactivity) out of five ABC subscales than ASD children with no frequent gastrointestinal symptoms [84]. The pain and discomfort caused by gastrointestinal distress can worsen the behaviour in people with ASD, more particularly in non-verbal individuals who cannot express their feelings. Mankad et al. (2015) reported significantly worsened externalizing behaviours in response to *n*-3 LCPUFA supplementation which could be attributed to higher gastrointestinal distress reported in the active treatment group compared with the placebo (8/19 vs. 1/19, respectively) [37]. Thus, it is important to consider the potential modulating effect of gastrointestinal symptoms over the course of study on behavioural changes in response to supplementation.

Additionally, a variety of assessment tools (ranging from one to six tools) were used in each study which complicated effective comparisons across studies resulting in the exclusion of three studies from the meta-analysis, and potentially compromised the validity of a study by increasing the likelihood of type 1 error [44]. With the exception of ABC, a widely-used tool to assess problem behaviours in pharmacological trials in ASD, the majority of assessment tools have been designed for diagnostic purposes and there is a lack of evidence regarding the sensitivity of these tools to slight changes in behaviour in response to intervention in ASD populations. It is also worth noting that the inappropriate speech subscale of ABC is not a comprehensive measure of communication compared to other tools like SRS (inappropriate speech subscale of ABC comprises of four questions while the SRS communication subscale consists of 22 questions). Thus, findings regarding communication (measured by ABC) should be interpreted with caution.

It is also worth noting that the small or lack of effect reported here could be due to large placebo response in many trials included in this review. The large placebo response may have limited our capacity to identify any differences in some behaviour across groups. It is documented that different factors [e.g., raters of outcome assessment tools (clinicians vs. parents), increased response to active intervention, location, pharmacological and adjunctive intervention, participants' age (younger vs. older), study duration (shorter vs. longer), and severity of condition (lower baseline severity vs. higher severity)] are associated with the increased placebo response in ASD and other neurodevelopment and psychiatric disorders [85–87]. However, the reason for observed improvement in placebo groups included in this review is unclear and could not be determined due to small number of studies included.

4.3. Potential Mechanistic Pathways

There are, though not very well understood, several potential biological pathways for a role of LCPUFA in ASD [88,89]. Approximately 60% of the brain's dry weight is fat, with DHA comprising 60% and 40% of the PUFA in the retina and brain, respectively [90], suggesting that it is structurally important. Evidence suggests that some individuals with ASD have abnormalities in the gray and white matter of brain regions that are involved in social interaction, RRB, and sensory processing [13,91–93]. Ingestion of DHA (through diet or supplementation) has been shown to be positively associated with gray matter volume and its functional integrity and with white matter microstructural integrity in healthy individuals [16,17,94].

At the cellular level, PUFA interact with and influence the functioning of integral membrane proteins, including enzymes, receptors, and ion channels [95,96]. Evidence suggests that the activity of Na^+/K^+-ATPase (an enzyme that controls ion transport produced by neurotransmission) and adenylate cyclase (an enzyme that catalyses the conversion of ATP to cyclic AMP and has been shown to modulate social behaviours [97]) is disturbed in individuals with ASD [14,98]. Ghezzo et al. (2013) reported children with ASD having a significant reduction in Na^+/K^+-ATPase activity, alterations in erythrocyte fatty acid membrane (a decrease in n-3 LCPUFA and consequently an increase in n-6 LCPUFA to n-3 LCPUFA ratio, and an increase in monounsaturated fatty acids), and a reduction in erythrocyte membrane fluidity [14]. These alterations correlated with clinical features of ASD, particularly hyperactivity scores [14].

Further evidence for a relationship between n-3 LCPUFA and ASD comes from studies investigating its role in neurogenesis and several neurotransmitter systems. LCPFA, particularly n-3 series DHA, has been shown to favourably affect neurite survival, outgrowth and myelination in animal cultured cortical [99–101], sensory [102], and hippocampal neurons [18,103,104]. The development of axons and dentrites as well as myelination in multiple brain areas (involved in social behaviours, emotions, and RRB) has been reported to be impaired in individuals with ASD [105,106]. Similarly, an abnormal level of brain derived neurotrophic factor (BDNF, a protein that promotes the survival of neurons) in the circulation has been reported in children with ASD, which was associated with the severity of condition [88,107,108]. Docosahexaenoic acid administration normalised BDNF in the hippocampus, increased the growth of uninjured corticospinal and serotonergic fibres, and enhanced synaptic plasticity in an animal model of spinal cord injury [101,109].

Autistic children have been shown to exhibit significantly higher levels of several dopamine derivatives (in urine), dopamine transporter binding proteins, and serotonin in brain, and lower levels of serotonin transporter binding protein (in brain), glutamine signal (in basal ganglia), and oxytocin than healthy controls [110–116]. Furthermore, within the ASD populations, basal ganglia glutamine signal and plasma oxytocin negatively correlated with impaired behaviour [114,116]. In response to an *n*-3 PUFA limited diet in rats, dopamine levels reduced and basal synaptic release of serotonin increased while the turn over metabolites of dopamine increased and those of serotonin decreased [19,117–119]. A DHA depleted diet also altered the glutamergic system in offspring female rats [120]. This alteration was associated with anxiety-like behaviours, memory deficit and exploratory behaviours during adulthood [120]. On the other hand, DHA treatment significantly increased synaptic plasticity in hippocampal neurons and enhanced glutamatergic activity [121].

Another plausible mechanism supporting the association between LCPUFA and ASD is the anti- and pro-inflammatory properties of LCPUFA metabolic products. Eicosanoids (a collective name for prostaglandins, thromboxanes, leukotrienes and a variety of hydroxyl and hydroproxy fatty acid) are the enzymatic metabolic products of PUFA, and have important roles in inflammation [20]. While EPA or DHA derived eicosanoids have anti-inflammatory properties, those derived from ARA have pro-inflammatory properties [20]. Elevated levels of several peripheral pro-inflammatory cytokines and nuclear factor Kappa B (NF-κB, a transcription factor involved in inflammatory signaling pathways) has been reported in children with ASD [122–124]. Brigandi et al. [24] reported children with ASD having significantly higher plasma levels of PGE2 than healthy controls, a finding confirmed by El-Ansary and Al-Ayadhi (2012) [125] who also reported higher levels of leukotriene and 8-isoprostane together with PGE2 in children with ASD. In addition, lower levels of antioxidant proteins and increased levels of oxidative stress markers was associated with more severe ASD symptoms, including sensory issues [14,124,126]. Supplementation with *n*-3 PUFA, on the other hand, decreased the gene expression of NF-κB, IL-12 and IL-13 [127], macrophage inflammatory protein-2 (MIP2), IL-6 [128] and tumor necrosis factor-α (TNF-α) [128–130].

Decreased antioxidant capacity and increased lipid peroxidation may result in RBC LCPUFA instability and decrease these fatty acids in autism [23,74]. Instability in RBC LCPUFA composition has been shown by a great loss in PUFA levels when the blood samples of autistic children were stored at −20 °C, a finding not observed in the blood sample of healthy controls [62]. The reason for such instability could be related to cellular phospholipase activity. Tostes et al. (2013) [68] and Bell et al. (2004) [66] reported children with ASD having significantly higher phospholipase A2 (PLA2) activity than typically developing controls that was reduced by EPA supplementation [66]. PLA2 is responsible for releasing fatty acids, more particularly ARA, from phospholipids [66].

Finally, the role of LCPUFA in ASD could be explained by defects in enzymes involved in the conversion of LCPUFA from their precursors or deficits in the process of incorporation of LCPUFA into the cell membrane [24–26]. Gene variants in fatty acid desaturase (FADS)—one of the strongest genome wide associated signals—have been shown to enhance the conversion of ARA from its precursor and to be sex- and ethnicity-specific [131,132]. The effect of FADS genotype has been shown to be more pronounced in African Americans than Europeans (approximately two fold higher) [131]. The higher frequency of this genetic variant, but not the allelic effect of G allele, explained such a difference [131]. Also, while in Caucasians, one FADS2 single nucleotide polymorphism (SNP) and multiple FADS2 SNP (two SNP in males and nine SNP in females) were associated with *n*-6 aggregate desaturase indices, it was associated with five FADS2 SNP in East Asian Females [132]. In addition, carriers of APOE4 allele seems to have altered long chain omega-3 metabolism [133]. Compared to the non APOE4-carriers, the carriers have higher β-oxidisation rates of *n*-3 LCPUFA [133]. Furthermore, Shimamoto et al. (2014) showed altered mRNA gene expression levels of fatty acid binding protein 7 (FABP7) in post-mortem ASD brains, and increased hyperactivity and anxiety-related phenotype (two common features in ASD) in FABP7 knockout mice [134]. Although the modifying role of genetic variants in enzymes involved in fatty acid metabolism in the LCPUFA-disease relationship has been well documented, in the context of ASD, it warrants further investigation.

5. Conclusions

The current meta-analysis of case-controls studies, to our knowledge, is the first to investigate fatty acid composition in populations with ASD. Future observational studies of *n*-3 LCPUFA in children with ASD are encouraged while including a uniform biomarker (e.g., omega-3 index or percentage of *n*-3 LCPUFA in RBC) and reporting method (e.g., relative or absolute), collecting dietary intake of both *n*-3 and *n*-6 LCPUFA, and matching cases and controls on potential modulating attributes (e.g., age, sex, severity, genotype, and medication use). It is also critical to know whether inadequate LCPUFA status in ASD is attributed to inefficient or disrupted metabolism or other factors like LCPUFA consumption.

Based on the current evidence, *n*-3 LCPUFA supplementation cannot be recommended as an alternative to support behavioural therapies for ASD children. However, it seems prudent that *n*-3 LCPUFA could be used to complement other therapies in ASD populations given its long-term tolerability and acceptability (up to six months), potentially inefficient or disrupted LCPUFA metabolic pathways in this population, and its critical role in brain function and development, and various body processes some of which are involved in the pathobiology of ASD. It should be noted that this recommendation is made cautiously because the results of this study are based on a very small sample of studies (with methodological differences and limitations) and short duration of the interventions. Therefore, the generated statistics should not be over-interpreted but seen as indicative of the need to study the issue further (while controlling for potential modifying and confounding variables) to pursue the trends observed in this study. The effect of *n*-3 LCPUFA on behaviour may be modulated by background diet and baseline LCPUFA status, sex, age, trial duration, and gastrointestinal stress at baseline and over the study period, all of which are recommended to be considered in future research. Furthermore, an investigation of the potential modulating effect of genotype (e.g., APOE) on behavioural changes in response to LCPUFA supplementation is warranted. It is also recommended that future studies include a uniform assessment tool that is sensitive to minor behavioural changes in response to complementary/nutritional therapies. Finally, the potential placebo effect and the reasons for such effects are encouraged to be investigated and accounted for in the design stage of RCTs.

Supplementary Materials:
Table S1: Study characteristics of open label trials and case-studies excluded from systematic literature review; Table S2: Quality appraisal of included case-control studies; Table S3: Quality appraisal of included RCTs; Figure S1: Risk of bias table showing judgments on each risk factor for each primary study included in both meta-analysis and overall interpretation.

Acknowledgments: No funding was received in support of this research work. Massey University provided funds for covering the costs to publish this research work in open access.

Author Contributions: H.M. conceived the manuscript idea, H.M. researched the manuscript and identified eligible studies, H.M. and M.D. extracted data and performed the quality appraisal of studies; H.M. performed the meta-analyses and drafted the manuscript, all other authors critically reviewed the manuscript.

References

1. Chakrabarti, S.; Fombonne, E. Pervasive developmental disorders in preschool children. *JAMA* **2001**, *285*, 3093–3099. [CrossRef] [PubMed]
2. New Zealand Guidelines Group. *What Does ASD Look Like? A Resource to Help Identify Autism Spectrum Disorder*; New Zealand Guidelines Group: Wellington, New Zealand, 2010.
3. Baio, J. Prevalence of Autism Spectrum Disorders—Autism and Developmental Disabilities Monitoring Network, 14 Sites, United States, 2008. *Surveill. Summ.* **2012**, *61*, 1–19.
4. Ghanizadeh, A. A preliminary study on screening prevalence of pervasive developmental disorder in schoolchildren in Iran. *J. Autism Dev. Disord.* **2008**, *38*, 759–763. [CrossRef] [PubMed]
5. Kogan, M.D.; Blumberg, S.J.; Schieve, L.A.; Boyle, C.A.; Perrin, J.M.; Ghandour, R.M.; Singh, G.K.; Strickland, B.B.; Trevathan, E.; van Dyck, P.C. Prevalence of Parent-Reported Diagnosis of Autism Spectrum Disorder Among Children in the US, 2007. *Pediatrics* **2009**, *124*, 1395–1403. [CrossRef] [PubMed]

6. Diagnostic and Statistical Manual of Mental Disorders. In *Diagnostic and Statistical Manual of Mental Disorders: DSM-5*; American Psychiatric Association: Washington, DC, USA, 2013.
7. Napolioni, V.; Ober-Reynolds, B.; Szelinger, S.; Corneveaux, J.J.; Pawlowski, T.; Ober-Reynolds, S.; Kirwan, J.; Perisco, A.M.; Melmed, R.D.; Craig, D.W.; et al. Plasma cytokine profiling in sibling pairs discordant for Autism Spectrum Disorder. *J. Neuroinflamm.* **2013**, *10*, 38. [CrossRef] [PubMed]
8. Rossignol, D.A.; Frye, R.E. Evidence linking oxidative stress, mitochondrial dysfunction, and inflammation in the brain of individuals with autism. *Front. Physiol.* **2014**, *5*, 150. [CrossRef] [PubMed]
9. Singh, V.K. Phenotypic expression of autoimmune autistic disorder (AAD): A major subset of autism. *Ann. Clin. Psychiatry* **2009**, *21*, 148–161. [PubMed]
10. Napoli, E.; Wong, S.; Hertz-Picciotto, I.; Giulivi, C. Deficits in Bioenergetics and Impaired Immune Response in Granulocytes From Children With Autism. *Pediatrics* **2014**, *133*, e1405–e1410. [CrossRef] [PubMed]
11. Rose, S.; Frye, R.E.; Slattery, J.; Wynne, R.; Tippett, M.; Pavliv, O.; Melnyk, S.; James, S.J. Oxidative Stress Induces Mitochondrial Dysfunction in a Subset of Autism Lymphoblastoid Cell Lines in a Well-Matched Case Control Cohort. *PLoS ONE* **2014**, *9*, e85436. [CrossRef] [PubMed]
12. Melnyk, S.; Fuchs, G.J.; Schulz, E.; Lopez, M.; Kahler, S.G.; Fussell, J.J.; Bellando, J.; Pavliv, O.; Rose, S.; Seidel, L.; et al. Metabolic imbalance associated with methylation dysregulation and oxidative damage in children with autism. *J. Autism Dev. Disord.* **2012**, *42*, 367–377. [CrossRef] [PubMed]
13. D'Mello, A.M.; Crocetti, D.; Mostofsky, S.H.; Stoodley, C.J. Cerebellar gray matter and lobular volumes correlate with core autism symptoms. *NeuroImage Clin.* **2015**, *7*, 631–639. [CrossRef] [PubMed]
14. Ghezzo, A.; Visconti, P.; Abruzzo, P.M.; Bolotta, A.; Ferreri, C.; Gobbi, G.; Malisardi, G.; Manfredini, S.; Marini, M.; Nanetti, L.; et al. Oxidative Stress and Erythrocyte Membrane Alterations in Children with Autism: Correlation with Clinical Features. *PLoS ONE* **2013**, *8*, e66418. [CrossRef] [PubMed]
15. Schaaf, C.P.; Zoghbi, H.Y. Solving the autism puzzle a few pieces at a time. *Neuron* **2011**, *70*, 806–808. [CrossRef] [PubMed]
16. McNamara, R.K.; Able, J.; Jandacek, R.; Rider, T.; Tso, P.; Eliassen, J.C.; Alfieri, D.; Weber, W.; Jarvis, K.; DelBello, M.P.; et al. Docosahexaenoic acid supplementation increases prefrontal cortex activation during sustained attention in healthy boys: A placebo-controlled, dose-ranging, functional magnetic resonance imaging study. *Am. J. Clin. Nutr.* **2010**, *91*, 1060–1067. [CrossRef] [PubMed]
17. Witte, A.V.; Kerti, L.; Hermannstädter, H.M.; Fiebach, J.B.; Schreiber, S.J.; Schuchardt, J.P.; Hahn, A.; Flöel, A. Long-Chain Omega-3 Fatty Acids Improve Brain Function and Structure in Older Adults. *Cereb. Cortex* **2013**, *24*, 3059–3068. [CrossRef] [PubMed]
18. Pu, H.; Guo, Y.; Zhang, W.; Huang, L.; Wang, G.; Liou, A.K.; Zhang, J.; Zhang, P.; Leak, R.K.; Wang, Y.; et al. Omega-3 polyunsaturated fatty acid supplementation improves neurologic recovery and attenuates white matter injury after experimental traumatic brain injury. *J. Cereb. Blood Flow Metab.* **2013**, *33*, 1474–1484. [CrossRef] [PubMed]
19. Tang, M.; Zhang, M.; Cai, H.; Li, H.; Jiang, P.; Dang, R.; Liu, Y.; He, X.; Xue, Y.; Cao, L.; et al. Maternal diet of polyunsaturated fatty acid altered the cell proliferation in the dentate gyrus of hippocampus and influenced glutamatergic and serotoninergic systems of neonatal female rats. *Lipids Health Dis.* **2016**, *15*, 71. [CrossRef] [PubMed]
20. Calder, P.C. *n*-3 Polyunsaturated fatty acids, inflammation, and inflammatory diseases. *Am. J. Clin. Nutr.* **2006**, *83*, S1505–S1519.
21. Serra-Majem, L.; Nissensohn, M.; Overby, N.C.; Fekete, K. Dietary methods and biomarkers of omega 3 fatty acids: A systematic review. *Br. J. Nutr.* **2012**, *107* (Suppl. 2), S64–S76. [CrossRef] [PubMed]
22. Spahis, S.; Vanasse, M.; Bélanger, S.A.; Ghadirian, P.; Grenier, E.; Levy, E. Lipid profile, fatty acid composition and pro- and anti-oxidant status in pediatric patients with attention-deficit/hyperactivity disorder. Prostaglandins Leukot. *Essent. Fatty Acids* **2008**, *79*, 47–53. [CrossRef] [PubMed]
23. Khan, M.M.; Evans, D.R.; Gunna, V.; Scheffer, R.E.; Parikh, V.V.; Mahadik, S.P. Reduced erythrocyte membrane essential fatty acids and increased lipid peroxides in schizophrenia at the never-medicated first-episode of psychosis and after years of treatment with antipsychotics. *Schizophr. Res.* **2002**, *58*, 1–10. [CrossRef]
24. Brigandi, S.; Shao, H.; Qian, S.; Shen, Y.; Wu, B.-L.; Kang, J. Autistic Children Exhibit Decreased Levels of Essential Fatty Acids in Red Blood Cells. *Int. J. Mol. Sci.* **2015**, *16*, 10061. [CrossRef]

25. Vancassel, S.; Durant, G.; Lejeune, B.; Martineau, J.; Guiloteau, D.; Andres, C.; Chalon, S. Plasma fatty acid levels of autistic children. *Prostaglandins Leukot. Essent. Fatty Acids* **2001**, *65*, 1–7. [CrossRef] [PubMed]
26. Mostafa, G.A.; Al-Ayadhi, L.Y. Reduced levels of plasma polyunsaturated fatty acids and serum carnitine in autistic children: Relation to gastrointestinal manifestations. *Behav. Brain Funct.* **2015**, *11*, 4. [CrossRef] [PubMed]
27. Bell, J.G.; Miller, D.; MacDonald, D.J.; MacKinlay, E.E.; Dick, J.R.; Cheseldine, S.; Boyle, R.M.; Graham, C.; O'Hare, A.E. The fatty acid compositions of erythrocyte and plasma polar lipids in children with autism, developmental delay or typically developing controls and the effect of fish oil intake. *Br. J. Nutr.* **2010**, *103*, 1160–1167. [PubMed]
28. Bu, B.; Ashwood, P.; Harvey, D.; King, I.B.; van de Water, J.; Jin, L.W. Fatty acid compositions of red blood cell phospholipids in children with autism. *Prostaglandins Leukot. Essent. Fatty Acids* **2006**, *74*, 215–221. [CrossRef] [PubMed]
29. Johnson, C.; Handen, B.; Zimmer, M.; Sacco, K. Polyunsaturated Fatty Acid Supplementation in Young Children with autism. *J. Dev. Phys. Disabil.* **2010**, *22*, 1–10. [CrossRef]
30. Meguid, N.A.; Atta, H.M.; Gouda, A.S.; Khalil, R.O. Role of polyunsaturated fatty acids in the management of Egyptian children with autism. *Clin. Biochem.* **2008**, *41*, 1044–1048. [CrossRef] [PubMed]
31. Meiri, G.; Bichovsky, Y.; Belmaker, R.H. Omega 3 fatty acid treatment in autism. *J. Child Adolesc. Psychopharmacol.* **2009**, *19*, 449–451. [CrossRef] [PubMed]
32. Ooi, Y.P.; Weng, S.J.; Jang, L.Y.; Low, L.; Seah, J.; Teo, S.; Ang, R.P.; Lim, C.G.; Liew, A.; Fung, D.S.; Sung, M. Omega-3 fatty acids in the management of Autism Spectrum Disorders: Findings from an open-label pilot study in Singapore. *Eur. J. Clin. Nutr.* **2015**, *69*, 969–971. [CrossRef] [PubMed]
33. Patrick, L.; Salik, R. The Effect Of Essential Fatty Acid Supplementation on Language Development and Learning Skills in Autism and Aspergers Syndrome. *Autism Asperger's Digest. Jan-Feb* **2005**, 36–37.
34. Politi, P.; Cena, H.; Comelli, M.; Marrone, G.; Allegri, C.; Emanuele, E.; Ucelli di Nemi, S. Behavioral Effects of Omega-3 Fatty Acid Supplementation in Young Adults with Severe Autism: An Open Label Study. *Arch. Med. Res.* **2008**, *39*, 682–685. [CrossRef] [PubMed]
35. Johnson, S.M.; Hollander, E. Evidence that eicosapentaenoic acid is effective in treating Autism. *J. Clin. Psychiatry* **2003**, *64*, 848–849. [CrossRef] [PubMed]
36. Amminger, G.P.; Berger, G.E.; Schäfer, M.R.; Klier, C.; Friedrich, M.H.; Feucht, M. Omega-3 Fatty Acids Supplementation in Children with Autism: A Double-blind Randomized, Placebo-controlled Pilot Study. *Biol. Psychiatry* **2007**, *61*, 551–553. [CrossRef] [PubMed]
37. Mankad, D.; Dupuis, A.; Smile, S.; Roberts, W.; Brian, J.; Lui, T.; Genore, L.; Zaghloul, D.; Iaboni, A.; Marcon, P.M.; et al. A randomized, placebo controlled trial of omega-3 fatty acids in the treatment of young children with autism. *Mol. Autism* **2015**, *6*, 18. [CrossRef]
38. Bent, S.; Bertoglio, K.; Hendren, R.L. Omega-3 fatty acids for Autistic Spectrum Disorder: A systematic review. *J. Autism Dev. Disord.* **2009**, *39*, 1145–1154. [CrossRef] [PubMed]
39. James, S.; Montgomery, P.; Williams, K. Omega-3 fatty acids supplementation for Autism Spectrum Disorders (ASD). *Cochrane Database Syst. Rev.* **2011**, *9*, CD007992.
40. Brondino, N.; Brondino, N.; Fusar-Poli, L.; Rocchetti, M.; Provenzani, U.; Barale, F.; Politi, P. Complementary and Alternative Therapies for Autism Spectrum Disorder. *Evid. Based Complement. Altern. Med. eCAM* **2015**, *2015*, 258589. [CrossRef] [PubMed]
41. Stonehouse, W. Does Consumption of LC Omega-3 PUFA Enhance Cognitive Performance in Healthy School-Aged Children and throughout Adulthood? Evidence from Clinical Trials. *Nutrients* **2014**, *6*, 2730–2758. [CrossRef] [PubMed]
42. LaChance, L.; McKenzie, K.; Taylor, V.H.; Vigod, S.N. Omega-6 to Omega-3 Fatty Acid Ratio in Patients with ADHD: A Meta-Analysis. *J. Can. Acad. Child Adolesc. Psychiatry* **2016**, *25*, 87–96. [PubMed]
43. Bolte, E.E.; Diehl, J.J. Measurement tools and target symptoms/skills used to assess treatment response for individuals with Autism Spectrum Disorder. *J. Autism Dev. Disord.* **2013**, *43*, 2491–2501. [CrossRef] [PubMed]
44. Leon, A.C. Implications of Clinical Trial Design on Sample Size Requirements. *Schizophr. Bull.* **2008**, *34*, 664–669. [CrossRef] [PubMed]
45. Sun, Q.; Ma, J.; Campos, H.; Hankinson, S.E.; Hu, F.B. Comparison between plasma and erythrocyte fatty acid content as biomarkers of fatty acid intake in US women. *Am. J. Clin. Nutr.* **2007**, *86*, 74–81. [PubMed]

46. Sergeant, S.; Ruczinski, I.; Ivester, P.; Lee, T.C.; Morgan, T.M.; Nicklas, B.J.; Mathias, R.A.; Chilton, F.H. Impact of methods used to express levels of circulating fatty acids on the degree and direction of associations with blood lipids in humans. *Br. J. Nutr.* **2016**, *115*, 251–261. [CrossRef] [PubMed]
47. Health Canada. *Guidance Document for Preparing a Submission for Food Health Claims, Bureau of Nutritional Sciences Food Directorate*; Health Products and Food Branch Health Canada: Ottawa, ON, Canada, 2009.
48. Higgins, J.P.T.; Green, S. Cochrane Handbook for Systematic Reviews of Interventions. Available online: http://training.cochrane.org/handbook (accessed on 11 February 2016).
49. Sliwinski, S.; Croonenberghs, J.; Christophe, A.; Deboutte, D.; Maes, M. Polyunsaturated fatty acids: Do they have a role in the pathophysiology of autism? *Neuro Endocrinol. Lett.* **2006**, *27*, 465–471. [PubMed]
50. El-Ansary, A.K.; Ben Bacha, A.G.; Al-Ayahdi, L.Y. Impaired plasma phospholipids and relative amounts of essential polyunsaturated fatty acids in autistic patients from Saudi Arabia. *Lipids Health Dis.* **2011**, *10*, 63. [CrossRef] [PubMed]
51. Jory, J. Abnormal fatty acids in Canadian children with autism. *Nutrition* **2016**, *32*, 474–477. [CrossRef] [PubMed]
52. Parletta, N.; Niyonsenga, T.; Duff, J. Omega-3 and Omega-6 Polyunsaturated Fatty Acid Levels and Correlations with Symptoms in Children with Attention Deficit Hyperactivity Disorder, Autistic Spectrum Disorder and Typically Developing Controls. *PLoS ONE* **2016**, *11*, e0156432. [CrossRef] [PubMed]
53. Yui, K.; Imataka, G.; Kawasak, Y.; Yamada, H. Increased omega-3 polyunsaturated fatty acid/arachidonic acid ratios and upregulation of signaling mediator in individuals with Autism Spectrum Disorders. *Life Sci.* **2016**, *145*, 205–212. [CrossRef] [PubMed]
54. Yui, K.; Koshiba, M.; Nakamura, S.; Kobayashim, Y.; Ohnishi, M. Efficacy of Adding Large Doses of Arachidonic Acid to Docosahexaenoic Acid against Restricted Repetitive Behaviors in Individuals with Autism Spectrum Disorders: A Placebo-Controlled Trial. *J. Addict. Res.Ther.* **2011**. [CrossRef]
55. Voigt, R.G.; Mellon, M.W.; Katusic, S.K.; Weaver, A.L.; Matern, D.; Mellon, B.; Jensen, C.L.; Barbaresi, W.J. Dietary docosahexaenoic acid supplementation in children with autism. *J. Pediatr. Gastroenterol. Nutr.* **2014**, *58*, 715–722. [PubMed]
56. Parellada, M.; Llorente, C.; Calvo, R.; Gutierrez, S.; Lazaro, L.; Graell, M.; Alvarez, M.; Guisasola, M.; Dulin, E.; Dorado, M.L.; et al. Double-blind crossed-over randomized controlled-trial with omega-3 fatty acids for Autism Spectrum Disorders. *Eur. Neuropsychopharmacol.* **2015**, *25*, S138. [CrossRef]
57. Yui, K.; Koshiba, M.; Nakamura, S.; Kobayashi, Y. Effects of Large Doses of Arachidonic Acid Added to Docosahexaenoic Acid on Social Impairment in Individuals With Autism Spectrum Disorders: A Double-Blind, Placebo-Controlled, Randomized Trial. *J. Clin. Psychopharmacol.* **2012**, *32*, 200–206. [CrossRef] [PubMed]
58. Esparham, A.E.; Smith, T.; Belmont, J.M.; Haden, M.; Wagner, L.E.; Evans, R.G.; Drisko, J.A. Nutritional and Metabolic Biomarkers in Autism Spectrum Disorders: An Exploratory Study. *Integr. Med.* **2015**, *14*, 40–53.
59. Wang, H.; Liang, S.; Wang, M.; Gao, J.; Sun, C.; Wang, J.; Xia, W.; Wu, S.; Sumner, S.J.; Zhang, F.; et al. Potential serum biomarkers from a metabolomics study of autism. *J. Psychiatry Neurosci.* **2016**, *41*, 27–37. [CrossRef] [PubMed]
60. Wiest, M.M.; German, J.B.; Harvey, D.J.; Watkins, S.M.; Hertz-Picciotto, I. Plasma fatty acid profiles in autism: A case-control study. *Prostaglandins Leukot. Essent. Fatty Acids* **2009**, *80*, 221–227. [CrossRef] [PubMed]
61. Pastural, É.; Ritchie, S.; Lu, Y.; Jin, W.; Kavianpour, A.; Khine, S.-M.K.; Heath, D.; Wood, P.L.; Fisk, M.; Goodenowe, D.B. Novel plasma phospholipid biomarkers of autism: Mitochondrial dysfunction as a putative causative mechanism. *Prostaglandins Leukot. Essent. Fatty Acids* **2009**, *81*, 253–264. [CrossRef] [PubMed]
62. Bell, J.G.; Sargent, J.R.; Tocher, D.R.; Dick, J.R. Red blood cell fatty acid compositions in a patient with Autistic Spectrum Disorder: A characteristic abnormality in neurodevelopmental disorders? *Prostaglandins Leukot. Essent. Fatty Acids* **2000**, *63*, 21–25. [CrossRef] [PubMed]
63. Yui, K.; Imataka, G.; Kawasaki, Y. Competitive Interaction Between Plasma Omega-3 Fatty Acids and Arachidonic Acid is Related to Down-Regulation of A Signaling Mediator. *Med. Chem.* **2016**, *12*, 318–327. [CrossRef] [PubMed]
64. Yui, K.; Imataka, G.; Kawasaki, Y.; Yamada, T. Down-regulation of Signaling Mediator in Related to Increased Ratio of Docosahexaenoic Acid/Arachidonic Acid in Individuals with Autism Spectrum Disorders. *J. Transl. Med. Dev. Disord.* **2015**, *2*, 1–9.

65. El-Ansary, A.K.; Ben Bacha, A.G.; Al-Ayahdi, L.Y. Plasma fatty acids as diagnostic markers in autistic patients from Saudi Arabia. *Lipids Health Dis.* **2011**, *10*. [CrossRef] [PubMed]
66. Bell, J.G.; MacKinlay, E.E.; Dick, J.R.; MacDonald, D.J.; Boyle, R.M.; Glen, A.C. Essential fatty acids and phospholipase A2 in Autistic Spectrum Disorders. *Prostaglandins Leukot. Essent. Fatty Acids* **2004**, *71*, 201–204. [CrossRef] [PubMed]
67. Al-Farsi, Y.M.; Waly, M.I.; Deth, R.C.; Al-Sharbati, M.M.; Al-Shafaee, M.; Al-Farsi, O.; Al-Khaduri, M.M.; Al-Adawi, S.; Hodgson, N.W.; Gupta, I.; et al. Impact of nutrition on serum levels of docosahexaenoic acid among Omani children with autism. *Nutrition* **2013**, *29*, 1142–1146. [CrossRef] [PubMed]
68. Tostes, M.H.; Polonini, H.C.; Mendes, R.; Brandao, M.A.; Gattaz, W.F.; Raposo, N.R. Fatty acid and phospholipase A2 plasma levels in children with autism. *Trends Psychiatry Psychother.* **2013**, *35*, 76–80. [CrossRef] [PubMed]
69. Bent, S.; Bertoglio, K.; Ashwood, P.; Bostrom, A.; Hendren, R.L. A pilot randomized controlled trial of omega-3 fatty acids for Autism Spectrum Disorder. *J. Autism Dev. Disord.* **2011**, *41*, 545–554. [CrossRef] [PubMed]
70. Bent, S.; Hendren, R.L.; Zandi, T.; Law, K.; Choi, J-E.; Widjaja, F.; Kalb, L.; Nestle, J.; Law, P. Internet-Based, Randomized, Controlled Trial of Omega-3 Fatty Acids for Hyperactivity in Autism. *J. Am. Acad. Child Adolesc. Psychiatry* **2014**, *53*, 658–666. [CrossRef] [PubMed]
71. Hawkey, E.; Nigg, J.T. Omega-3 fatty acid and ADHD: Blood level analysis and meta-analytic extension of supplementation trials. *Clin. Psychol. Rev.* **2014**, *34*, 496–505. [CrossRef] [PubMed]
72. Harris, W.S.; Pottala, J.V.; Varvel, S.A.; Borowski, J.J.; Ward, J.N.; McConnell, J.P. Erythrocyte omega-3 fatty acids increase and linoleic acid decreases with age: Observations from 160,000 patients. *Prostaglandins Leukot Essent Fatty Acids* **2013**, *88*, 257–263. [CrossRef] [PubMed]
73. Laryea, M.; Cieslicki, P.; Diekmann, E.; Wendel, U. Age-dependent fatty acid composition of erythrocyte membrane phospholipids in healthy children. *Z. Ernahrungswiss.* **1990**, *29*, 284–294. [CrossRef] [PubMed]
74. Evans, D.R.; Parikh, V.V.; Khan, M.M.; Coussons, C.; Buckley, P.F.; Mahadik, S.P. Red blood cell membrane essential fatty acid metabolism in early psychotic patients following antipsychotic drug treatment. *Prostaglandins Leukot. Essent. Fatty Acids* **2003**, *69*, 393–399. [CrossRef] [PubMed]
75. Castano, A.; Cutanda, F.; Esteban, M.; Part, P.; Navarro, C.; Gomez, S.; Rosado, M.; Lopez, A.; Lopez, E.; Exley, K.; et al. Fish consumption patterns and hair mercury levels in children and their mothers in 17 EU countries. *Environ. Res.* **2015**, *141*, 58–68. [CrossRef] [PubMed]
76. Flock, M.R.; Skulas-Ray, A.C.; Harris, W.S.; Etherton, T.D.; Fleming, J.A.; Kris-Etherton, P.M. Determinants of erythrocyte omega-3 fatty acid content in response to fish oil supplementation: A dose-response randomized controlled trial. *J. Am. Heart Assoc.* **2013**, *2*, e000513. [CrossRef] [PubMed]
77. Lagerstedt, S.A.; Hinrichs, D.R.; Batt, S.M.; Magera, M.J.; Rinaldo, P.; McConnell, J.P. Quantitative determination of plasma c8-c26 total fatty acids for the biochemical diagnosis of nutritional and metabolic disorders. *Mol. Genet. Metab.* **2001**, *73*, 38–45. [CrossRef] [PubMed]
78. Alessandri, J.M.; Extier, A.; Al-Gubory, K.H.; Harbeby, E.; Lallemand, M.S.; Linard, A.; Lavialle, M.; Guesnet, P. Influence of gender on DHA synthesis: The response of rat liver to low dietary alpha-linolenic acid evidences higher omega3 4-desaturation index in females. *Eur. J. Nutr.* **2012**, *51*, 199–209. [CrossRef] [PubMed]
79. Katan, M.B.; Deslypere, J.P.; van Birgelen, A.P.; Penders, M.; Zegwaard, M. Kinetics of the incorporation of dietary fatty acids into serum cholesteryl esters, erythrocyte membranes, and adipose tissue: An 18-month controlled study. *J. Lipid Res.* **1997**, *38*, 2012–2022. [PubMed]
80. Raine, A.; Portnoy, J.; Liu, J.; Mahoomed, T.; Hibbeln, J.R. Reduction in behavior problems with omega-3 supplementation in children aged 8–16 years: A randomized, double-blind, placebo-controlled, stratified, parallel-group trial. *J. Child Psychol. Psychiatry* **2015**, *56*, 509–520. [CrossRef] [PubMed]
81. Sun, C.; Xia, W.; Zhao, Y.; Li, N.; Zhao, D.; Wu, L. Nutritional status survey of children with autism and typically developing children aged 4–6 years in Heilongjiang Province, China. *J. Nutr. Sci.* **2013**, *2*, e16.
82. Wang, L.W.; Tancredi, D.J.; Thomas, D.W. The prevalence of gastrointestinal problems in children across the United States with Autism Spectrum Disorders from families with multiple affected members. *J. Dev. Behav. Pediatr.* **2011**, *32*, 351–360. [CrossRef] [PubMed]

83. Mazurek, M.O.; Vasa, R.A.; Kalb, L.G.; Kanne, S.M.; Rosenberg, D.; Keefer, A.; Murray, D.S.; Freedman, B.; Lowery, L.A. Anxiety, sensory over-responsivity, and gastrointestinal problems in children with Autism Spectrum Disorders. *J. Abnorm. Child Psychol.* **2013**, *41*, 165–176. [CrossRef] [PubMed]
84. Chaidez, V.; Hansen, R.L.; Hertz-Picciotto, I. Gastrointestinal problems in children with autism, developmental delays or typical development. *J. Autism Dev. Disord.* **2014**, *44*, 1117–1127. [CrossRef] [PubMed]
85. Agid, O.; Siu, C.O.; Potkin, S.G.; Kapur, S.; Watsky, E.; Vanderburg, D.; Zipursky, R.B.; Remington, G. Meta-regression analysis of placebo response in antipsychotic trials, 1970–2010. *Am. J. Psychiatry* **2013**, *170*, 1335–1344. [CrossRef] [PubMed]
86. Masi, A.; Lampit, A.; Glozier, N.; Hickie, I.B.; Guastella, A.J. Predictors of placebo response in pharmacological and dietary supplement treatment trials in pediatric Autism Spectrum Disorder: A meta-analysis. *Transl. Psychiatry* **2015**, *5*, e640. [CrossRef] [PubMed]
87. King, B.H.; Dukes, K.; Donnelly, C.L.; Sikich, L.; McCracken, J.T.; Scahill, L.; Hollander, E.; Bregman, J.D.; Anagnostou, E.; Robinson, F.; et al. Baseline factors predicting placebo response to treatment in children and adolescents with Autism Spectrum Disorders: A multisite randomized clinical trial. *JAMA Pediatr.* **2013**, *167*, 1045–1052. [CrossRef] [PubMed]
88. Das, U.N. Autism as a disorder of deficiency of brain-derived neurotrophic factor and altered metabolism of polyunsaturated fatty acids. *Nutrition* **2013**, *29*, 1175–1185. [CrossRef] [PubMed]
89. Das, U.N. Nutritional factors in the pathobiology of autism. *Nutrition* **2013**, *29*, 1066–1069. [CrossRef] [PubMed]
90. Singh, M. Essential fatty acids, DHA and human brain. *Indian J. Pediatr.* **2005**, *72*, 239–242. [CrossRef] [PubMed]
91. Petropoulos, H.; Friedman, S.D.; Shaw, D.W.; Artru, A.A.; Dawson, G.; Dager, S.R. Gray matter abnormalities in Autism Spectrum Disorder revealed by T2 relaxation. *Neurology* **2006**, *67*, 632–636. [CrossRef] [PubMed]
92. Rojas, D.C.; Peterson, E.; Winterrowd, E.; Reite, M.L.; Rogers, S.J.; Tregellas, J.R. Regional gray matter volumetric changes in autism associated with social and repetitive behavior symptoms. *BMC Psychiatry* **2006**, *6*, 56. [CrossRef] [PubMed]
93. Pryweller, J.R.; Schauder, K.B.; Anderson, A.W.; Heacock, J.L.; Foss-Feig, J.H.; Newsom, C.R.; Loring, W.A.; Cascio, C.J. White matter correlates of sensory processing in autism spectrum disorders. *NeuroImage Clin.* **2014**, *6*, 379–387. [CrossRef] [PubMed]
94. Conklin, S.M.; Gianaros, P.J.; Brown, S.M.; Yao, J.K.; Hariri, A.R.; Manuck, S.B.; Muldoon, M.F. Long-chain omega-3 fatty acid intake is associated positively with corticolimbic gray matter volume in healthy adults. *Neurosci. Lett.* **2007**, *421*, 209–212. [CrossRef] [PubMed]
95. Murphy, M.G. Dietary fatty acids and membrane protein function. *J. Nutr. Biochem.* **1990**, *1*, 68–79. [CrossRef]
96. Ibarguren, M.; López, D.J.; Escribá, P.V. The effect of natural and synthetic fatty acids on membrane structure, microdomain organization, cellular functions and human health. *Biochim. Biophys. Acta* **2014**, *1838*, 1518–1528. [CrossRef] [PubMed]
97. Donahue, R.J.; Venkataraman, A.; Carroll, F.I.; Meloni, E.G.; Carlezon, W.A., Jr. Pituitary adenylate cyclase activating polypeptide disrupts motivation, social interaction, and attention in male Sprague-Dawley rats. *Biol. Psychiatry* **2016**, *80*, 955–964. [CrossRef] [PubMed]
98. Abu Shmais, G.A.; Al-Ayadhi, L.Y.; Al-Dbass, A.M.; El-Ansary, A.K. Mechanism of nitrogen metabolism-related parameters and enzyme activities in the pathophysiology of autism. *J. Neurodev. Disord.* **2012**, *4*, 4. [CrossRef] [PubMed]
99. Cao, D.; Xue, R.; Xu, J.; Liu, Z. Effects of docosahexaenoic acid on the survival and neurite outgrowth of rat cortical neurons in primary cultures. *J. Nutr. Biochem.* **2005**, *16*, 538–546. [CrossRef] [PubMed]
100. Mita, T.; Mayanagi, T.; Ichijo, H.; Fukumoto, K.; Otsuka, K.; Sakai, A.; Sobue, K. Docosahexaenoic acid promotes axon outgrowth by translational regulation of tau and collapsin response mediator protein 2 expression. *J. Biol. Chem.* **2016**, *291*, 4955–4965. [CrossRef] [PubMed]
101. Liu, Z.-H.; Yip, P.K.; Adams, L.; Davies, M.; Lee, J.W.; Michael, G.J.; Priestley, J.V.; Michael-Titus, A.T. A single bolus of docosahexaenoic acid promotes neuroplastic changes in the innervation of spinal cord interneurons and motor neurons and improves functional recovery after spinal cord injury. *J. Neurosci.* **2015**, *35*, 12733–12752. [CrossRef]

102. Robson, L.G.; Dyall, S.; Sidloff, D.; Michael-Titus, A.T. Omega-3 polyunsaturated fatty acids increase the neurite outgrowth of rat sensory neurones throughout development and in aged animals. *Neurobiol. Aging* **2010**, *31*, 678–687. [CrossRef] [PubMed]
103. Calderon, F.; Kim, H.Y. Docosahexaenoic acid promotes neurite growth in hippocampal neurons. *J. Neurochem.* **2004**, *90*, 979–988. [CrossRef] [PubMed]
104. Nakato, M.; Matsuo, M.; Kono, N.; Arita, M.; Arai, H.; Ogawa, J.; Kioka, N.; Ueda, K. Neurite outgrowth stimulation by *n*-3 and *n*-6 PUFAs of phospholipids in apoE-containing lipoproteins secreted from glial cells. *J. Lipid Res.* **2015**, *56*, 1880–1890. [CrossRef] [PubMed]
105. Zikopoulos, B.; Barbas, H. Changes in prefrontal axons may disrupt the network in autism. *J. Neurosci.* **2010**, *30*, 14595–14609. [CrossRef] [PubMed]
106. Zikopoulos, B.; Barbas, H. Altered neural connectivity in excitatory and inhibitory cortical circuits in autism. *Front. Hum. Neurosci.* **2013**, *7*, 609. [CrossRef] [PubMed]
107. Kasarpalkar, N.J.; Kothari, S.T.; Dave, U.P. Brain-derived neurotrophic factor in children with autism spectrum disorder. *Ann. Neurosci.* **2014**, *21*, 129–133. [CrossRef] [PubMed]
108. Bryn, V.; Halvorsen, B.; Ueland, T.; Isaksen, J.; Kolkova, K.; Ravn, K.; Skjeldal, O.H. Brain derived neurotrophic factor (BDNF) and Autism Spectrum Disorders (ASD) in childhood. *Eur. J. Paediatr. Neurol.* **2015**, *19*, 411–414. [CrossRef] [PubMed]
109. Wu, A.; Ying, Z.; Gomez-Pinilla, F. Dietary omega-3 fatty acids normalize BDNF levels, reduce oxidative damage, and counteract learning disability after traumatic brain injury in rats. *J. Neurotrauma* **2004**, *21*, 1457–1467. [CrossRef] [PubMed]
110. Martineau, J.; Barthelemy, C.; Jouve, J.; Muh, J.P.; Lelord, G. Monoamines (serotonin and catecholamines) and their derivatives in infantile autism: Age-related changes and drug effects. *Dev. Med. Child Neurol.* **1992**, *34*, 593–603. [CrossRef] [PubMed]
111. Nakamura, K.; Sekine, Y.; Ouchi, Y.; Tsujii, M.; Yoshikawa, E.; Futatsubashi, M.; Tsuchiya, K.J.; Sugihara, G.; Iwata, Y.; Suzuki, K.; et al. Brain serotonin and dopamine transporter bindings in adults with high-functioning autism. *Arch. Gen. Psychiatry* **2010**, *67*, 59–68. [CrossRef] [PubMed]
112. Chugani, D.C.; Muzik, O.; Behen, M.; Rothermel, R.; Janisse, J.J.; Lee, J.; Chugani, H.T. Developmental changes in brain serotonin synthesis capacity in autistic and nonautistic children. *Ann. Neurol.* **1999**, *45*, 287–295. [CrossRef]
113. Mulder, E.J.; Anderson, G.M.; Kema, I.P.; de Bildt, A.; van Lang, N.D.; den Boer, J.A.; Minderaa, R.B. Platelet serotonin levels in pervasive developmental disorders and mental retardation: Diagnostic group differences, within-group distribution, and behavioral correlates. *J. Am. Acad. Child Adolesc. Psychiatry* **2004**, *43*, 491–499. [CrossRef] [PubMed]
114. Husarova, V.M.; Lakatosova, S.; Pivovarciova, A.; Babinska, K.; Bakos, J.; Durdiakova, J.; Kubranska, A.; Ondrejka, I.; Ostatnikova, D. Plasma oxytocin in children with autism and its correlations with behavioral parameters in children and parents. *Psychiatry Investig.* **2016**, *13*, 174–183. [CrossRef] [PubMed]
115. Modahl, C.; Green, L.; Fein, D.; Morris, M.; Waterhouse, L.; Feinstein, C.; Levin, H. Plasma oxytocin levels in autistic children. *Biol. Psychiatry* **1998**, *43*, 270–277. [CrossRef]
116. Horder, J.; Lavender, T.; Mendez, M.A.; O'Gorman, R.; Daly, E.; Craig, M.C.; Lythgoe, D.J.; Barker, G.J.; Murphy, D.G. Reduced subcortical glutamate/glutamine in adults with Autism Spectrum Disorders: A [lsqb]1H[rsqb]MRS study. *Transl. Psychiatry* **2013**, *3*, e279. [CrossRef] [PubMed]
117. Delion, S.; Chalon, S.; Herault, J.; Guilloteau, D.; Besnard, J.C.; Durand, G. Chronic dietary alpha-linolenic acid deficiency alters dopaminergic and serotoninergic neurotransmission in rats. *J. Nutr.* **1994**, *124*, 2466–2476. [PubMed]
118. Zimmer, L.; Hembert, S.; Durand, G.; Breton, P.; Guilloteau, D.; Besnard, J.C.; Chalon, S. Chronic *n*-3 polyunsaturated fatty acid diet-deficiency acts on dopamine metabolism in the rat frontal cortex: A microdialysis study. *Neurosci. Lett.* **1998**, *240*, 177–181. [CrossRef]
119. Kodas, E.; Galineau, L.; Bodard, S.; Vancassel, S.; Guilloteau, D.; Besnard, J.C.; Chalon, S. Serotoninergic neurotransmission is affected by *n*-3 polyunsaturated fatty acids in the rat. *J. Neurochem.* **2004**, *89*, 695–702. [CrossRef] [PubMed]

120. Moreira, J.D.; Knorr, L.; Ganzella, M.; Thomazi, A.P.; de Souza, C.G.; de Souza, D.G.; Pitta, C.F.; Mello e Souza, T.; Wofchuk, S.; Elisabetsky, E.; et al. Omega-3 fatty acids deprivation affects ontogeny of glutamatergic synapses in rats: Relevance for behavior alterations. *Neurochem. Int.* **2010**, *56*, 753–759. [CrossRef] [PubMed]
121. Kim, H.-Y.; Spector, A.A.; Xiong, Z.-M. A synaptogenic amide *N*-docosahexaenoylethanolamide promotes hippocampal development. *Prostaglandins Other Lipid Mediat.* **2011**, *96*, 114–120. [CrossRef] [PubMed]
122. Naik, U.S.; Gangadharan, C.; Abbagani, K.; Nagalla, B.; Dasari, N.; Manna, S.K. A Study of nuclear transcription factor-kappa b in childhood autism. *PLoS ONE* **2011**, *6*, e19488. [CrossRef] [PubMed]
123. Inga Jácome, M.; Morales ChacÈn, L.M.; Vera Cuesta, H.; Maragoto Rizo, C.; Whilby Santiesteban, M.; Ramos Hernandez, L.; Noris García, E.; González Fraguela, M.E.; Fernandez Verdecia, C.I.; Vegas Hurtado, Y.; et al. Peripheral Inflammatory Markers Contributing to Comorbidities in Autism. *Behav. Sci.* **2016**, *6*, 29. [CrossRef] [PubMed]
124. El-Ansary, A.; Hassan, W.M.; Qasem, H.; Das, U.N. Identification of biomarkers of impaired sensory profiles among autistic patients. *PLoS ONE* **2016**, *11*, e0164153. [CrossRef] [PubMed]
125. El-Ansary, A.; Al-Ayadhi, L. Lipid mediators in plasma of autism spectrum disorders. *Lipids Health Dis.* **2012**, *11*, 1–9. [CrossRef] [PubMed]
126. Adams, J.B.; Baral, M.; Geis, E.; Mitchell, J.; Ingram, J.; Hensley, A.; Zappia, I.; Newmark, S.; Gehn, E.; Rubin, R.A.; et al. The severity of autism is associated with toxic metal body burden and red blood cell glutathione levels. *J. Toxicol.* **2009**, *2009*, 532640. [CrossRef] [PubMed]
127. SalLam, M.M.; Motaleb, F.I.A.; Ahmed, M.B.; Mahmoud, A.A. Anti-inflammatory effect of omega-3 polyunsaturated fatty acids in children with bronchial asthma; relation to nuclear factor-kappa B (NF-κB) and inflammatory cytokines IL-12 and IL-13. Egypt. *J. Biochem. Mol. Biol.* **2010**, *28*, 51–66.
128. Zhang, R.; He, G.-Z.; Wang, Y.-K.; Zhou, K.-G.; Ma, E.-L. Omega-3 polyunsaturated fatty acids inhibit the increase in cytokines and chemotactic factors induced in vitro by lymph fluid from an intestinal ischemia-reperfusion injury model. *Nutrition* **2015**, *31*, 508–514. [CrossRef] [PubMed]
129. Zhao, Y.; Joshi-Barve, S.; Barve, S.; Chen, L.H. Eicosapentaenoic acid prevents LPS-induced TNF-α expression by preventing NF-κB activation. *J. Am. Coll. Nutr.* **2004**, *23*, 71–78. [CrossRef] [PubMed]
130. Allam-Ndoul, B.; Guénard, F.; Barbier, O.; Vohl, M.-C. Effect of *n*-3 fatty acids on the expression of inflammatory genes in THP-1 macrophages. *Lipids Health Dis.* **2016**, *15*, 69. [CrossRef] [PubMed]
131. Mathias, R.A.; Sergeant, S.; Ruczinski, I.; Torgerson, D.G.; Hugenschmidt, C.E.; Kubala, M.; Vaidya, D.; Suktitipat, B.; Ziegler, J.T.; Ivester, P.; et al. The impact of FADS genetic variants on ω6 polyunsaturated fatty acid metabolism in African Americans. *BMC Genet.* **2011**, *12*, 50. [CrossRef] [PubMed]
132. Abdelmagid, S.A.; Clarke, S.E.; Roke, K.; Nielsen, D.E.; Badawi, A.; El-Sohemy, A.; Mutch, D.M.; Ma, D.W.L. Ethnicity, sex, FADS genetic variation, and hormonal contraceptive use influence delta-5- and delta-6-desaturase indices and plasma docosahexaenoic acid concentration in young Canadian adults: A cross-sectional study. *Nutr. Metab. (Lond.)* **2015**, *12*, 14. [CrossRef] [PubMed]
133. Chouinard-Watkins, R.; Plourde, M. Fatty acid metabolism in carriers of apolipoprotein e epsilon 4 allele: Is it contributing to higher risk of cognitive decline and coronary heart disease? *Nutrients* **2014**, *6*, 4452–4471. [CrossRef] [PubMed]
134. Shimamoto, C.; Ohnishi, T.; Maekawa, M.; Watanabe, A.; Ohba, H.; Arai, R.; Iwayama, Y.; Hisano, Y.; Toyota, T.; Toyoshima, M.; et al. Functional characterization of FABP3, 5 and 7 gene variants identified in schizophrenia and autism spectrum disorder and mouse behavioral studies. *Hum. Mol. Genet.* **2014**, *23*, 6495–6511. [CrossRef] [PubMed]

14

Combined Longitudinal Effect of Physical Activity and Screen Time on Food and Beverage Consumption in European Preschool Children: The ToyBox-Study

María L. Miguel-Berges [1,2,*], Alba M. Santaliestra-Pasias [1,2,3,4], Theodora Mouratidou [1], Pilar De Miguel-Etayo [1,2,4], Odysseas Androutsos [5], Marieke De Craemer [6], Sonya Galcheva [7], Berthold Koletzko [8], Zbigniew Kulaga [9], Yannis Manios [5] and Luis A. Moreno [1,2,3,4] on behalf of the ToyBox-study group

1 Growth, Exercise, Nutrition and Development (GENUD) Research Group, University of Zaragoza, C/Pedro Cerbuna 12, 50009 Zaragoza, Spain; albasant@unizar.es (A.M.S.-P.); theodoramouratidou@icloud.com (T.M.); pilardm@unizar.es (P.D.M.-E.); lmoreno@unizar.es (L.A.M.)
2 Instituto Agroalimentario de Aragón (IA2), 50009 Zaragoza, Spain
3 School of Health Science (EUCS), University of Zaragoza, C/Domingo Miral s/n, 50009 Saragossa, Spain
4 Centro de Investigación Biomédica en Red de Fisiopatología de la Obesidad y Nutrición (CIBERObn), 50009 Zaragoza, Spain
5 Department of Nutrition and Dietetics, School of Health Science and Education, Harokopio University, 17671 Athens, Greece; oandrou@hua.gr (O.A.); manios.toybox@hua.gr (Y.M.)
6 Department of Movement and Sports Sciences, Ghent University, Watersportlaan 2, 9000 Ghent, Belgium; marieke.decraemer@ugent.be
7 Department of paediatrics. Medical University Varna, 55 Marin Drinov Str., 9002 Varna, Bulgaria; sonya_galcheva@mail.bg
8 Dr von Hauner Children's Hospital, University of Munich Medical Centre, 80337 Munich, Germany; berthold.koletzko@med.uni-muenchen.de
9 The Children's Memorial Health Institute, 04-730 Warsaw, Poland; z.kulaga@ipczd.pl
* Correspondence: mlmiguel@unizar.es

Abstract: Lifestyle behavioral habits such as excess screen time (ST), a lack of physical activity (PA), and high energy-dense food consumption are associated with an increased risk of children being overweight or obese. This study aimed to (1) track longitudinal adherence to PA and ST recommendations at baseline (T0) and follow-up (T1) and (2) assess the association between changes in adherence to PA and ST recommendations and food and beverage consumption at follow-up. The present study included 2321 preschool children (3.5 to 6) participating in the multicenter ToyBox-study. A lineal mixed effects model was used to examine the association between different types of food and beverages and their relationship with changes in adherence to PA and ST recommendations. Approximately half of the children (50.4%) did not meet the PA and ST recommendations at both baseline and follow-up. However, only 0.6% of the sample met both PA and ST recommendations. Preschool children who met both recommendations consumed fewer fizzy drinks, juices, sweets, desserts, and salty snacks and consumed more water, fruits and vegetables, and dairy products than did those not meeting both recommendations. In conclusion, the proportion of European preschool children adhering to both PA and ST recommendations was very low and was associated with a low consumption of energy-dense foods.

Keywords: screen time; physical activity; preschool children; food and beverage consumption

1. Introduction

Being overweight or obese during childhood and adolescence is a major public health challenge [1]. Excess weight gain during childhood is associated with long-term health risks and adult diseases such as cardiovascular disease, type 2 diabetes, and hypertension [2]. Behaviors such as excessive screen time (ST), a lack of physical activity (PA), and high consumption of energy-dense foods have been shown to be independently associated with increased risks of being overweight or obese in children, adolescents, and adults [3]. Individually and combined, high sugar-sweetened beverage and low fruit and vegetable consumption are associated with an increased obesity risk [4,5], while behaviors such as PA appear to be protective [6,7]. Hence, it is crucial that interventions during childhood target lifestyle behaviors such as diet, physical activity, and sedentary behavior, which are established in early years and track into adulthood [8].

PA guidelines for preschool children recommend that preschool children should spend at least 180 min per day doing PA [9]. Limited evidence suggests that a total daily physical activity volume of 10,000–14,000 steps per day is associated with 60–100 min of moderate vigorous PA in preschool children [10]. De Craemer et al. [11] proposed using 11,500 steps per day as an attainable and realistic cut-off for PA recommendations, helping to promote PA among preschool children. Regarding ST, established guidelines for preschool children (one- to five-year-olds) state that they should limit TV viewing and use of other electronic media such as computers, DVDs, and other electronic games to less than one hour per day [9].

ST has been shown to be associated with increased energy-dense food and beverage consumption and decreased fruit and vegetable (F & V) consumption in preschool children [12]. In European children participating in the IDEFICS study, low time spent on moderate to vigorous physical activity (MVPA) was associated with a low consumption of vegetables and yogurt and high fast food consumption [13]. A low socioeconomic status was also associated with consumption of high energy-dense foods, increased ST, and low levels of PA [14,15].

To the authors' knowledge, there are no studies that have investigated the individual and combined effects of PA and ST on food consumption in preschool children. For this reason, the current study aimed to (1) track longitudinal adherence to PA and ST recommendations at baseline (T0) and follow-up (T1) and (2) assess the association between changes in the adherence to PA and ST recommendations and food and beverage consumption at follow-up (T1).

2. Methods

2.1. Study Design

The ToyBox-study (www.toybox-study.eu) was were a cluster-randomized clinical trial aiming to prevent obesity in preschool children. It was conducted in six European countries, namely Belgium, Bulgaria, Germany, Greece, Poland, and Spain. The detailed protocol is described elsewhere [16,17]. In total, 309 kindergarteners and 7056 children aged 3.5–6 years were recruited at baseline (T0), and 5529 children continued at follow-up (T1) [18]. The ToyBox intervention aimed to promote preschool children's water consumption, healthy snacking, and PA and limit/interrupt their sedentary time by improving the children's physical and social environment both in kindergarten and at home. In this study, 2321 (33% of the baseline sample) preschool children were included with complete information from a parental questionnaire and also pedometer information at baseline (T0) and follow-up (T1). Data collection was carried out in May–June 2012 (T0) and May–June 2013 (T1). The ToyBox-study adhered to the Declaration of Helsinki and the conventions of the Council of Europe on human rights and biomedicine. In all countries, ethical approval was obtained from their respective ethical committees and local authorities.

2.2. Socioeconomic Variables

Maternal education level (years of education) was recorded in five categories: less than 7 years, 7–12 years, 13–14 years, 15–16 years, and more than 16 years of education. For the purposes of the analysis, this was then recategorized into three categories: less than 7 years to 12 years, between 13 and 16 years, and more than 16 years of education. The selection of this indicator was based on its identification as the best proxy indicator of socioeconomic status [19].

2.3. Anthropometric Measures

Body weight was measured in underwear and without shoes using an electronic scale (Type SECA 861 or SECA 813) to the nearest 0.1 kg, and body height was measured with a telescopic height instrument (Type SECA 225 or SECA 214) to the nearest 0.1 cm. Body mass index (BMI) was calculated as weight (kg) divided by squared height (m^2). BMI z-scores (zBMI) were computed to classify children as being of a normal weight, being overweight, or being obese, for which the Cole et al. criteria were considered [20]. The intra- and interobserver reliability for weight and height was excellent (greater than 99% and 98%) in all participating countries [21].

2.4. Diet Assessment

Food and beverage consumption was assessed via a parentally reported semiquantitative food frequency questionnaire (FFQ) [22]. Low to moderate relative validity was observed, which varied by food and beverage group [23]. Estimated correlations ranged from 0.52 to 0.79. Food and beverage consumption was expressed as the number of portions per week. In the FFQ, 37 items were included, and in the current analysis they were merged into 21 groups according to their nutritional content (the main nutrient being proteins, carbohydrates, or fats). Of those 21, 10 were chosen and entered into the current analysis because they were considered to be associated with obesity development [24]: (1) water; (2) fizzy drinks (soft drinks and light drinks); (3) fresh fruit juices and packed juices; (4) dried, canned, and fresh fruits; (5) dairy products (milk, yogurt, and cheese); (6) sweets (chocolate and chocolate spreads, cakes, biscuits, and pastries); (7) desserts (smoothies, milk-based desserts, and sugar desserts); (8) meat and processed meat; (9) salty snacks; and (10) pasta and rice.

2.5. Physical Activity

In all of the countries except Belgium, PA was assessed by means of pedometers (Omron Walking Style Pro pedometers (HJ-720IT-E2)) assessing the number of steps per day. In Belgium, steps were measured using ActiGraph (Pensacola, FL, USA) accelerometers. Step counts from the accelerometers and pedometers were comparable. Evidence of their validity in preschool children indicated high correlations (daily, $r = 0.89$). In addition, evidence has suggested that the Omron Walking Style Pro pedometer is a valid and accurate measure to assess preschoolers' steps per hour [25]. The devices were worn on the right hip (secured by an elastic waistband) for six consecutive days, including two weekend days [22]. The steps were further categorized into two categories, including ≥11,500 steps per day (if children followed the PA recommendations) and <11,500 steps per day (if children did not follow the PA recommendations). The selected step count cut-off was based on Reilly et al. [26] and De Craemer et al. [11].

2.6. Screen Time

Data on children's screen time was collected via a standardized proxy-administered parental questionnaire (i.e., the Primary Caregivers' Questionnaire). Screen time was used as a proxy indicator of sedentary behavior. The behaviors assessed included watching TV and DVDs and playing computer/video games. Parents/caregivers reported frequency for both weekdays and weekend days. The frequency categories included "never", "less than 30 min/day", "30 min to 1 h/day", "1–2 h/day", "3–4 h/day", "5–6 h/day", "7–8 h/day", "8 h/day", and "more than 8 h/day". Average hours per day of TV/video viewing and personal computer use (separately for weekdays and weekend days) were summed up to obtain the screen time. To obtain the daily screen time, the average minutes per day, both for week- and weekend days, were summed up and divided by 7 days. The answers were further aggregated into two categories, including ≤1 h per day (if children followed the recommendations) and >1 h per day (if children did not follow the recommendations). These categories were based on the Australian and Canadian sedentary behavior recommendations, which state that preschool children should limit their screen time to a maximum of 1 h per day [9,27,28].

2.7. Statistical Analysis

Statistical analyses were performed using Statistical Package for the Social Sciences (version 21.0; SPSS, Inc., Chicago, IL, USA). Analysis was done for the whole sample, as there were no differences by sex in all of the included variables as tested using a *t*-test for continuous variables and a chi-squared test for categorical variables. In order to evaluate possible changes in the adherence to both behaviors (ST and PA) between T0 and T1, seven groups were established, reflecting differential combinations of meeting or not meeting the ST and/or PA recommendations. Figure 1 shows the seven groups derived from possible combinations of ST and/or PA recommendations. Two of them included children who got worse in their behaviors from T0 to T1 (meeting both recommendations at T0 and meeting one of the recommendations at T1; meeting one of the recommendations at T0 and not meeting any recommendations at T1). Two groups included children who improved in their behaviors from T0 to T1 (not meeting any recommendations at T0 and meeting one of the recommendations at T1; meeting one of the recommendations at T0 and meeting both recommendations at T1). The last three groups included children who maintained their behaviors from T0 to T1 (meeting both recommendations at T0 and T1; meeting one of the recommendations at T0 and T1; and not meeting any recommendations at T0 and T1). After establishing the potential combinations of ST and PA recommendations, a lineal mixed effects model with random effects for country and food consumption at T1 as predictor variables and z-BMI, maternal education, and intervention versus control region at T1 as covariates were analyzed. Marginal means and standard deviations (SE) were used to show differences in food and beverage consumption by PA and ST recommendation combinations. All statistical tests and corresponding *p*-values lower than 0.05 were considered statistically significant.

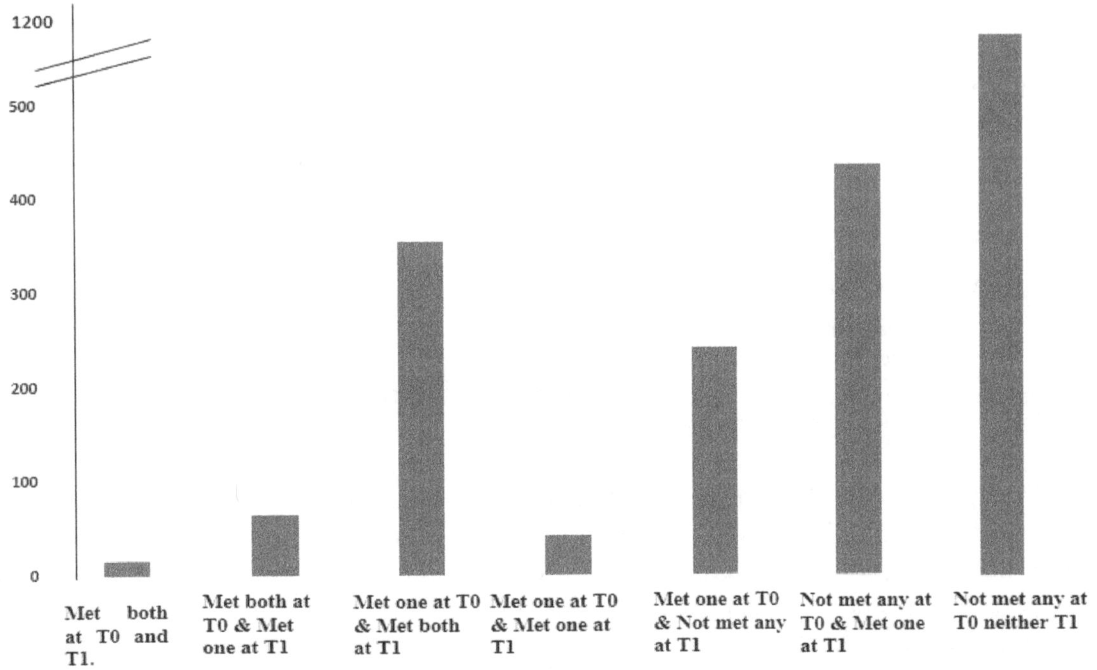

Figure 1. Proportion of European preschool children in each group. Groups are according to whether they met physical activity (PA) and/or screen time (ST) recommendations.

3. Results

Table 1 presents descriptive information on age, gender, BMI categories, z-BMI scores, maternal education, and country for the total sample, both at the T0 and T1 periods. According to BMI, 2.8% of the sample at T0 was obese and 10.6% was overweight, while 3.2% of the sample at T1 was obese and 10.3% was overweight.

Table 1. Descriptive characteristics of European preschool children participating in the ToyBox-study.

		T0	T1	*P*-Figvalue
		Mean (SE)	**Mean (SE)**	
Age (years)		4.74 (0.4)	5.72 (0.4)	<0.001
Sex	Boys	1209 (52.1)	1210 (52.1)	0.152
	Girls	1111 (47.9)	1111 (47.9)	
BMI status *	Normal weight	1988 (85.7)	1980 (85.3)	
	Overweight	245 (10.6)	240 (10.3)	<0.001
	Obese	64 (2.8)	75 (3.2)	
zBMI		0.20 (1.0)	0.27 (1.0)	<0.001
		n (%)		
Maternal education	<7–12	337 (14.5)		
(years)	13–16	947 (40.8)		0.104
	>16	965 (41.6)		
Center	Belgium	522 (22.5)		
	Bulgaria	74 (3.2)		
	Germany	284 (12.2)		0.645
	Greece	317 (13.7)		
	Poland	688 (29.6)		
	Spain	435 (18.7)		

Abbreviations: BMI, body mass index; zBMI, body mass index z-score; T0, baseline period; T1, follow-up period; * BMI according to Cole's cut-off [20].

Table 2 presents the proportion of the sample adhering to PA and ST recommendations for preschool children at both time points. Only 12.4% of children at T0 and 8.8% at T1 met the PA recommendation. In terms of ST, 30.2% of children at T0 and 27.7% at T1 met the recommendations.

Table 2. Number (%) of European preschool children participating in the ToyBox study that met or did not meet the physical activity and screen time recommendations at baseline (T0) and follow-up (T1) ($n = 2321$).

		T0 *n* (%)	T1 *n* (%)
Physical activity recommendations *	<11,500 steps/day	2033 (87.6)	2117 (91.2)
	≥11,500 steps/day	288 (12.4)	204 (8.8)
Screen time recommendations **	≤1 h/day	701 (30.2)	644 (27.7)
	>1 h/day	1620 (69.8)	1670 (72.3)

* Recommendations according to Reilly et al. [26] and De Craemer et al. [11] ** Recommendations on healthy eating and physical activity guidelines for early childhood settings in Australia [9,27,28].

Derived from the general linear model, Figure 2 presents the marginal means and SDs of eight food and beverage groups (F & V, dairy products, desserts, sweets, water, salty snacks, juices, and fizzy drinks), according to several grouping combinations for meeting or not meeting PA and ST recommendations at baseline (T0) and follow-up (T1). In general, preschool children who met both recommendations (PA and ST) consumed less dessert (Figure 2c), sweets (Figure 2d), salty snacks (Figure 2f), juices (Figure 2g), and fizzy drinks (Figure 2h) and more F & V (Figure 2a), dairy products (Figure 2b), and water (Figure 2e). In contrast, preschool children who failed to meet the recommendations over time had a higher consumption of desserts (Figure 2c), sweets (Figure 2d), juices (Figure 2g), and fizzy drinks (Figure 2h), and lower consumption of F & V (Figure 2a) and water (Figure 2e).

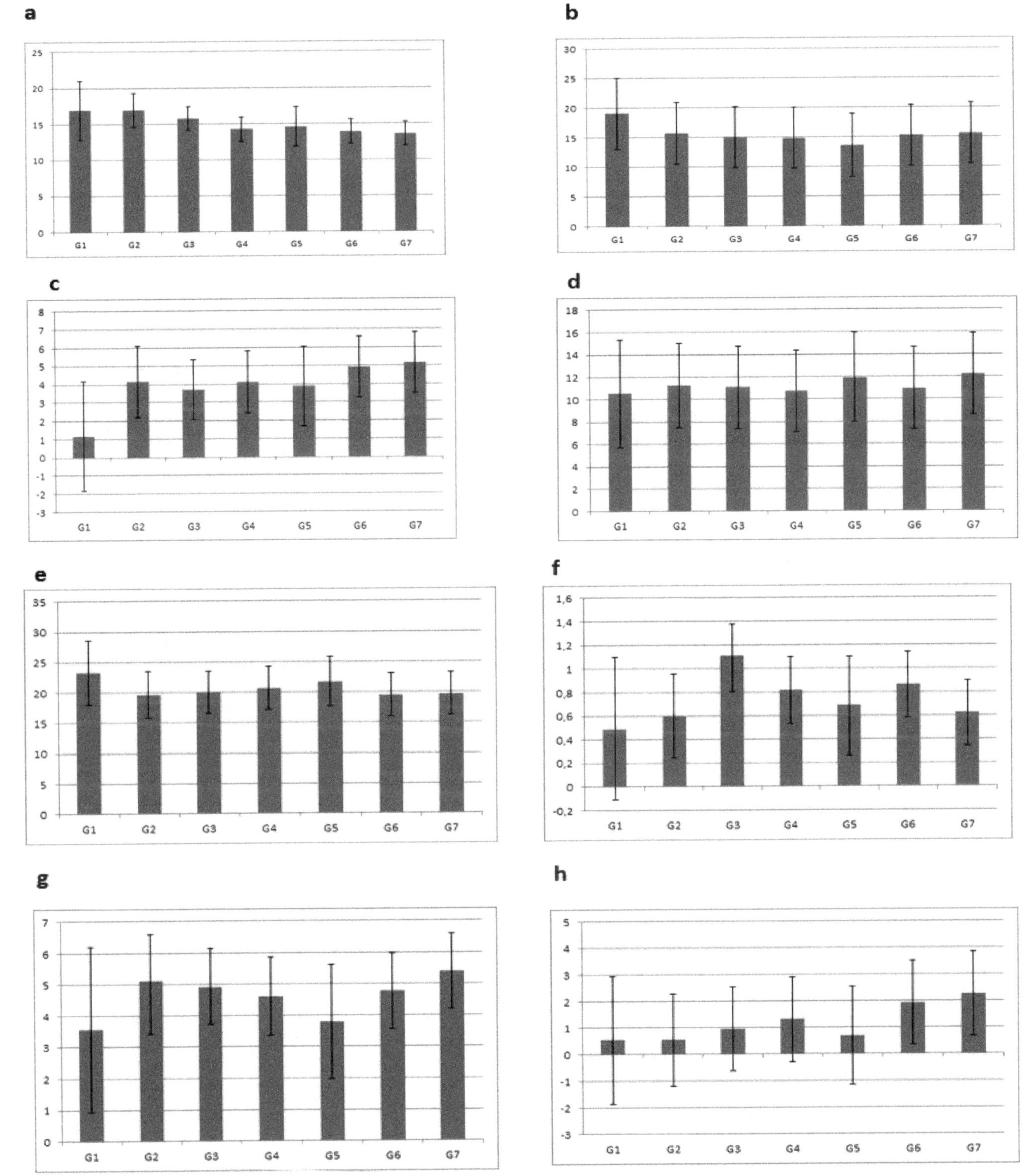

Figure 2. Marginal means and SD of food and beverage consumption (number of portions per week) according to PA and ST recommendations. G1: met both recommendations at T0 and met both recommendations at T1; G2: met both recommendations at T0 and met one of the recommendations at T1; G3: met one of the recommendations at T0 and met both recommendations at T1; G4: met one of the

recommendations at T0 and met one of the recommendations at T1; G5: met one of the recommendations at T0 and did not meet any recommendations at T1; G6: did not meet any recommendations at T0 and met one of the recommendations at T1; G7: did not meet any recommendations at T0 and did not meet any recommendations at T1. Adjusted for maternal education, body mass index z-score at T1, sex, and center. Abbreviations: PA, physical activity; ST, screen time; SD, standard deviation; T0, baseline period; T1, follow-up period; F & V, fruits and vegetables; dairy products (milk, yogurt and cheese); desserts (smoothies, milk-based desserts and sugar desserts); sweets (chocolate and chocolate spreads, cakes, biscuits and pastries); juices (fresh fruit juices and packed juices); fizzy drinks (soft drinks and light drinks). (**a**) F & V, (**b**) dairy products, (**c**) dessert, (**d**) sweets, (**e**) water, (**f**) salty snacks, (**g**) juices, (**h**) fizzy drinks.

Table 3 presents the associations between several grouping combinations of meeting or not meeting the PA and ST recommendations at T0 and at follow-up T1 and food and beverage consumption at follow up (T1). Seven possible combinations were identified. Approximately half of the sample (50.4%) did not meet either the PA or the ST recommendations in either period. With the opposite, only 0.6% of the sample met both PA and ST recommendations at both T0 and T1. Those who did not meet either recommendation at either time point (T0 and T1) were used as the reference group for analysis. Those children who met both recommendations at T0 and T1 consumed significantly fewer milk-based desserts and salty snacks in comparison to those who did not meet either recommendation at either time point. Those who met both recommendations at T0 and only one at T1 had a significantly lower consumption of fizzy drinks and salty snacks and higher consumption of F & V in comparison to the reference group. In addition, those children who met one of the recommendations at T0 and T1 had a significantly lower consumption of fizzy drinks, sweets, desserts, and salty snacks, and higher consumption of F & V. Those children who did not adhere to the recommendations at T0 and met one of them at T1 had a lower consumption of fizzy drinks, juices, sweets, desserts, and salty snacks in comparison to the reference group. At the same time, those children who met one of the recommendations at T0 and both at T1 had a lower consumption of fizzy drinks, juices, and salty snacks in comparison to not meeting either recommendation at either time point. Lastly, a significantly low consumption of juices, sweets, and salty snacks was observed in those children who met one of the recommendations at T0 and did not meet any recommendations at T1 in comparison to those who did not meet the PA and ST recommendations over time.

Table 3. Results of the lineal mixed effects model between food consumption and adherence to physical activity and screen time recommendations at baseline (T0) and follow-up (T1) periods (n = 2321).

PA and ST Recommendations at T0	PA and ST Recommendations at T1	n %	Water	Fizzy Drinks	Juices	F & V	Dairy Products	Sweets	Desserts	Meat and Processed Meat	Salty Snacks	Pasta and Rice
			β (95% CI)	β (95% CI)	β (95% CI)	β (95% CI)	β (95% CI)	β (95% CI)	β (95% CI)	β (95% CI)	β (95% CI)	β (95% CI)
Met both recommendations	Met both recommendations	15 (0.6)	3.41 (−1.22; 8.04)	−1.65 (−3.71; 0.41)	−1.84 (−4.32; 0.65)	3.32 (−0.62; 7.25)	3.43 (−0.77; 7.63)	−1.69 (−5.43; 2.04)	−4.03 (−6.75; −1.29) *	−2.38 (−5.06; 0.29)	−0.60 (−1.18; −0.02) *	0.49 (−0.51; 1.49)
Met both recommendations	Met one of the recommendations	64 (2.8)	0.25 (−2.16; 2.67)	−1.75 (−2.80; −0.69) *	−0.38 (−1.67; 0.90)	3.42 (1.41; 5.44) *	0.078 (−2.07; 2.23)	−0.93 (−2.84; 0.98)	−1,04 (−2.44; 0.35	−0.33 (−1.66; 0.99)	−0.51 (−0.80; −0.20) *	−0.26 (−0.77; 0.25)
Met one of the recommendations	Met both recommendations	354 (15.3)	1.76 (−1.09; 4.62)	−1.47 (−2.78; −0.16) *	−1.60 (−3.18; −0.02) *	0.99 (−1.50; 3.49)	−2.07 (−4.73; 0.59)	−0.32 (−2.69; 2.05)	−1.32 (−3.05; 0.40)	−0.10 (−1.77; 1.56)	−0.41 (−0.78; −0.04) *	−0.09 (−0.73; 0.55)
Met one of the recommendations	Met one of the recommendations	41 (1.8)	0.58 (−0.49; 1.66)	−1.34 (−1.82; −0.86) *	−0.47 (−1.05; 011)	2.29 (1.36; 3.20) *	−0.58 (−1.56; 0.40)	−1.15 (−2.03; −0.27) *	−1,45 (−2.08; −0.81) *	−0.56 (−1.17; 0.05)	−0.49 (−0.62; −0.35) *	0.01 (−0.22; 0.25)
Met one of the recommendations	Did not meet any recommendations	241 (10.4)	0.07 (−1.06; 1.21)	−0.34 (−0.85; 0.16)	−0.63 (−1.24; −0.01) *	0.38 (−0.58; 1.34)	−0.34 (−1.37; 0.69)	−1.24 (−2.15; −0.31) *	−0.24 (−0.90; 0.43)	−0.28 (−0.92; 0.35)	−0.24 (−0.38; −0.09) *	−0.21 (−0.46; 0.03)
Did not meet any recommendations	Met one of the recommendations	436 (18.8)	1.05 (−0.30; 2.41)	−0.97 (−1.55; −0.38) *	−0.78 (−1.49; −0.07) *	0.67 (−0.45; 1.79)	−0.74 (−1.92; 0.45)	−1.46 (−2.52; −0.40) *	−1.05 (−1.82; −0.27) *	−0.57 (−1.31; 0.17)	−0.29 (−0.46; −0.12) *	0.03 (−0.26; 0.31)
Did not meet any recommendations	Did not meet any recommendations	1170 (50.4)	REF	REF	REF	REF	REF	REF	REF	REF	REF	REF

Adjusted for maternal education, body mass index z-score at T1, sex, and center. Abbreviations: PA, physical activity; ST, screen time; REF, reference group not meeting any recommendations at either T0 or T1; CI, confidence interval; fizzy drinks (soft drinks and light drinks); juices (fresh fruit juices and packed juices); F & V, fruits and vegetables; dairy products (milk, yogurt, and cheese); sweets (chocolate and chocolate spreads, cakes, biscuits, and pastries); desserts (smoothies, milk-based desserts, and sugar desserts). * $P < 0.001$.

4. Discussion

In this study, associations between lifestyle behaviors, i.e., PA and ST and food and beverage consumption in preschool children, were investigated. The novelty of this report included examining adherence to both PA and ST recommendations across two time points and its relationship with food and beverage consumption in a large sample of European preschool children. The main finding of our study suggests that meeting both PA and ST recommendations at T0 and T1 was associated with a high consumption of foods considered healthy (F & V and water) and a lower consumption of energy-dense products (fizzy drinks, sweets, desserts, and salty snacks). In addition, we also observed a low proportion of children adhering to both recommendations during the follow-up.

The high proportion of children who failed to meet individual PA and ST recommendations at both periods agreed with results from other longitudinal studies, which observed similar trends. To our knowledge, there is no study reporting the proportion of preschool children meeting both PA and ST recommendations at the same time. Studies focusing on PA have reported that the percentage compliance with MVPA recommendations for European children is generally low [29]. The Health Behavior in School-Aged Children (HBSC) Study found that only 26% of its sample spent at least 1 h per day in MVPA [30]. Regarding ST, the HBSC study reported that 39% of the children complied with screen time recommendations [31]. In European children, approximately one-third of the children failed to meet current screen time recommendations [32]. An Australian study with a follow-up of three years reported that less than 20% of the sample met the ST recommendations and that screen time increased over the three-year follow-up. In addition, in an Australian study, participants were less likely to meet ST recommended guidelines as they got older [33].

In our sample, we found low levels of PA and high levels of ST in preschool children. The preschool age is an important period, as lifestyle behaviors such as PA and ST are established. However, different studies have observed that PA decreases during early childhood and adolescence [34,35] and even more so during the transition period from adolescence to adulthood [35,36]. Regarding ST, studies have observed an increase in ST during early childhood and also during the transition from primary to secondary school [37]. Both low PA and high ST have been associated with unfavorable body composition indicators such as BMI and waist circumference [38–40], both being determinants of obesity development in adulthood [33]. It has been suggested that ST, particularly TV, has an important role in the etiology of obesity due to its relationship with other unhealthy behaviors and its displacement of PA [41]. However, there is little evidence about the relationship between PA and ST on the one hand and food and beverage consumption on the other hand.

Previously, several cross-sectional studies analyzed the effects of PA or ST (alone) on food and beverage consumption. In European children (2–10 years old), boys and girls spending less time doing MVPA were more likely to consume fast food and less likely to consume vegetables and yogurt than those spending more time doing MVPA [13]. Similar associations were observed in European adolescents [42]: Those adolescents with the lowest PA levels consumed fewer fruits and dairy products compared to active adolescents. In a previous publication of the ToyBox study, those exceeding baseline ST recommendations had a higher consumption of energy-dense foods (sugar-based desserts, salty snacks, pastries, cakes, and biscuits) and beverages (fizzy drinks, sweet milk, and juices) than those complying with ST recommendations [12]. Another study reported that high TV viewing was related to less healthy food options (consumption of sweets and soft drinks) in children from different countries [43]. A study carried out in Brazil [44] in children less than two years old observed a positive association between time spent watching TV and the consumption of soft drinks. Santaliestra-Pasias et al. [45] reported that increased TV viewing and computer and internet use were associated with higher odds of sugar-sweetened beverage consumption and lower odds of fruit consumption in European adolescents. In an Australian adolescent sample, TV viewing was positively associated with energy-dense snack consumption and with higher availability of energy-dense snack foods at home [46].

There is consistent evidence to show that consumption of energy-dense foods is positively associated with low PA and high ST levels. However, research assessing the relationship between combinations of both PA and ST and food and beverage consumption is very scarce. Although high levels of both PA and ST have been observed in children [5], no studies have observed the combined effects of adherence to PA and ST recommendations on food and beverage consumption in preschool children.

This study had limitations. First, the generalizability of the findings is limited to the specific age group studied in the current study. The method used to assess PA was a pedometer, aside from Belgium. However, pedometers are not the gold standard in measuring preschool child PA, and therefore our results should be interpreted with caution. Nevertheless, the use of a pedometer provided objective information on PA, specifically in this age group. Information on food and beverage consumption and ST were collected via parental self-reported questionnaires, which are prone to over- or underreporting. However, the questionnaires used were developed/adapted and validated for the purposes of the study [22].

The main strengths of our study included the use of a large and culturally and socioeconomically diverse sample of preschool children from six different countries across Europe and its longitudinal design. Information through questionnaires was assessed via standardized and harmonized procedures [22].

5. Conclusions

This study examined the relationship between adherence to PA and ST recommendations and food and beverage consumption. In this sample of preschool children, we found that low PA levels and high ST were associated with an unhealthy food and beverage consumption profile. Preschool children and their parents should try to increase family time spent at activities promoting physical activity and to minimize the time they spend on screen time or being sedentary. In addition, public health interventions should focus on activities aimed at increasing movement in preschool children. Enabling healthier food and physical activity environments, together with the promotion of positive parental role modeling, should be prioritized to achieve higher rates of adherence to PA and ST recommendations.

Author Contributions: Y.M. and O.A. designed research; formal analysis, M.L.M.-B.; investigation M.L.M.-B., writing—original draft preparation, M.L.M.-B.; writing—review and editing, M.L.M.-B.; visualization, A.M.S.-P., T.M. and P.D.M.-E.; supervision, L.A.M.; funding acquisition, Y.M. All authors revised the manuscript for important intellectual content, read and approved the final manuscript.

References

1. *Obesity: Preventing and Managing the Global Epidemic: Report of a WHO Consultation*; World Health Organization: Geneva, Switzerland, 1999.
2. Dietz, W.H. Health consequences of obesity in youth: Childhood predictors of adult disease. *PEDIATRICS* **1998**, *101*, 518–525.
3. Van Stralen, M.M.; Velde, S.J.T.; Van Nassau, F.; Brug, J.; Grammatikaki, E.; Maes, L.; De Bourdeaudhuij, I.; Verbestel, V.; Galcheva, S.; Iotova, V.; et al. Weight status of European preschool children and associations with family demographics and energy balance-related behaviours: A pooled analysis of six European studies. *Obes. Rev.* **2012**, *13*, 29–41. [CrossRef] [PubMed]
4. Paes, V.M.; Hesketh, K.; O'Malley, C.; Moore, H.; Summerbell, C.; Griffin, S.; Van Sluijs, E.M.F.; Ong, K.K.; Lakshman, R. Determinants of sugar-sweetened beverage consumption in young children: A systematic review. *Obes. Rev.* **2015**, *16*, 903–913. [CrossRef] [PubMed]

5. Santaliestra-Pasías, A.M.; Mouratidou, T.; Reisch, L.; Pigeot, I.; Ahrens, W.; Mårild, S.; Molnár, D.; Siani, A.; Sieri, S.; Tornatiris, M.; et al. Clustering of lifestyle behaviours and relation to body composition in European children. The IDEFICS study. *Eur. J. Clin. Nutr.* **2015**, *69*, 811–816. [CrossRef] [PubMed]
6. Kimm, S.Y.; Glynn, N.W.; Obarzanek, E.; Kriska, A.M.; Daniels, S.R.; Barton, B.A.; Liu, K. Relation between the changes in physical activity and body-mass index during adolescence: A multicentre longitudinal study. *Lancet* **2005**, *366*, 301–307. [CrossRef]
7. Miguel-Berges, M.L.; Reilly, J.J.; Moreno Aznar, L.A.; Jimenez-Pavon, D. Associations Between Pedometer-Determined Physical Activity and Adiposity in Children and Adolescents: Systematic Review. *Clin. J. Sport Med.* **2017**, *28*, 64–75. [CrossRef] [PubMed]
8. Brug, J.; Van Stralen, M.M.; Velde, S.J.T.; Chinapaw, M.J.M.; De Bourdeaudhuij, I.; Lien, N.; Bere, E.; Maskini, V.; Singh, A.S.; Maes, L.; et al. Differences in Weight Status and Energy-Balance Related Behaviors among Schoolchildren across Europe: The ENERGY-Project. *PLoS ONE* **2012**, *7*, e34742. [CrossRef]
9. Australian Department of Health and Aging. *Get Up and Grow: Healthy Eating and Physical Activity for Early Childhood*. Available online: https://www.health.gov.au/internet/main/publishing.nsf/Content/2CDB3A000FE57A4ECA257BF0001916EC/$File/HEPA%20-%20B5%20Book%20-%20Staff%20and%20Carer%20Book_LR.pdf (accessed on 9 May 2019).
10. Tudor-Locke, C.; Craig, C.L.; Beets, M.W.; Belton, S.; Cardon, G.M.; Duncan, S.; Hatano, Y.; Lubans, D.R.; Olds, T.S.; Raustorp, A.; et al. How many steps/day are enough? for children and adolescents. *Int. J. Behav. Nutr. Phys. Act.* **2011**, *8*, 78. [CrossRef]
11. De Craemer, M.; De Decker, E.; De Bourdeaudhuij, I.; Verloigne, M.; Manios, Y.; Cardon, G. The translation of preschoolers' physical activity guidelines into a daily step count target. *J. Sports Sci.* **2014**, *33*, 1051–1057. [CrossRef]
12. Miguel-Berges, M.L.; on behalf of the ToyBox-study Group; Santaliestra-Pasias, A.M.; Mouratidou, T.; Androutsos, O.; De Craemer, M.; Pinket, A.-S.; Birnbaum, J.; Koletzko, B.; Iotova, V.; et al. Associations between food and beverage consumption and different types of sedentary behaviours in European preschoolers: The ToyBox-study. *Eur. J. Nutr.* **2016**, *56*, 1939–1951. [CrossRef]
13. Santaliestra-Pasías, A.M.; Dios, J.E.L.; Sprengeler, O.; Hebestreit, A.; De Henauw, S.; Eiben, G.; Felső, R.; Lauria, F.; Tornaritis, M.; Veidebaum, T.; et al. Food and beverage intakes according to physical activity levels in European children: The IDEFICS (Identification and prevention of Dietary and lifestyle induced health EFfects In Children and infantS) study. *Public Health Nutr.* **2018**, *21*, 1717–1725. [CrossRef] [PubMed]
14. Fernández-Alvira, J.M.; Mouratidou, T.; Bammann, K.; Hebestreit, A.; Barba, G.; Sieri, S.; Reisch, L.; Eiben, G.; Hadjigeorgiou, C.; Kovacs, E.; et al. Parental education and frequency of food consumption in European children: The IDEFICS study. *Public Health Nutr.* **2017**, *16*, 487–498. [CrossRef] [PubMed]
15. Miguel-Berges, M.L.; Zachari, K.; Santaliestra-Pasias, A.M.; Mouratidou, T.; Androutsos, O.; Iotova, V.; Galcheva, S.; De Craemer, M.; Cardon, G.; Koletzko, B.; et al. Clustering of energy balance-related behaviours and parental education in European preschool children: The ToyBox study. *Br. J. Nutr.* **2017**, *118*, 1089–1096. [CrossRef] [PubMed]
16. Androutsos, O.; Apostolidou, E.; Iotova, V.; Socha, P.; Birnbaum, J.; Moreno, L.; De Bourdeaudhuij, I.; Koletzko, B.; Manios, Y. Process evaluation design and tools used in a kindergarten-based, family-involved intervention to prevent obesity in early childhood. The ToyBox-study. *Obes. Rev.* **2014**, *15*, 74–80. [CrossRef] [PubMed]
17. Manios, Y. The 'ToyBox-study' obesity prevention programme in early childhood: An introduction. *Obes. Rev.* **2012**, *13*, 1–2. [CrossRef] [PubMed]
18. Manios, Y.; Androutsos, O.; Katsarou, C.; Iotova, V.; Socha, P.; Geyer, C.; Moreno, L.; Koletzko, B.; De Bourdeaudhuij, I. Designing and implementing a kindergarten-based, family-involved intervention to prevent obesity in early childhood: The ToyBox-study. *Obes. Rev.* **2014**, *15*, 5–13. [CrossRef] [PubMed]
19. Nixon, C.A.; Moore, H.J.; Douthwaite, W.; Gibson, E.L.; Vögele, C.; Kreichauf, S.; Wildgruber, A.; Manios, Y.; Summerbell, C. Identifying effective behavioural models and behaviour change strategies underpinning preschool- and school-based obesity prevention interventions aimed at 4–6-year-olds: A systematic review. *Obes. Rev.* **2012**, *13*, 106–117. [CrossRef]
20. Cole, T.J.; Bellizzi, M.C.; Flegal, K.M.; Dietz, W.H. Establishing a standard definition for child overweight and obesity worldwide: International survey. *BMJ* **2000**, *320*, 1240. [CrossRef]

21. De Miguel-Etayo, P.; Mesana, M.I.; Cardon, G.; De Bourdeaudhuij, I.; Góźdź, M.; Socha, P.; Lateva, M.; Iotova, V.; Koletzko, B.V.; Duvinage, K.; et al. Reliability of anthropometric measurements in European preschool children: The ToyBox-study. *Obes. Rev.* **2014**, *15*, 67–73. [CrossRef]
22. Mouratidou, T.; Miguel, M.L.; Androutsos, O.; Manios, Y.; De Bourdeaudhuij, I.; Cardon, G.; Kulaga, Z.; Socha, P.; Galcheva, S.; Iotova, V.; et al. Tools, harmonization and standardization procedures of the impact and outcome evaluation indices obtained during a kindergarten-based, family-involved intervention to prevent obesity in early childhood: The ToyBox-study. *Obes. Rev.* **2014**, *15*, 53–60. [CrossRef]
23. Mouratidou, T.; Graffe, M.I.M.; Huybrechts, I.; De Decker, E.; De Craemer, M.; Androutsos, O.; Manios, Y.; Galcheva, S.; Lateva, M.; Gurzkowska, B.; et al. Reproducibility and relative validity of a semiquantitative food frequency questionnaire in European preschoolers: The ToyBox study. *Nutrition* **2019**, *65*, 60–67. [CrossRef] [PubMed]
24. Commission of the European Communities. Green Paper: Promoting Healthy Diets and Physical Activity: A European Dimension for the Prevention of Overweight, Obesity, and Chronic Disease. 2005. Available online: https://publications.europa.eu/en/publication-detail/-/publication/fb6264c8-c756-47c4-944d-6d10bc9fce10/language-en (accessed on 9 May 2019).
25. De Craemer, M.; De Decker, E.; Santos-Lozano, A.; Verloigne, M.; De Bourdeaudhuij, I.; Deforche, B.; Cardon, G. Validity of the Omron pedometer and the actigraph step count function in preschoolers. *J. Sci. Med. Sport* **2015**, *18*, 289–293. [CrossRef] [PubMed]
26. Reilly, J.J.; Coyle, J.; Kelly, L.; Burke, G.; Grant, S.; Paton, J.Y. An Objective Method for Measurement of Sedentary Behavior in 3- to 4-Year Olds. *Obes. Res.* **2003**, *11*, 1155–1158. [CrossRef] [PubMed]
27. Leblanc, A.G.; Choquette, L.; Dillman, C.; Duggan, M.; Gordon, M.J.; Hicks, A.; Kho, M.E.; Latimer-Cheung, A.E.; Murumets, K.; Okely, A.D.; et al. Canadian Sedentary Behaviour Guidelines for the Early Years (aged 0–4 years). *Appl. Physiol. Nutr. Metab.* **2012**, *37*, 370–380. [CrossRef] [PubMed]
28. *Guidelines on Physical Activity, Sedentary Behaviour and Sleep for Children under 5 Years of Age*; World Health Organization: Geneva, Switzerland, 2019.
29. Konstabel, K.; on behalf of the IDEFICS consortium; Veidebaum, T.; Verbestel, V.; Moreno, L.A.; Bammann, K.; Tornaritis, M.; Eiben, G.; Molnár, D.; Siani, A.; et al. Objectively measured physical activity in European children: The IDEFICS study. *Int. J. Obes.* **2014**, *38*, S135–S143. [CrossRef] [PubMed]
30. Inequalities in Young People's Health: Health Behaviour in School-Aged Children (HBSC) Study. International Report from the 2005/2006 Survey. Available online: http://www.euro.who.int/__data/assets/pdf_file/0005/53852/E91416.pdf (accessed on 9 May 2019).
31. Sigmundová, D.; Sigmund, E.; Bucksch, J.; Bad'ura, P.; Kalman, M.; Hamřík, Z. Trends in Screen Time Behaviours in Czech Schoolchildren between 2002 and 2014: HBSC Study. *Cent. Eur. J. Public Health* **2017**, *25*, S15–S20. [CrossRef]
32. Santaliestra-Pasias, A.M.; Mouratidou, T.; Verbestel, V.; Bammann, K.; Molnar, D.; Sieri, S.; Siani, A.; Veidebaum, T.; Marild, S.; Lissner, L.; et al. Physical activity and sedentary behaviour in European children: The IDEFICS study. *Public Health Nutr.* **2014**, *17*, 2295–2306. [CrossRef]
33. Hesketh, K.; Wake, M.; Graham, M.; Waters, E. Stability of television viewing and electronic game/computer use in a prospective cohort study of Australian children: Relationship with body mass index. *Int. J. Behav. Nutr. Phys. Act.* **2007**, *4*, 60. [CrossRef]
34. Dumith, S.C.; Gigante, D.P.; Domingues, M.R.; Kohl, H.W., 3rd. Physical activity change during adolescence: A systematic review and a pooled analysis. *Int. J. Epidemiol.* **2011**, *40*, 685–698. [CrossRef] [PubMed]
35. Jones, R.A.; Hinkley, T.; Okely, A.D.; Salmon, J. Tracking Physical Activity and Sedentary Behavior in Childhood: A Systematic Review. *Am. J. Prev. Med.* **2013**, *44*, 651–658. [CrossRef]
36. Telama, R. Tracking of Physical Activity from Childhood to Adulthood: A Review. *Obes. Facts* **2009**, *2*, 187–195. [CrossRef] [PubMed]
37. Pearson, N.; Haycraft, E.; Johnston, J.P.; Atkin, A.J. Sedentary behaviour across the primary-secondary school transition: A systematic review. *Prev. Med.* **2017**, *94*, 40–47. [CrossRef]
38. Tremblay, M.S.; Leblanc, A.G.; Kho, M.E.; Saunders, T.J.; Larouche, R.; Colley, R.C.; Goldfield, G.; Gorber, S.C. Systematic review of sedentary behaviour and health indicators in school-aged children and youth. *Int. J. Behav. Nutr. Phys. Act.* **2011**, *8*, 98. [CrossRef] [PubMed]
39. Biddle, S.J.; Petrolini, I.; Pearson, N. Interventions designed to reduce sedentary behaviours in young people: A review of reviews. *Br. J. Sports Med.* **2014**, *48*, 182–186. [CrossRef]

40. Strong, W.B.; Malina, R.M.; Blimkie, C.J.; Daniels, S.R.; Dishman, R.K.; Gutin, B.; Hergenroeder, A.C.; Must, A.; Nixon, P.A.; Pivarnik, J.M.; et al. Evidence Based Physical Activity for School-age Youth. *J. Pediatr.* **2005**, *146*, 732–737. [CrossRef] [PubMed]
41. Birch, L.L.; Davison, K.K. Childhood overweight: A contextual model and recommendations for future research. *Obes. Rev.* **2001**, *2*, 159–171.
42. Ottevaere, C.; Huybrechts, I.; Béghin, L.; Cuenca-Garcia, M.; De Bourdeaudhuij, I.; Gottrand, F.; Hagströmer, M.; Kafatos, A.; Le Donne, C.; Moreno, L.A.; et al. Relationship between self-reported dietary intake and physical activity levels among adolescents: The HELENA study. *Int. J. Behav. Nutr. Phys. Act.* **2011**, *8*, 8. [CrossRef]
43. Vereecken, C.A.; Todd, J.; Roberts, C.; Mulvihill, C.; Maes, L. Television viewing behaviour and associations with food habits in different countries. *Publish Health Nutr.* **2006**, *9*, 244–250. [CrossRef]
44. Jaime, P.C.; Prado, R.R.D.; Malta, D.C. Family influence on the consumption of sugary drinks by children under two years old. *Rev. Saude Publica* **2017**, *51*, 13. [CrossRef]
45. Santaliestra-Pasías, A.M.; Mouratidou, T.; Verbestel, V.; Huybrechts, I.; Gottrand, F.; Donne, C.L.; Cuenca-García, M.; Díaz, L.E.; Kafatos, A.; Manios, Y.; et al. Food Consumption and Screen-Based Sedentary Behaviors in European Adolescents: The HELENA Study. *Arch. Pediatr. Adolesc. Med.* **2012**, *166*, 1010–1020. [CrossRef] [PubMed]
46. Pearson, N.; Biddle, S.J.; Williams, L.; Worsley, A.; Crawford, D.; Ball, K. Adolescent television viewing and unhealthy snack food consumption: The mediating role of home availability of unhealthy snack foods. *Public Health Nutr.* **2014**, *17*, 317–323. [CrossRef] [PubMed]

Permissions

All chapters in this book were first published by MDPI; hereby published with permission under the Creative Commons Attribution License or equivalent. Every chapter published in this book has been scrutinized by our experts. Their significance has been extensively debated. The topics covered herein carry significant findings which will fuel the growth of the discipline. They may even be implemented as practical applications or may be referred to as a beginning point for another development.

The contributors of this book come from diverse backgrounds, making this book a truly international effort. This book will bring forth new frontiers with its revolutionizing research information and detailed analysis of the nascent developments around the world.

We would like to thank all the contributing authors for lending their expertise to make the book truly unique. They have played a crucial role in the development of this book. Without their invaluable contributions this book wouldn't have been possible. They have made vital efforts to compile up to date information on the varied aspects of this subject to make this book a valuable addition to the collection of many professionals and students.

This book was conceptualized with the vision of imparting up-to-date information and advanced data in this field. To ensure the same, a matchless editorial board was set up. Every individual on the board went through rigorous rounds of assessment to prove their worth. After which they invested a large part of their time researching and compiling the most relevant data for our readers.

The editorial board has been involved in producing this book since its inception. They have spent rigorous hours researching and exploring the diverse topics which have resulted in the successful publishing of this book. They have passed on their knowledge of decades through this book. To expedite this challenging task, the publisher supported the team at every step. A small team of assistant editors was also appointed to further simplify the editing procedure and attain best results for the readers.

Apart from the editorial board, the designing team has also invested a significant amount of their time in understanding the subject and creating the most relevant covers. They scrutinized every image to scout for the most suitable representation of the subject and create an appropriate cover for the book.

The publishing team has been an ardent support to the editorial, designing and production team. Their endless efforts to recruit the best for this project, has resulted in the accomplishment of this book. They are a veteran in the field of academics and their pool of knowledge is as vast as their experience in printing. Their expertise and guidance has proved useful at every step. Their uncompromising quality standards have made this book an exceptional effort. Their encouragement from time to time has been an inspiration for everyone.

The publisher and the editorial board hope that this book will prove to be a valuable piece of knowledge for researchers, students, practitioners and scholars across the globe.

List of Contributors

Sarah Browne
School of Public Health, Physiotherapy & Sports Science, University College Dublin, Dublin 4, Ireland

Carol Barron, Anthony Staines and Mary Rose Sweeney
School of Nursing, Psychotherapy and Community Health, Dublin City University, Dublin 9, Ireland

Oh Yoen Kim
Department of Health Science, Graduate School, Dong-A University, Busan 49315, Korea
Department of Food Science and Nutrition, Dong-A University, Busan 49315, Korea

Eun Mi Kim
Dietetic Department, Kangbuk Samsung Hospital, Seoul 03181, Korea

Sochung Chung
Department of Pediatrics, Konkuk University Medical Center, Konkuk University School of Medicine, Seoul 05030, Korea

Dominika Guzek and Marzena Jezewska-Zychowicz
Department of Organization and Consumption Economics, Faculty of Human Nutrition and Consumer Sciences, Warsaw University of Life Sciences (SGGW-WULS), 159C Nowoursynowska Street, 02-787 Warsaw, Poland

Dominika Głąbska and Ewa Lange
Department of Dietetics, Faculty of Human Nutrition and Consumer Sciences, Warsaw University of Life Sciences (SGGW-WULS), 159C Nowoursynowska Street, 02-787 Warsaw, Poland

Zhenru Huang, Runying Gao, Nadila Bawuerjiang, Yali Zhang, Xiaoxu Huang and Meiqin Cai
School of Public Health, Shanghai Jiao Tong University, 227 South Chongqing Rd, Huangpu Qu, Shanghai 200025, China

Kristin Manz, Gert B. M. Mensink, Jonas D. Finger, Marjolein Haftenberger, Anna-Kristin Brettschneider, Clarissa Lage Barbosa, Susanne Krug and Anja Schienkiewitz
Department of Epidemiology and Health Monitoring, Robert Koch Institute, 13353 Berlin, Germany

Samira Khan and Thomas G. Hurley
Statewide Cancer Prevention and Control Program (CPCP), Arnold School of Public Health, University of South Carolina, 915 Greene Street, Columbia, SC 29208, USA
Connecting Health Innovations, LLC, Columbia, SC 29201, USA

Nitin Shivappa and James R. Hebert
Statewide Cancer Prevention and Control Program (CPCP), Arnold School of Public Health, University of South Carolina, 915 Greene Street, Columbia, SC 29208, USA
Connecting Health Innovations, LLC, Columbia, SC 29201, USA
Epidemiology and Biostatistics, Arnold School of Public Health, University of South Carolina, 915 Greene Street, Columbia, SC 29208, USA

Andrew Ortaglia
Epidemiology and Biostatistics, Arnold School of Public Health, University of South Carolina, 915 Greene Street, Columbia, SC 29208, USA

Christian R. Alvarado
Statewide Cancer Prevention and Control Program (CPCP), Arnold School of Public Health, University of South Carolina, 915 Greene Street, Columbia, SC 29208, USA
Epidemiology and Biostatistics, Arnold School of Public Health, University of South Carolina, 915 Greene Street, Columbia, SC 29208, USA

Michael D. Wirth
Statewide Cancer Prevention and Control Program (CPCP), Arnold School of Public Health, University of South Carolina, 915 Greene Street, Columbia, SC 29208, USA
Connecting Health Innovations, LLC, Columbia, SC 29201, USA
Epidemiology and Biostatistics, Arnold School of Public Health, University of South Carolina, 915 Greene Street, Columbia, SC 29208, USA
College of Nursing, University of South Carolina, Columbia, SC 29208, USA

Alice Rosi, Maria Vittoria Calestani, Furio Brighenti and Francesca Scazzina
Human Nutrition Unit, Department of Food and Drug, University of Parma, 43125 Parma, Italy

Liborio Parrino and Giulia Milioli
Sleep Disorders Center, Department of Medicine and Surgery, University of Parma, 43126 Parma, Italy

Luigi Palla
Department of Medical Statistics, Faculty of Epidemiology and Population Health, London School of Hygiene and Tropical Medicine, London WC1E 7HT, UK

Elio Volta
Giocampus Steering Committee, 43124 Parma, Italy

Norashikin Mustafa, Zoi Toumpakari, Harriet Amy Carroll and Laura Johnson
Centre for Exercise Nutrition and Health Sciences, School for Policy Studies, University of Bristol, Bristol BS8 1TZ, UK

Nabilla Al Sadat
Centre for Population Health (CePH) and Department of Social & Preventive Medicine, Faculty of Medicine, University of Malaya, 50603 Kuala Lumpur, Malaysia

Hazreen Abd Majid
Centre for Population Health (CePH) and Department of Social & Preventive Medicine, Faculty of Medicine, University of Malaya, 50603 Kuala Lumpur, Malaysia
Faculty of Public Health, Universitas Airlangga, Surabaya 60115, Indonesia

Muhammad Yazid Jalaludin
Department of Paediatrics, Faculty of Medicine, University of Malaya, 50603 Kuala Lumpur, Malaysia

Victoria Srbely, and Genevieve Newton
Department of Human Health & Nutritional Science, University of Guelph, Guelph, ON N1G2W1, Canada

Imtisal Janjua
Department of Biomedical Sciences, University of Guelph, Guelph, ON N1G2W1, Canada

Andrea C. Buchholz
Department of Family Relations and Applied Nutrition, University of Guelph, Guelph, ON N1G2W1, Canada

Patrícia de Fragas Hinnig, Adriana Soares Lobo, Patrícia Faria Di Pietro and Francilene Kunradi Vieira
Post Graduate Program in Nutrition, Health Sciences Center, Federal University of Santa Catarina, CCS/UFSC, Campus Trindade, Florianopolis 88040-900, Brazil

Danielle Biazzi Leal and Maria Alice Altenburg de Assis
Post Graduate Program in Nutrition, Health Sciences Center, Federal University of Santa Catarina, CCS/UFSC, Campus Trindade, Florianopolis 88040-900, Brazil
Post Graduate Program in Physical Education, Sports Center, Federal University of Santa Catarina, CDS/UFSC, Campus Trindade, Florianopolis 88040-900, Brazil

Jeovani Schmitt and Pedro Henrique de Moura Araujo
Post Graduate Program in Production Engineering, Technological Center, Federal University of Santa Catarina, University Campus Trindade, Florianopolis 88040-900, Brazil

France Bellisle
Equipe de Recherche en Epidémiologie Nutritionnelle, Centre de Recherche en Epidémiologie et Statistiques, Université Paris 13, Inserm (U1153), Inra (U1125), Cnam, COMUE Sorbonne Paris Cité, Bobigny 93017, France

Dalton Francisco de Andrade
Informatics and Statistics Department, Technological Center, Federal University of Santa Catarina, University Campus Trindade, Florianopolis 88040-900, Brazil

Silvia Bel-Serrat, Mirjam M. Heinen, Celine M. Murrin and Cecily C. Kelleher
National Nutrition Surveillance Centre, School of Public Health, Physiotherapy and Sports Science, University College Dublin, D4 Dublin, Ireland

Ana Ojeda-Rodríguez
National Nutrition Surveillance Centre, School of Public Health, Physiotherapy and Sports Science, University College Dublin, D4 Dublin, Ireland
Department of Nutrition, Food Science and Physiology, University of Navarra, 31008 Pamplona, Spain

Marta Buoncristiano and João Breda
Division of Noncommunicable Diseases and Promoting Health through the Life-course, WHO European Office for Prevention and Control of Noncommunicable Diseases, 125009 Moscow, Russia

Shynar Abdrakhmanova
National Center of Public Health, Ministry of Health of the Republic of Kazakhstan, 010000 Astana, Kazakhstan

Vesselka Duleva
National Center of Public Health and Analyses, 1431 Sofia, Bulgaria

Victoria Farrugia Sant'Angelo
Primary Health Care, 1940 Floriana, Malta

Anna Fijałkowska
Department of Cardiology, Institute of Mother and Child, 01-211 Warsaw, Poland

Tatjana Hejgaard
Danish Health Authority, 2300 Kobenhavn, Denmark

Constanta Huidumac
National Institute of Public Health, 050463 Bucharest, Romania

Jolanda Hyska
Institute of Public Health, 1001 Tirana, Albania

Enisa Kujundzic
Institute of Public Health of Montenegro, 8100 Podgorica, Montenegro

Sanja Musić Milanović
Croatian Institute of Public Health, 10000 Zagreb, Croatia
School of Medicine, School of Public Health Andrija Štampar, University of Zagreb, 10000 Zagreb, Croatia

Guljemal Ovezmyradova
WHO Country Office in Turkmenistan, 744000 Ashgabat, Turkmenistan

Napoleón Pérez-Farinós
Spanish Agency for Food Safety and Nutrition (AESAN), 28071 Madrid, Spain

Ausra Petrauskiene
Department of Preventive Medicine, Lithuanian University of Health Sciences, 44307 Kaunas, Lithuania

Ana Isabel Rito
National Institute of Health Doutor Ricardo Jorge, I.P., 1649-016 Lisbon, Portugal

Lela Shengelia
National Center for Disease Control and Public Health of Georgia, 0186 Tbilisi, Georgia

Radka Taxová Braunerová
Obesity Management Centre, Institute of Endocrinology, 113 94 Prague, Czech Republic

Harry Rutter
Department of Social and Policy Sciences, University of Bath, Claverton Down, Bath BA2 7AY, UK

Lydia Morell-Azanza and Ana Ojeda-Rodríguez
Department of Nutrition, Food Sciences and Physiology, University of Navarra, c/Irunlarrea, 1. 31008 Pamplona, Spain
IdiSNA, Instituto de Investigación Sanitaria de Navarra, c/Irunlarrea, 3. 31008 Pamplona, Spain

Johanna Giuranna, Johannes Hebebrand and Anke Hinney
Department of Child and Adolescent Psychiatry, Psychosomatics and Psychotherapy, University Hospital Essen, University of Duisburg-Essen, Virchowstr. 174, D-45147 Essen, Germany

Azcona-SanJulián
IdiSNA, Instituto de Investigación Sanitaria de Navarra, c/Irunlarrea, 3. 31008 Pamplona, Spain
Department of Paediatrics, Clínica Universidad de Navarra, Paediatric Endocrinology Unit, c/Piío XII, 36. 31008 Pamplona, Spain

M[a] Cristina Azcona-SanJulián and Amelia Marti
Department of Nutrition, Food Sciences and Physiology, University of Navarra, c/Irunlarrea, 1. 31008 Pamplona, Spain
Idi SNA, Instituto de Investigación Sanitaria de Navarra, c/Irunlarrea, 3. 31008 Pamplona, Spain
Biomedical Research Centre Network on Obesity and Nutrition (CIBERobn), Physiopathology of Obesity and Nutrition, Institute of Health Carlos III, Av. Monforte de Lemos, 3-5. 28029 Madrid, Spain

Hajar Mazahery, Maryam Delshad, Cathryn A. Conlon, Kathryn L. Beck and Pamela R. von Hurst
Massey Institute of Food Science and Technology, School of Food and Nutrition, Massey University, Auckland 0745, New Zealand

Welma Stonehouse
Commonwealth Scientific Industrial Research Organisation (CSIRO) Food, Nutrition and Bioproducts, Adelaide SA 5000, Australia

Marlena C. Kruger
Massey Institute of Food Science and Technology, School of Food and Nutrition, Massey University, Palmerston North 4410, New Zealand

Theodora Mouratidou
Growth, Exercise, Nutrition and Development (GENUD) Research Group, University of Zaragoza, C/Pedro Cerbuna 12, 50009 Zaragoza, Spain

María L. Miguel-Berges
Growth, Exercise, Nutrition and Development (GENUD) Research Group, University of Zaragoza, C/Pedro Cerbuna 12, 50009 Zaragoza, Spain
Instituto Agroalimentario de Aragón (IA2), 50009 Zaragoza, Spain

Alba M. Santaliestra-Pasias and Luis A. Moreno
Growth, Exercise, Nutrition and Development (GENUD) Research Group, University of Zaragoza, C/Pedro Cerbuna 12, 50009 Zaragoza, Spain
Instituto Agroalimentario de Aragón (IA2), 50009 Zaragoza, Spain
School of Health Science (EUCS), University of Zaragoza, C/Domingo Miral s/n, 50009 Saragossa, Spain
Centro de Investigación Biomédica en Red de Fisiopatología de la Obesidad y Nutrición (CIBERObn), 50009 Zaragoza, Spain

Pilar De Miguel-Etayo
Growth, Exercise, Nutrition and Development (GENUD) Research Group, University of Zaragoza, C/Pedro Cerbuna 12, 50009 Zaragoza, Spain
Instituto Agroalimentario de Aragón (IA2), 50009 Zaragoza, Spain
Centro de Investigación Biomédica en Red de Fisiopatología de la Obesidad y Nutrición (CIBERObn), 50009 Zaragoza, Spain

Odysseas Androutsos and Yannis Manios
Department of Nutrition and Dietetics, School of Health Science and Education, Harokopio University, 17671 Athens, Greece

Marieke De Craemer
Department of Movement and Sports Sciences, Ghent University, Watersportlaan 2, 9000 Ghent, Belgium

Sonya Galcheva
Department of paediatrics. Medical University Varna, 55 Marin Drinov Str., 9002 Varna, Bulgaria

Berthold Koletzko
Dr von Hauner Children's Hospital, University of Munich Medical Centre, 80337 Munich, Germany

Zbigniew Kulaga
The Children's Memorial Health Institute, 04-730 Warsaw, Poland

Index

M

N

O

P

S

T

W

Z

www.ingramcontent.com/pod-product-compliance
Lightning Source LLC
LaVergne TN
LVHW060527210926
848485LV00005B/1160